Piezoelectric as Smart Biomaterials for Cardiovascular Tissue Regeneration

This book covers the range of piezoelectric biomaterials having the potential for applications in cardiac tissue engineering (CTE) and addresses the recent developments, trends, and challenges of piezoelectric biomaterials for targeted cardiovascular disease (CVD) therapies.

It covers the applications of engineered piezoelectric biomaterials including recent developments in piezoelectric biomaterials and their possible impact on treating CVDs and CTE. Main points discussed in the book are:

- Focusses on piezoelectric biomaterials for the treatment of cardiovascular diseases
- Covers imitation of mechanoelectrical transduction system as in cardiac tissues
- Comprehensively covers functional piezoelectric biomaterials preparation and applications
- Reviews engineered piezoelectric biomaterials applications for better healthcare
- Discusses elastomer actuators for heart tissues

This book is aimed at graduate students and researchers in tissue engineering, regenerative medicine, biophysics, and biomaterials.

Advances in Bionanotechnology

Series Editors: Ravindra Pratap Singh, *Department of Biotechnology, Indira Gandhi National Tribal University, Anuppur, Madhya Pradesh, India,* Jay Singh, *Department of Chemistry, Institute of Science, Banaras Hindu University, Varanasi, Uttar Pradesh, India* and Charles Oluwaseun Adetunji, *Department of Microbiology, Edo State University Uzairue, Iyamho, Edo State, Nigeria*

Bionanotechnology is a multi-disciplinary field that shows immense applicability in different domains, namely chemistry, physics, material sciences, biomedical, agriculture, environment, robotics, aeronautics, energy, electronics, and so forth. This book series will explore the enormous utility of bionanotechnology for biomedical, agricultural, environmental, food technology, space industry, and many other fields. It aims to highlight all the spheres of bionanotechnological applications and its safety and regulations for using biogenic nanomaterials that are a key focus of the researchers globally.

Bionanotechnology Towards Sustainable Management of Environmental Pollution
Edited by Naveen Dwivedi and Shubha Dwivedi

Natural Products and Nano-formulations in Cancer Chemoprevention
Edited by Shiv Kumar Dubey

Bionanotechnology towards Green Energy: Innovative and Sustainable Approach
Edited by Shubha Dwivedi and Naveen Dwivedi

Biotic Stress Management of Crop Plants Using Nanomaterials
Edited by Krishna Kant Mishra and Santosh Kumar

Bionanotechnology for Advanced Applications
Edited by Ajaya Kumar Singh and Bhawana Jain

Nanoarchitectonics for Brain Drug Delivery
Edited by Anurag Kumar Singh, Vivek K. Chaturvedi, and Jay Singh

Functional Fluorescent Materials: Applications in Sensing, Bioimaging, and Optoelectronics
Edited by Vivek Mishra, Syed Sibtay Razi, and Ajit Kumar

Nanotherapeutics for Inflammatory Arthritis: Design, Diagnosis, and Treatment
Edited by Vivek Mishra, Ramendrapati Pandey, Anjali Priyadarshini, Chung-Ming Chang, and Elcio Leal

Piezoelectric as Smart Biomaterials for Cardiovascular Tissue Regeneration
Edited by Rakesh Bhaskar, Santosh Kumar, and Mukesh Kumar Gupta

For more information about this series, please visit: www.routledge.com/Advances-in-Bionanotechnology/book-series/CRCBIONAN

Piezoelectric as Smart Biomaterials for Cardiovascular Tissue Regeneration

Edited by
Rakesh Bhaskar, Santosh Kumar, and
Mukesh Kumar Gupta

CRC Press
Taylor & Francis Group
Boca Raton London New York

CRC Press is an imprint of the
Taylor & Francis Group, an **informa** business

Designed cover image: Rakesh Bhaskar, Soon Mo Choi and Sung Soo Han

First edition published 2026
by CRC Press
2385 NW Executive Center Drive, Suite 320, Boca Raton FL 33431

and by CRC Press
4 Park Square, Milton Park, Abingdon, Oxon, OX14 4RN

CRC Press is an imprint of Taylor & Francis Group, LLC

ISBN: 978-1-032-68981-4 (hbk)
ISBN: 978-1-041-13681-1 (pbk)
ISBN: 978-1-003-67099-5 (ebk)

DOI: 10.1201/9781003670995

Typeset in Times
by KnowledgeWorks Global Ltd.

Contents

About the Editors

Rakesh Bhaskar is an Assistant Professor (International Faculty Member) specializing in polymers and biomaterials in the School of Chemical Engineering at Yeungnam University, Gyeongsan, South Korea. He received his doctoral degree in the field of neuroendocrine science from Allahabad University, India. Then moved to NIT Rourkela, as a postdoctoral fellow, during which tenure he worked in the areas of tissue engineering and regenerative medicine. He has published more than 102 scientific papers in SCI/SCIE-grade journals and has also published five book chapters. His work has received more than 2200 citations, with an h-index of 23. He is also a reputed reviewer for several peer-reviewed international journals. His research interests are in stem cells, cardiac regeneration, tissue engineering, cultured meat production, and in vitro spermatogenesis.

Santosh Kumar is currently working as an Associate Professor in the Department of Chemistry, Harcourt Butler Technical University, Kanpur, India. He also served as Research Professor in the Department of Organic and Nano System Engineering, Division of Chemical Engineering, Konkuk University, Seoul, South Korea. Dr. Kumar received his B.Sc and M.Sc. in Chemistry and his D.Phil. in Organic Chemistry from University of Allahabad, India. He worked as a Research Associate (CSIR) at the Department of Chemistry, Motilal Nehru National Institute of Technology, Allahabad, India. He was awarded CAS-TWAS Postdoctoral Fellowship in 2008 and worked in the Changchun Institute of Applied Chemistry, Chinese Academy of Sciences, Changchun, China. Later he joined as a KU Brain Pool professor and researcher at Konkuk University, Seoul, South Korea (2010–2013). He was awarded the FCT Postdoctoral Fellowship in 2012 and worked in the Chemistry Centre, University of Coimbra, Coimbra, Portugal (2013–2017). During his career, Dr. Kumar has published more than 115 research papers, three international patents, edited four books, and contributed 19 book chapters. He has also served as a member of different organizing committees and as an editorial board member and reviewer for numerous scientific journals. His current research interests involve source apportionment of chemical modification, optical and biological properties of chitosan biopolymer for biomedical applications, hydrogel, aerogel, nanomaterials, drug and gene delivery, and environmental chemistry.

Mukesh Kumar Gupta is a Professor of Biotechnology and Medical Engineering at the National Institute of Technology, Rourkela. He is currently Director of the ICMR-National Animal Resource Facility for Biomedical Research, Hyderabad, India. He earned his Ph.D. in interdisciplinary Biotechnology, Nanotechnology and Information Technology from the Department of Advanced Fusion Technology at Konkuk University, South Korea in 2007. He served as Assistant/Associate Professor in the College of Biosciences and Bioresources at Konkuk University, South Korea, and as Participating Faculty at the Institute of Biomedical Science and

Technology, South Korea during 2007-2011. He has also been a visiting scientist to the Instituto Superior Técnico, Portugal; Warsaw Institute of Technology, Poland; and the University of Malaysia, Malaysia. He has more than 15 years of research and teaching experience, has published more than 85 publications in various SCI-indexed journals, and has 18 patents to his credit. He has also written more than 15 book chapters and has edited one book. He is an editorial board member of eight international journals and a reviewer for several peer-reviewed SCI-indexed journals. He is a founding member of the Council of Asian Science Editors (CASE) and is an Elected Fellow of the Royal Society of Biology, U.K.; National Academy of Agricultural Sciences, India; National Academy of Biological Sciences, India; National Academy of Dairy Sciences, India; National Environment Science Academy, India; Society of Applied Biotechnology, India; Academy of Environment and Life Sciences, India; and the Indian Association for Advancement of Veterinary Research, India, amongst others. He is a Board Member of the Animal Welfare Board of India and the Committee for Control and Supervision of Experiments in Animals, Government of India. He is also a subject expert of the National Testing Agency (NTA); Union Public Service Commission (UPSC); National Board of Accreditation (NBA); and the All India Council for Technical Education (AICTE), India.

Contributors

Rakesh Bhaskar
School of Chemical Engineering, Yeungnam University, Gyeongsan 38541, South Korea
Research Institute of Cell Culture, Yeungnam University, Gyeongsan 38541, South Korea

Soon Mo Choi
School of Chemical Engineering, Yeungnam University, Gyeongsan 38541, South Korea
Research Institute of Cell Culture, Yeungnam University, Gyeongsan 38541, South Korea

Shampa Ghosh
GloNeuro, Sector 107, Vishwakarma Road, Noida 201301, Uttar Pradesh, India

Mukesh Kumar Gupta
Department of Biotechnology and Medical Engineering, National Institute of Technology Rourkela, Rourkela 769008, Odisha, India
CMR-National Animal Resource Facility for Biomedical Research, Genome Valley, Shamirpet, Hyderabad, 500 078 India

Banalata Mohanty
Department of Zoology, University of Allahabad, Allahabad, 211001, Utter Pradesh, India

Sung Soo Han
School of Chemical Engineering, Yeungnam University, Gyeongsan 38541, South Korea
Research Institute of Cell Culture, Yeungnam University, Gyeongsan 38541, South Korea

H. G. Jayasinghe
Mathematics, Physical and Natural Sciences Division, University of New Mexico-Gallup, 705 Gurley Ave., Gallup, NM 87301, USA

P. Kumar
Department of Physics and Astronomy, National Institute of Technology Rourkela, Rourkela 769008, Odisha, India

Santosh Kumar
Department of Chemistry, School of Basic & Applied Science, Harcourt Butler Technical University, Kanpur 208002, Uttar Pradesh, India

U.S.K. Madduma-Bandarage
Department of Chemistry, New Mexico Institute of Mining and Technology, Socorro, NM 87801, USA

S.V. Madihally
School of Chemical Engineering, Oklahoma State University, Stillwater, OK 74078, USA

Aarti Nagayach
Department of Cancer Biology, College of Medicine, University of Cincinnati, Cincinnati, OH 45267, USA

Kannan Badri Narayanan
School of Chemical Engineering, Yeungnam University, Gyeongsan 38541, South Korea
Research Institute of Cell Culture, Yeungnam University, Gyeongsan 38541, South Korea

Surya Prakash Pandey
Department of Zoology, School of Science, IFTM University, Moradabad 211002, Uttar Pradesh, India

Ira Singh
Department of Chemistry, School of Basic and Applied Sciences, Harcourt Butler Technical University, Kanpur 208002, Uttar Pradesh, India

Jitendra Kumar Sinha
GloNeuro, Sector 107, Vishwakarma Road, Noida 201301, Uttar Pradesh, India

Krishna Kumar Singh
Symbiosis Centre for Information Technology, Symbiosis International (Deemed University), Pune 411057, Maharashtra, India

Priya Singh
Department of Chemistry, Harcourt Butler Technical University, Kanpur 208002, Uttar Pradesh, India

Shalinee Singh
Department of Chemistry, School of Basic and Applied Sciences, Harcourt Butler Technical University, Kanpur 208002, Uttar Pradesh, India

Sujata Swain
Department of Physics and Astronomy, National Institute of Technology Rourkela, Odisha 769008, India

Preface

Cardiovascular diseases (CVDs) resulting from myocardial infarction (MI), atherosclerosis, arrhythmia, cardiomyopathies, heart valve disease, long–QT syndromes (LQTS), etc., cause millions of deaths worldwide. They account for approximately 7.4 million annual deaths, and this number is predicted to increase to around 23 million by 2030. The World Health Organization (WHO) estimates that CVDs are responsible for annually causing 17.5 million global deaths. Ischemic heart disease and stroke alone are responsible for 21.1% of all deaths among CVDs. Although there has been significant research into the treatment of CVDs, including heart surgery, heart transplant, and ventricular assist device implantation, it remains a major therapeutic challenge. Most CVDs damage cardiac and vascular cells through apoptotic and necrotic processes, leading to the death and loss of functional cardiomyocytes. As the self-renewal or regenerative potential of adult cardiomyocytes is extremely limited, cardiac tissue constructs seeded with different stem and progenitor cells are increasingly viewed as an alternative therapy for end-stage CVDs. The field of cardiac tissue engineering (CTE) is rapidly advancing with the design of novel scaffolds and bioreactors, new analytical techniques, and advances in stem cell biology.

The choice of biomaterials is a pivotal factor for developing cardiac tissue constructs. Appropriate biomaterials should provide physical support to cells, enable cellular interactions between cells, and release growth factors while preventing anoikis or programmed cell death of cells after detaching from the ECM. Smart piezoelectric materials can potentially offer alternative substrates and promote cell-biomaterial interactions. Piezoelectric materials have the ability to imitate the mechanoelectrical transduction system found in cardiac tissues, but their study has primarily focused on bone and cartilage tissue engineering. Therefore, piezoelectric biomaterials are expected to receive more attention in future treatment of CVDs. However, none of the published books so far cover the range of piezoelectric biomaterials having the potential for applications in CTE. The currently available book does not address the recent developments, trends, and challenges of piezoelectric biomaterials for targeted CVD therapies.

Chapter 1 discussed with function anatomy of the human heart, Chapter 2 discussed with cellular sources and biomechanical conditioning for cardiac tissue engineering, Chapter 3 discussed with biomaterials for cardiac tissue engineering, Chapter 4 discussed with electroconductive biomaterials for cardiac tissue engineering, Chapter 5 discussed with piezoelectric fundamental and property, Chapter 6 discussed with piezoelectric materials in cardiac patches for cardiovascular disease, Chapter 7 discussed with biomaterial-driven differentiation and maturation of cardiomyocytes: Advancements in cardiac tissue engineering, Chapter 8 discussed with piezoelectric biomaterials for the development of cardiac sensors and actuators, and Chapter 9 discussed with elastomer actuators: for heart tissue.

This proposed book aims to cover the numerous applications of engineered piezoelectric biomaterials for better healthcare. More specifically, this book aims to cover recent developments in piezoelectric biomaterials and their possible impact on treating CVDs and CTE.

1 Function Anatomy of the Human Heart

Shalinee Singh and Santosh Kumar

1.1 INTRODUCTION

Heart is the origin of life; it is the source of every action as it supplies blood throughout the body, as written by William Harvey in 1673 [1]. The anatomy of the heart is not simple. With two separate functioning units connected by a specific conduction system, the mammalian heart is a complex organ (Figure 1.1). These units are always changing in the opposite direction. More important in terms of function is the ventricular component, which is inherently complex. Although it is split into two chambers that support two essentially independent circulatory systems, it functions as a single unit both physically and functionally.

While blood and oxygen are delivered to the tissues by the circulatory system, waste products are eliminated from the body by the kidneys, liver, and lungs, among other organs (Figure 1.2). The cardiovascular system's main job is to transfer waste products and nutrients throughout the body. The heart circulates blood via a complex system of blood veins, supplying different organs with oxygen and nutrients at the same time. Understanding blood flow in both healthy and unhealthy circumstances is essential to understanding cardiovascular health. The complex mixture of cells, proteins, lipoproteins, and ions that makes up blood helps carry waste and nutrients through the body. About 40% of blood's content is made up of red blood cells, which are tiny, semi-solid particles that increase blood viscosity and affect fluid dynamics [2].

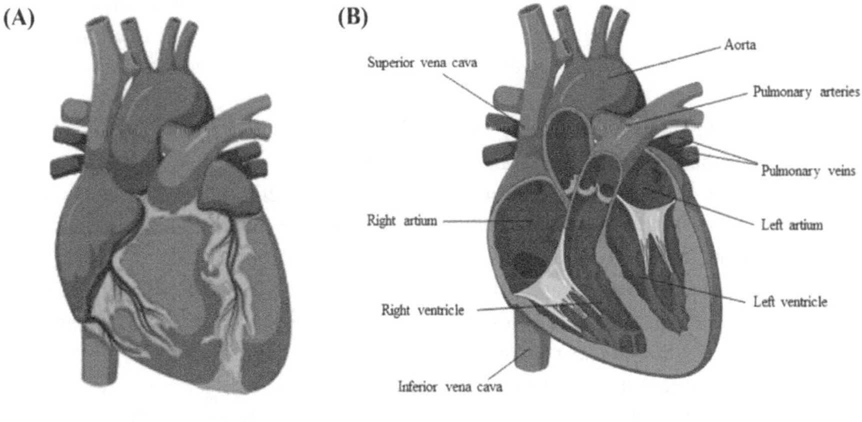

FIGURE 1.1 (A) Human heart and (B) cross-sectional picture of human heart.

DOI: 10.1201/9781003670995-1

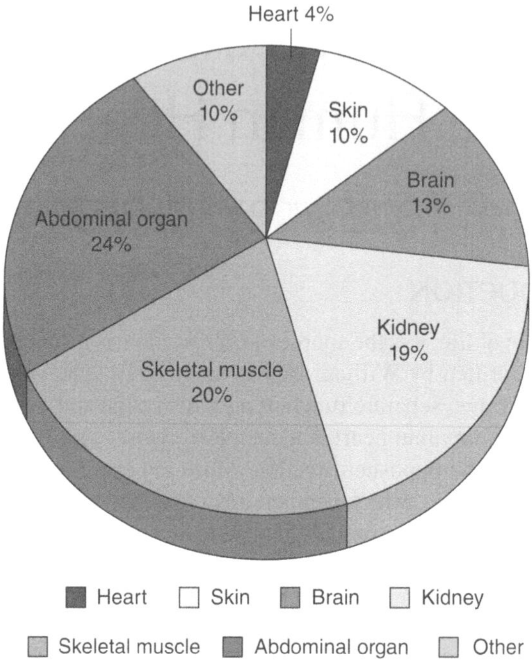

FIGURE 1.2 Systemic blood flow in various organs of human body.

The heart is powered by electrical impulses that control the sequential filling and emptying of ventricles, acting as a muscle pump to circulate blood throughout the body. The normal function of ventricles is depicted in Figure 1.3. It starts with an isovolumic contraction phase to increase pre-ejection tension, isovolumic relaxation phase, ejection phase, and ultimately rapid and slow filling phases. Echoing the rapid early rise in the flow curve, the left ventricular (LV) volume declines rapidly, early in systole and more slowly thereafter. The volume increases more slowly in late filling and more quickly in early filling, suggesting that the heart passively dilated to fill after witnessing cadaver dissections and contracted to expel blood. There are three main issues with this conventional understanding of heart function, though:

i. It is predicated on the idea that the LV muscle is homogeneous and that every fiber contracts or relaxes at the same time. This false belief stems from the outdated application of 2D imaging methods such as echocardiography and angiography, which only recorded global alterations in the myocardium and form of the heart.
ii. The intricate fiber architecture of ventricles, especially the spiral muscular bands that create a partial loop at the apex, was not taken into consideration by traditional theories of ventricular function.
iii. The examination of the twisting motions observed during ventricular emptying and filling was limited by 2D approaches. Spiral muscle fibers, which rotate in both clockwise and counterclockwise directions, can be used to

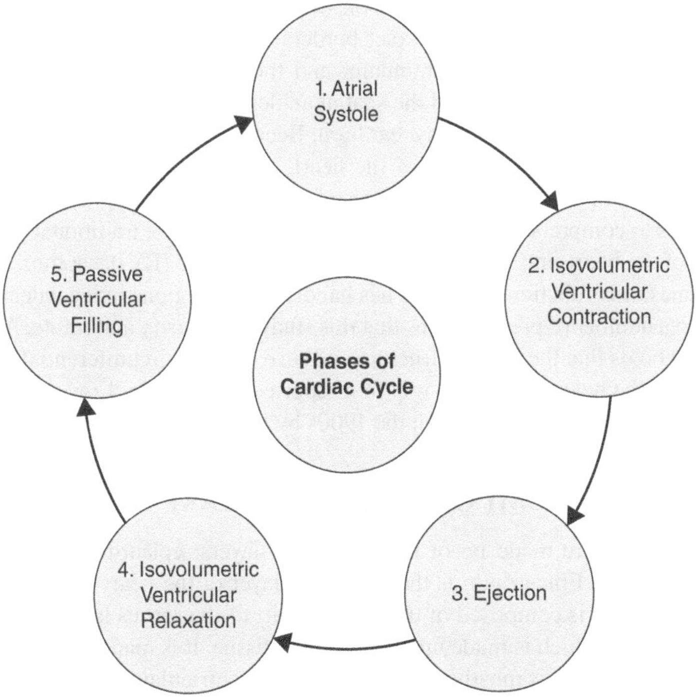

FIGURE 1.3 Different phases of cardiac cycle.

explain these twisting actions. This muscle structure has been described by anatomists before, and tensor MRI has confirmed it. However, there has been little comprehensive correlation between anatomy and physiology.

The significance of the predominant circumferential fibers has occasionally been eclipsed by the increased attention paid to spiral fibers. Investigating the interactions between these two sets of fibers is one of our objectives [3]. Both blood pressure and flow are erratic. All arteries are pulsatile due to the heart's cyclic pumping function. The heart pumps blood out during systole and none at all during diastole when the heart rests. Both flow and pressure exhibit distinctive pulsatile patterns that vary across the vascular system. The heart pumps blood sporadically, which stops completely when the aortic valve closes. In order to keep blood pressure from falling to zero during diastole, the aorta functions as a compliance chamber by holding high pressure during both systole and diastole. Certain arteries, such as the brachial, femoral, and external carotid, have substantial downstream resistance when at rest, which can cause blood flow to stop or even reverse during diastole, resulting in an on/off flow pattern with each cardiac cycle [2].

The concept of a compound unit inside a compound organ is encapsulated in the term "ventricular complex" [4]. The muscular ventricular myocardium and the collagenous tissue connected to its four orifices make up the ventricular complex's structural components. The base of the heart is where these two anatomical parts merge, and it is here that one must look intently in order to accurately characterize the ventricular complex. The exact borders of the ventricular mass are defined in this region by the fibrous continuum, and the exact planes of the collagenous structures at the four orifices and the spatial angles between them are defined by the three-dimensional shape of the myocardium. Because many intracardiac procedures involve the tissues at the bottom of the heart, this area is significant not only for comprehension of cardiac anatomy but also for cardiac surgeons [4]. Nowadays, most approaches to comprehending cardiac dynamics center on the traditional topographical split of the heart into ventricles (LV and right ventricle [RV]), septum, and heart. Many times, this functional analysis has handled these regions independently, which has led to a number of presumptions that this study will clarify and refute. A different viewpoint holds that the helical structure and surrounding circumferential wrap form the mass of the heart muscle, as was first reported in 1600s by Lower, in the 1700s by Senac, in the 1800s by Krehl, in the 1900s by Mall, and latterly by Guasp [5–7].

1.2 BASIC ANATOMY OF THE HUMAN HEART

The heart walls are made up of three different layers: epicardium, endocardium, and myocardium. Epicardium is the outermost layer of the heart wall that contains blood vessels and is composed of the visceral part of the serous layer. Myocardium, the middle layer which is made up of contractile tissue. It is made up of three different muscle layers and is mostly present in the interventricular septum (IVS) and left ventricle (LV). The subendocardial layer, middle concentric layer, and subepicardial layer are some of these layers. The subepicardial and subendocardial layers make up the majority of the remaining cardiac tissue. The conducting system and nodal tissue are two more vital components located in the myocardium. The endothelium and subendothelial are the connective tissue that make up the endocardium, which is the deepest layer and forms the inner lining of the chambers and the valves, and it also contains nerves [8–10].

1.2.1 Heart Chambers and the Heart Valves

The human heart is made up of four separate chambers, each having a different wall thickness. The smaller, thinner-walled chambers are known as the left atrium (LA) and right atrium (RA). These are placed just above the RV and LV, respectively (Figures 1.1 and 1.4).

Larger, thicker-walled chambers called ventricles carry out the majority of the heart's function. After taking in blood from the lungs and venous system, the atria contract to force blood into the ventricles, which subsequently pump it to the lungs or throughout the body. The fibrous framework of the heart is composed of the membranous septum, an aortic intervalvular, the right and left fibrous trigones, and the annuli of the valves, which together support the four valves of the heart. The bundle of His passes through the central fibrous structure, which is made up of the membranous septum (the fibrous part) and right trigone. The heart is structurally supported by the fibrous skeleton, which also functions to electrically divide the ventricles from the atria. For physiological homeostasis to be maintained, each valve is essential [8, 9, 11, 12].

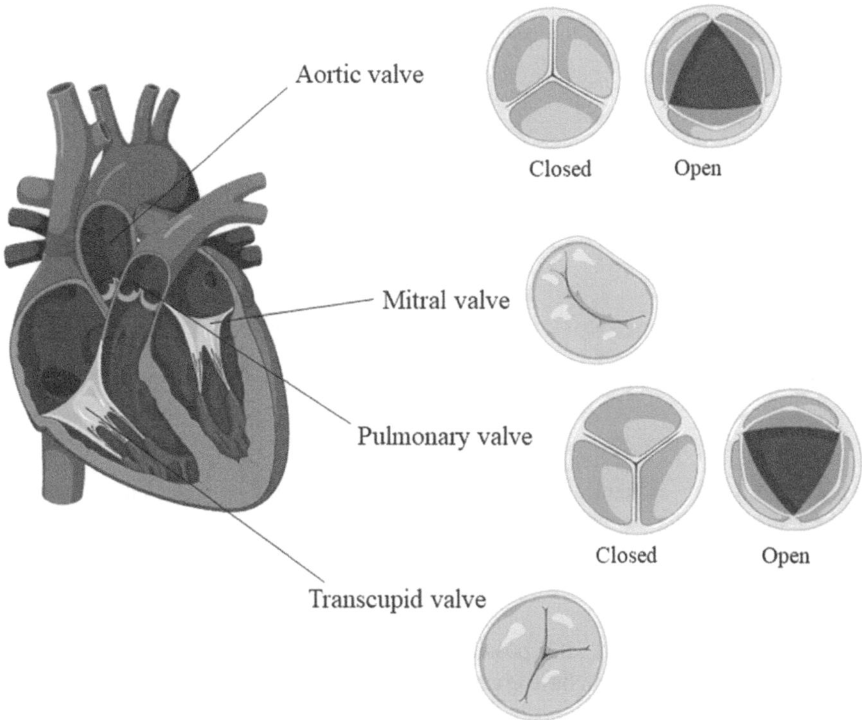

FIGURE 1.4 An anatomy of valves in human heart.

1.2.2 Anatomy of Mitral Valve

The valvar complex is fused of the leaflets, annulus, papillary muscles, and tendinous cords. The left atrial muscle that runs into the leaflets and the myocardium where the papillary muscles enter are also critical to its proper operation. The valve and the aortic valve are closely related and situated obliquely in the heart. The mitral valve is located right next to the aortic valve, in contrast to the tricuspid valve, which is separated from its equivalent, the pulmonary valve, by muscle (Figure 1.5) [13].

With an anterior and a posterior cusp, the MV is bileaflet (Figure 1.5). Every leaflet enters the mitral annulus at its base. The anterior mitral leaflet rests somewhat medially, and the posterior mitral leaflet lies somewhat laterally; the leaflets are not precisely anterior-posterior oriented. Each leaflet has roughly the same surface area, but the posterior leaflet (PL) is longer and thinner than the anterior leaflet (AL), with twice the annular attachment and just half the AL's base-to-tip length. Both anterolateral and posteromedial commissures are where the valvar leaflets unite. Between the two commissures during systole, a curved coaptation line emerges when the leaflet tips are opposed. During systole, there is often 3–5 mm of overlap between the leaflets along the coaptation line. Along with the noncoronary leaflet and, to a lesser extent, the left cusp of the AV, the AL is in fibrous continuity. The anterolateral, middle, and posteromedial are the three separate anatomic scallops or

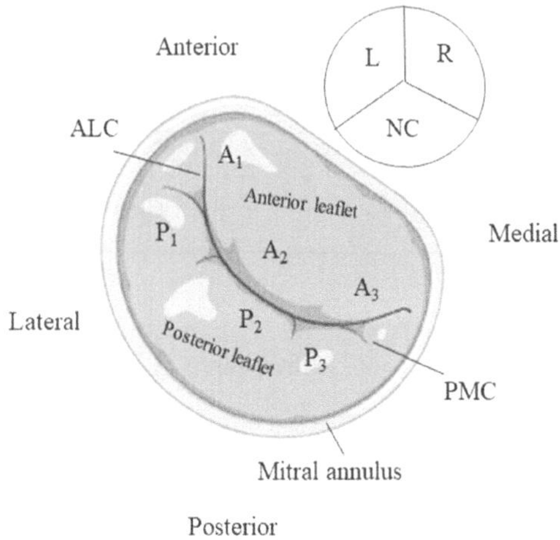

FIGURE 1.5 An anatomical view of mitral valve, showing anterolateral commissure (ALC), posteromedial commissure (PMC), and leaflets. MV is viewed from bottom of the heart looking toward left ventricle apex with the position of left (L), noncoronary (NC), and right (R) AV leaflets relative to mitral valve.

pieces that make up the PL. It is possible to spot little scallops near the commissures. Both Carpentier and Duran have created classification schemes for the mitral leaflets (Figures 1.5 and 1.6).

In anatomical view, when atria are removed, the valve is seen from the bottom of the heart or the LA side of the valve. The AL and PL appear in their proper locations, and the patient's left and right align with the observer's left and right, making this the most naturally occurring view. The medial (or septal) aspect of the valve is on the right, whereas the lateral aspect is on the left. From surgeon's view, the LA is opened, and the surgeon may see the valve from his or her position on the patient's right side. The LA appendage is visible at the 9 o'clock position, whereas the AV and the bottom of the anterior MV leaflet can be seen at the

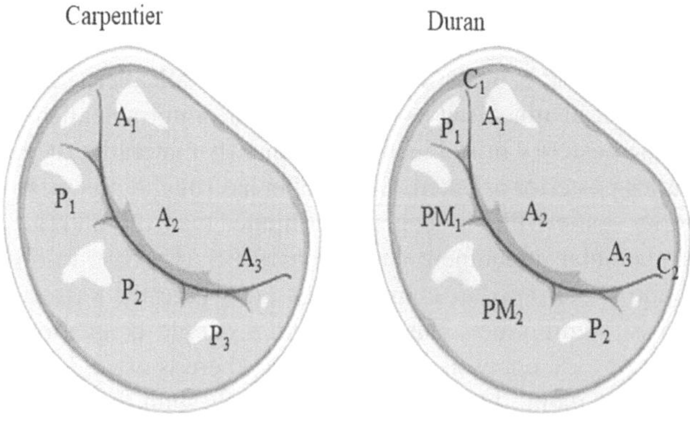

FIGURE 1.6 Carpentier and Duran naming of mitral valve segments.

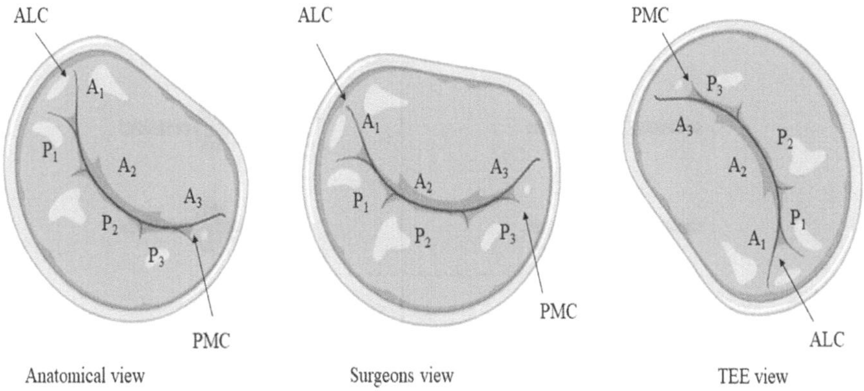

FIGURE 1.7 Different orientations of mitral valve: anatomic view (left), surgeons view (middle), transesophageal echocardiography (TEE) view (right).

12 o'clock position. The most popular orientation for viewing MV 3-D datasets is the surgeon's view. The TEE view is created by rotating the anatomic view 180 degrees, which flips the observer's left and right directions with respect to the patient. This is consistent with the MV's orientation in the trans-gastric basal shorter axial view (Figure 1.7). The Doppler-based echocardiographic recording of the first trans-mitral inflow into the LV is known as mitral valve opening (MVO). The anterior mitral leaflet moves most quickly during this event, which happens when LV pressure drops below the atrial pressure. MVO is a commonly used term that can be found in textbooks and academic articles. The only real prerequisite for MVO is the physically separating the mitral leaflets. A position that has been expressed by others who have also questioned the validity of MVO is that it is the mitral valve anomalies that correlate with the E point in echocardiogram of the mitral but are not directly related to the real opening of the mitral valve, as stated by Lee in 1990 [14, 15].

1.2.3 Cardiac Muscles and Cardiac Cells

The sarcolemma, a cell membrane, encloses each cardiac myocyte, which has a single nucleus. Mitochondria are abundant in the cells, supplying the constant flow of Adenosine Triphosphate (ATP) needed to maintain heart contraction. Similar to skeletal muscle, cardiac myocytes are made up of regulatory proteins (tropomyosin and troponin) as well as contractile proteins (actin the thin filaments and myosin thick filaments). Although the pattern of striating in cardiac muscle is not as organized as in skeletal muscle, it nevertheless occurs. The configuration of the thick and thin filaments is displayed in Figure 1.8. Sarcoplasmic reticulum sleeves encircle the myofilaments inside the myocyte; these sleeves are comparable to the endoplasmic reticulum present in other cells. The transverse tubules, or T tubules, are distinct tubular structures that traverse the cell. The sarcoplasmic reticulum envelops myofibrils, bundles of protein strands seen in cardiac cells. Cisternae, or dilated terminals, are part of this reticulum. The myofibril contractile units, or

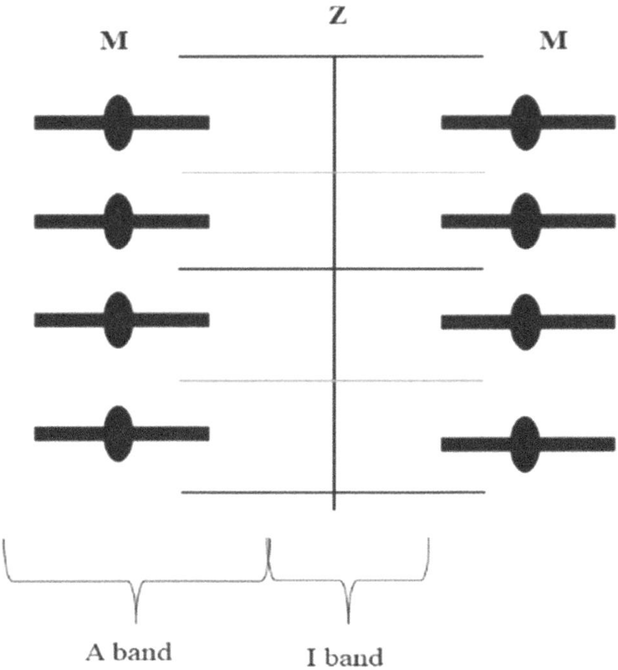

FIGURE 1.8 Cardiac muscle contractile units.

sarcomeres, collaborate with T tubules, which are cell membrane extensions that are situated close to the Z-lines and carry action potentials into the interior of the cell (Figure 1.8). T tubules link the sarcoplasmic reticulum and sarcolemma in cardiac and skeletal muscle [9].

Heart muscle is an involuntarily striated mononucleated muscle. Z-lines serve as anchors for the alternating lengths of dense and slender filaments of the protein that produce the cross-striations in cardiac muscle. Myosin and actin are the primary structural proteins of heart muscle, and it is comparatively shorter than skeletal muscle (Figures 1.8 and 1.9). Under the microscope, the thinner actin filaments in the heart muscle are seen as lighter bands, whereas the larger myosin filaments are seen as darker bands [16].

According to Ganong, the bright bands represent the actin filament region, while the dark bands represent the area where the actin and myosin filaments intersect (Figures 1.8 and 1.9). Tropomyosin and troponin, the two other proteins found in the weaker actin filaments, are crucial for contraction. Additionally, intercalated discs, which are composed of a transverse and a lateral component, are dense bands (specialized cell junctions) seen in cardiac muscle that divide each cell from one another at their ends. The peripheral part of the disc functions performs as a traversing channel, which takes part in the transmission of electrical signals between the proximate cardiac cells, allowing each heart cells to function as a syncytium. While transverse part of the disc performs as a firm contact zone and a track of transmission of constrictive force [16, 17].

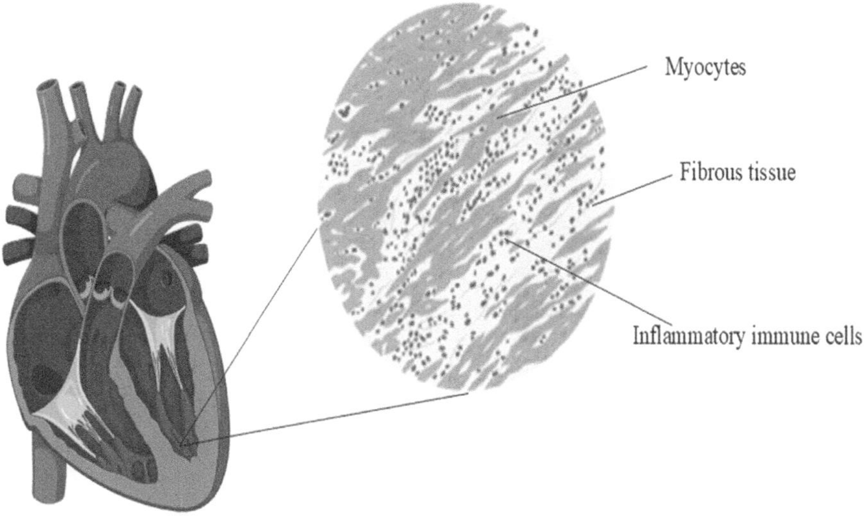

FIGURE 1.9 Systematic diagram of cardiac muscle.

1.2.4 Coronary Arteries

The aorta's initial branches, known as the coronary arteries, often emerge from two of the three Valsalva aortic sinuses. First to stress the value of attitudinally accurate nomenclature for professionals working in the therapeutic situation was the electrophysiology community. That holds comparable significance when explaining the coronary arteries. The aortic sinuses of Valsalva, which contain the aortic valve leaflets and are limited distally by the sinutubular junction, occupy the first part of the aortic root [18, 19]. The primary coronary arteries, which are the left main stem of the coronary artery and the right coronary artery (RCA), emanate from the two sinuses next to the pulmonary trunk in a typical human heart (Figure 1.10). These arteries can have rather different beginnings depending on how close they are to the sinutubular junction and the zones where the valvar leaflets appoint, or what are known as commissures. In this regard, variations of normal are defined as take-off deviations within 1 cm of the adult heart's sinutubular junction, whereas ectopic origin, also known as high take-off, is defined as origins deviating more than 1 cm from the junction [19, 20]. An extremely uncommon large coronary artery stems from the aortic sinus far from the pulmonary trunk. Thus, the aortic sinuses of Valsalva can be referred to as the left coronary, right coronary, and noncoronary sinuses, respectively, based on these origins (Figure 1.10). The RCA comes from the aortic sinus of right coronary in the top region of the right anterior surface of the aortic root. In nine-tenths of individuals, this artery supplies the majority of the diaphragmatic surface of the ventricular mass. This sinus frequently has two arterial orifices; the second orifice usually gives rise to the conal, or infundibular, artery; however, it can also occasionally give rise to the sinus node artery [18, 20, 21]. The RCA is located in the right atrioventricular (AV) groove after emerging from the aortic sinus. Similar to the RCA, the left coronary artery's main stem typically emerges from left coronary aortic sinus, which is

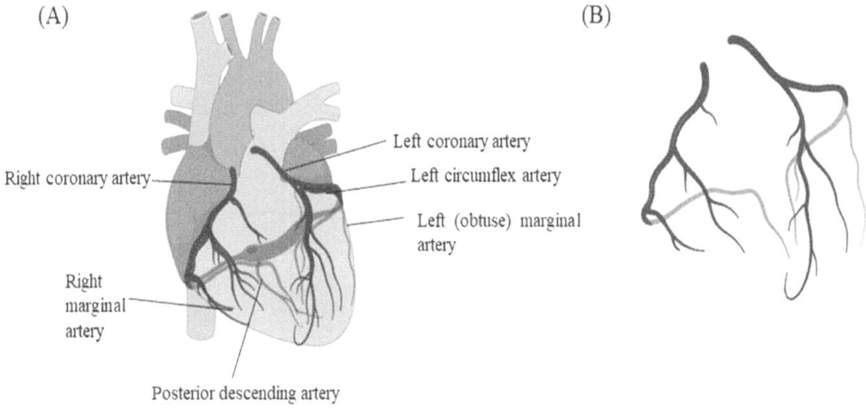

FIGURE 1.10 (A) Coronary arteries and (B) simplified diagram of coronary arteries.

located just below the sinutubular ridge. It leaves the aortic sinus and enters the transverse sinus's leftward edge, where it is situated between the pulmonary trunk and the left atrial appendage. In adults, its length rarely exceeds 1 or 2 cm, beyond which it splits into the circumflex and the anterior interventricular branches [20].

The right coronary arteries and left coronary arteries (RCA and LCA, respectively) supply blood to the heart. A single, left mainstem (short main artery), LCA emerges from the left aortic. The left circumflex (LCf) and left anterior descending (LAD) arteries are formed by the bifurcation of the LCA [22]. The PDA (posterior descending artery) is an offshoot of the RCA and the LAD anastomoses [22, 23]. The apex, anterior sections of the right and LVs, and the IVS (anterior two-thirds) are all supplied by the LAD. The left marginal artery is the main branch of the LCf, and in 10–15% of people, the LCf is interconnected with the RCA to form PDA. Generally, the LCf serves the superior part of the LV and the dorsal section of the LA. The right marginal artery, which supplies blood to the inferior LV wall, and both surfaces of the RV, is one of the major branches of the right coronary artery (RCA), originates from right aortic sinus. Other major branches include the sinoatrial nodal artery, which supplies the RA and the SA node, and the PDA, which supplies the posterior third of the AV and node of the IVS [22]. About 80–90% of the time, the AV node, a vital component of the heart's electrical system receives blood from the RCA. The AV node regulates the timing of heartbeats by transferring signals between the ventricles and atria. The coronary arteries terminate in end arteries, which particularly give blood to the myocardial tissue (the heart's muscular tissue), ensuring that the heart muscle gets enough oxygen and nutrients. The coronary arteries then branch off into smaller arteries and arterioles. When it comes to coronary artery dominance, the RCA is considered the dominant artery in approximately 60–65% of people [22, 23]. Approximately in 10–15% of cases, the LCf generates the PDA (left predominant circulation). And in 20–25% of cases, the RCA supplies the diaphragmatic surface of the LV (right predominance), followed by the PDA by spanning the posterior IVS as far as the obtuse marginal artery [22]. Even so, balanced coronary circulation is not differentiated by this condition.

1.3 ANATOMICAL VERSUS TOPOGRAPHICAL HEART

The heart's anatomy is accurately described by the classic morphological description, which divides the organ into two ventricles and a central muscular septum. However, this description does not shed any light on the functions of these three parts. Another structural theory, which has been around for the last 500 years, suggests that the architecture of the heart consists of a helix made up of both left- and right-handed fibers and is encircled by a circumferential wrap. This idea predates Torrent Guasp's discovery of interwoven architecture, which allowed him to solve the long-standing puzzle of cardiac anatomy by untangling the development of muscle bundles. The HVMB (helical ventricular myocardial band), as depicted by G. Torrent, is characterized by a vortex at the peak of his macroscopic anatomical pattern. This pattern shows how the circumferential wrap, the transverse muscle (located at the bottom of the heart), arching to bottom to form the inner descending helical limb (IDHL), and then turns upward to produce the outer ascending helical limb (OAHL), which ends at the aortic root, to form an apex. G. Torrent macroscopic observations were questioned by Grant, Lev, and Simkins, as well as by Anderson, especially in light of this complex helical structure [7, 24].

A detailed comprehension of the anatomical and functional relationship of the heart is necessary to comprehend the mechanical causes of its actions. Recent HVMB dissections have addressed concerns surrounding dissection accuracy in cadaver investigations, specifically with reference to the posterior papillary muscle. There is still debate, though, since Anderson's colleague MacIver has proposed that the concept of the "unique myocardial band" may not be sufficient because two-dimensional histology is unable to characterize it [25–28].

1.4 NORMAL FUNCTIONAL DYNAMICS OF STRUCTURAL COMPONENTS

Among these three architectural elements, the muscle with the greatest strength or dominance determines the direction of motion, and its contractions happen at varying intervals. In the pre-ejection isovolumic period, for instance, the wrapping muscle contracts and expands the ventricle to counteract the effect of the inner descending helix contracting simultaneously, which usually shortens the ventricle [29]. On the other hand, on the duration of ejection the shortening process points up the IDHL supremacy. Motivated by the greater lever radius of the OAHL, the ventricle twisting occurs as the base spins rightwards and the apex rotates leftwards. Given that its longitudinal strain signal shows elongation, the outer helical coil does not contribute to shortening. However, both helical arms are important in twisting: the OAHL turns the apex leftwards, while the inner descending coil shortens and propagates two times more longitudinal strain. Recent imaging technologies offer an understanding of this process by displaying the septal line generated by echo, which is formed by the echo beam tracking along the upward and downward muscle masses [30–32].

The wrap reverses its pre-ejection counterclockwise motion during the post-ejection isovolumic phase by starting a dexter global recoil. The helix's outer ascending arm continues to constrict, preventing it from taking part in this recoil. But the clockwise motion of the main circumferential wrap overwhelms its counterclockwise movement. When the dominant IDHL stops contracting, the contracting OAHL starts to straighten, causing the ventricle to lengthen simultaneously. Its helical muscles' reciprocal fiber orientation is reflected in the septum's apparent opposing motion, and measurements of global longitudinal strain are consistent with those obtained by sono-micrometry. About 60 ms after the IDHL's earlier contraction, the OAHL starts to contract. The timing difference between the termination of the IDHL and OAHL shortening is shown by a following ~90 ms gap. The idea that repolarization begins earlier in the AHL than in the DHL is mechanically contradicted by this hiatus betwixt the termination of contraction in the AHL and DHL [3, 27, 33, 34].

1.5 FUNCTION ANATOMY OF RIGHT VENTRICLE

The RV is disparate from the LV because of its complex anatomy and low-pressure function. The distinct anatomy, ultrafine structure of myocardium, and coronary functioning of the RV are engineered to operate as a low-pressure and high-volume pump under normal circumstances. The RV was characterized as a passive conduit with restricted pumping capacity in early research by Starr and others [35]. But thanks to advances in functional imaging, we now know that diastolic load and RV systolic function—which are influenced by ventricular interdependence—are important factors in pulmonary hypertension, congenital heart disease, cardiac transplantation, congestive heart failure prognosis, and LV assist device use [36, 37]. Three-dimensional analysis of magnetic resonance imaging has shed light on the intricate geometry of the ventricles within the pericardium as well as their interactions. Unlike the ellipsoidal, concentric structure of the LV and the RV is composed of an outflow tract and a sinus (body). The RV has approximately one-sixth of the muscle mass of the LV and has chamber looking like crescent. Both ventricles are linked by spiraling muscular bundles that encircle them in a complex, interwoven way, effectively generating a single functional unit despite their noticeably different muscle masses and chamber shapes. The prominent interest is the outflow tract, or RV conus. The RV conus was recognized by Keith in 1924 as physically separate from the RV's main body. It was proved that in every vertebrate embryo that is in developing phase, the S-shaped bulbus cordis exists as a distinct distal part to common ventricle. The bulbus cordis vanishes as the LV grows, but it continues to form the infundibulum or outflow tract in the RV [38]. Later research by Armour and Randall demonstrated that in nine distinct mammalian species, including humans, the muscle fibers of the RV conus go parallelly from the epicardium to the endocardium [39]. On the other hand, the muscle fibers of the RV sinus have a fiber orientation akin to the LV's as they progressively shift at right angles from the epicardium to the endocardium [35–37].

1.6 FUNCTION ANATOMY OF LEFT VENTRICLE

The LV has notable regional variation throughout its long axis, which extends from the apex to the base and is normally formed like a thick-walled prolate ellipsoid. The circumferential and longitudinal radii of the LV wall curvature vary significantly, according to tagging magnetic resonance (TMR) imaging. The LV wall becomes flatter toward the apex, and the LV cavity appears more oval along the short axis. Furthermore, the LV wall gradually thins as it gets closer to the apex, and the posterolateral wall is noticeably thicker than the septum all around the LV. The large variance in LV wall thickness has been explained by the law of Laplace and differences in the orientation of longitudinal and circumferential muscle fibers. According to the majority of research, the oblique helical fibrous arrangement is found in the LV's myocardial structure, with a clockwise helix in the subendocardial area and a left-handed helix that progressively changes into the subepicardial zone [40, 41]. Myocardial fibers are predominantly orientated circumferentially in the mid-layer of the LV wall, whereas endocardial fibers spiral obliquely toward the base and epicardial fibers spiral obliquely toward the apex. Mathematical simulations support the idea that this counter-directional helical arrangement of cardiac fibers is very energy-efficient and essential for the uniform redistribution of stress and strain inside the heart. With diffusion tensor cardiac magnetic resonance (CMR) imaging, a helical configuration of ventricular myocardial fibers that is remarkably consistent in mammalians was validated later. This imaging method detects regional anisotropic dispersion of water molecules, which enables accurate determination of the three-dimensional alignment of myocytes. Poveda et al. followed the ventricular myocardium's continuous helical structure from the pulmonary artery to the aorta using a streamlined tracto-graphic reconstruction technique. A counter-directional helical arrangement around the ventricles was revealed by following the helical structure that encircles the basal ring further into the LV and tracing it toward the apex [40–43].

1.6.1 Left Ventricle Torsional Deformation

The LV twists during systole and untwists during diastole due to the shortening and lengthening of myocardial fibers organized in a helical pattern. A brief clockwise rotation occurs prior to the LV apex's counterclockwise rotation around its longitudinal axis during systole, which is caused by the subendocardial fibers early shortening during isovolumic contraction. On the other hand, during cardiac contraction, the LV base rotates in reverse direction. It rotates clockwise during LV ejection and briefly counterclockwise during isovolumic contraction [41]. The net result is a twisting of the LV that enhances the mechanical efficiency of blood ejection into the aorta. The twisting of the LV is thought to be caused by the mechanical advantage of the subepicardial fibers, which produce more torque than the inner layers because of their longer lever arm. This motion is commonly compared to the process of wringing out a wet towel. Apical rotation is the primary factor that determines LV twist because the systole, the base rotation is smaller than the diastole, the apical rotation. Because the subepicardial fibers are farther from the LV axis and have a bigger lever arm than the endocardial fibers, it is thought that their mechanical advantage over the inner layer's accounts for the direction of LV twist. Effective LV systolic performance depends on systolic twist because it permits higher intraventricular pressure while decreasing ventricular transmural strain and oxygen consumption. Early diastole sees a quick unwinding of the LV after systolic LV twist as the potential energy is stocked as the contracted elastic components of myocardium during systole are unleashed. With the LV apex acting as the main catalyst for LV recoil, the majority of this untwisting takes place during isovolumic relaxation. Because it creates an early DIvPg (diastolic intraventricular pressure gradient) that facilitates diastolic suction, swift diastolic untwisting is necessary for a swift drop in LV pressure. Additionally, a sequence of diastolic events has been observed, with peak diastolic untwisting occurring before peak DIvPg and peak diastole filling velocity. Consequently, stroke volume, LV filling (while diastole, LA fills blood in LV), and LV end-diastolic volume can all be severely compromised by any disease that affects the rate of untwisting [40–44].

1.7 VENTRICULAR FUNCTIONING OF HEART

There is constant contact between the right and LVs due to their intimate physical connection, which includes their shared coronary blood flow, interlaced muscle bundles, and interatrial and interventricular septa. In terms of functionality, the ventricles function similarly to two piston pumps operating in a row, one linked to the less flexible systemic circulation and the other to extremely flexible pulmonary vasculature. The pericardium, which surrounds both ventricles, does not enlarge much in response to abrupt stress. When the vascular load on one of the pumps is altered by an acute or chronic hemodynamic disturbance, these anatomical and functional linkages allow for both series and direct interactions. Many people believe that Bernheim was the first to propose that modifications in one ventricle might have an impact on the other. He postulated in 1910 that compression of the RV due to LV hypertrophy and dilatation may result in decreased RV function, venous congestion, and heart failure [45]. Eventually, Henderson and Prince (1914) showed that applying pressure or volume to one ventricle decreased the function and output of the other ventricle using a model of an isolated cat heart. Dexter noted a decrease in LV performance in patients who experienced RV pressure and volume overload in 1956 when they had atrial septal abnormalities [36, 46]. The anticlockwise motion of the septum decreases LV filling and function; this is known as the reverse Bernheim effect. Since then, it has been established that variations in one chamber's compliance can have an impact on the other's filling, a diastolic interaction that is mostly mediated via the pericardium. Even in the absence of the pericardium, this interaction still occurs, suggesting additional contributory variables. The pericardial sac shields the heart from external structures by holding it in place and attaching it to the diaphragm, sternum, spinal column, and major vessels. The pericardium lubricates the heart to reduce friction and avoids acute cardiac overdistention, although it is not necessary for survival. The pericardium, which is made up of collagen fibrils and elastin fibers, is extremely resilient to acute distention. The J-shaped pressure-volume (rapid and slow effusion) and stress-strain curves indicate a rapid increase in stiffness following an initial phase of compliant behavior. The pericardium has anisotropic qualities due to the three layers of collagen fibers that are organized in distinct orientations. On the other hand, chronic arteriovenous fistulas have been demonstrated in animal models to exhibit creep and stress relaxation (increase in strain under constant stress is called creep, while the decrease in stress under constant strain is referred as stress relaxation) characteristics of the pericardium, hence diminishing their restraining function with time. Cardiac growth adapted by pericardium is due to creep (increase in volume with constant stretch) and cellular hypothermia.

1.7.1 Function of Interventricular Septum

Over the course of evolution, vertebrates modified the composition and functionality of their hearts to better suit their environments. Since the transition from aquatic to terrestrial life requires more oxygen and energy, vertebrates have developed a pulmonary circulation and septated the heart into venous and arterial segments to enable the flow of oxygenated blood to the peripheral parts. The three distinct septa-muscular, outlet, and inlet separately merge to form the IVS by the fifth week of embryonic development [47, 48]. There are two parts to the IVS: a muscle and a membrane. The common ventricle's endocardial surface is the source of the muscular IVS component, which has a typical thickness of roughly 9 mm in women and 10 mm in men. Between the LV and RV's outflow tracts is the relatively small membranous component of the IVS, known as the fibrous component. The studies on animals that examined the transmural and biaxial properties of the IVS revealed that the myofiber angle changed from a longitudinal orientation on the LV-side to a circumferential orientation in the mid-wall and back to a longitudinal orientation on the RV-side of the septum. Anisotropy, or the orientation of the myofibers, was the primary transmural alteration in the septum; it had nothing to do with the tissue's composition or mechanical characteristics. During this study, Truong and his coworkers discovered that the septum had substantially less collagen than the ventricular walls and that both of its sides were noticeably softer than the corresponding ventricular walls. This study suggested that at low strains, the LV and RV side of the septum showed a comparable anisotropic behavior with a stiffer material property in the longitudinal direction as opposed to the circumferential direction. A symmetric distribution of the fiber orientations was also observed. Both LV and RV sides exhibited isotropic behavior at high stresses. There was comparable intrinsic elasticity on both septal sides [48]. The larger volume of the blood supply to the IVS is provided by penetrating arteries that arrive from the LAD artery, with the exception of the posterior region of the IVS, which receives blood supply from branches of the PDA. In the human heart, the IVS is one of the collateral circulation channels. The inferior IVS is drained by the middle cardiac vein (also known as inferior interventricular vein), which flows into the CS (coronary sinus) from inferior interventricular sulcus.

The IVS undergoes thickening and advances towards LV during systole when electrical depolarization starts, and it briefly "shudders" toward the end of systole. In contrast, during diastole, it reverts to its initial thickness and location. Collagen content is lower in the IVS sides than in the equivalent ventricular free walls, and the IVS sides are noticeably softer. Furthermore, both sides exhibit comparable anisotropic behavior at low stresses, whereas both exhibit isotropic behavior at high strains. While "ventricular interdependence" refers to the functional interaction between the LV and RV through IVS, twisting and normal septal location are necessary for functioning of ventricular. The IVS is involved in both LV and RV functions because of its position. Studies examining the septum's role in LV and RV stroke output are, nevertheless, scarce. Molaug and colleagues investigated the lengths of myocardial cords using piezoelectric crystals placed along the longitudinal section of the IVS in which IVS seems roughly triangular and the free walls of the right and LVs during saline infusion in open-chest dogs. They discovered that end-diastolic cord lengths and also enhancement in myocardial shortening similarly in the free walls and the septum as end-diastolic pressures approached

10 mmHg in both ventricles. After peri-cardiotomy, end-diastolic pressures dropped by 1–2 mmHg, but myocardial shortening and end-diastolic segment lengths continued to rise in the free walls and IVS. Both transverse and longitudinal septal diameters reacted similarly in a group of dogs. These results imply that the IVS activates the Frank-Starling mechanism and that, rather than a change in septal position, the rise in left and right ventricular end-diastolic pressures is caused by the pericardium's restraining action during volume expansion. However, this conclusion cannot be conclusively proven without measuring septal curvature [36, 47–49].

1.8 CONDUCTION SYSTEM IN HEART

The ability of cardiac myocytes to spontaneously generate impulses that result in rhythmic contractions is a unique feature. SA node regulates the rhythm of heart as well as it also generates fastest impulse, which is usually where the electrical impulse begins. Subsequently, the impulse propagates via the right atrial walls, passes through interatrial conducting fibers to the LA, and ultimately arrives at the AV junctional tissue. Before the impulse travels across the AV bundle of His and Purkinje fibers and enters the ventricular myocardium, it is delayed by the AV node (Figures 1.11 and 1.12).

Excitation from the Purkinje fibers travels to the subendocardial surface via myocardial cells that are not part of the specialized conduction pathway. Both ventricles contract in unison as a result of the quick, synchronized diffusion of stimulation across the ventricles, which guarantees effective blood pumping to the pulmonary and systemic circulations.

The potassium (K^+) conductance is the primary element of the constant resting membrane potential of the ventricles, atria, and Purkinje system, which is maintained at around –90 mV. These cells have an action potential that lasts approximately 300 ms, which is a lot longer than the action potential of the majority of other body cells. The upstroke of the action potential, sometimes referred to as phase 0 (Figures 1.13 and 1.14),

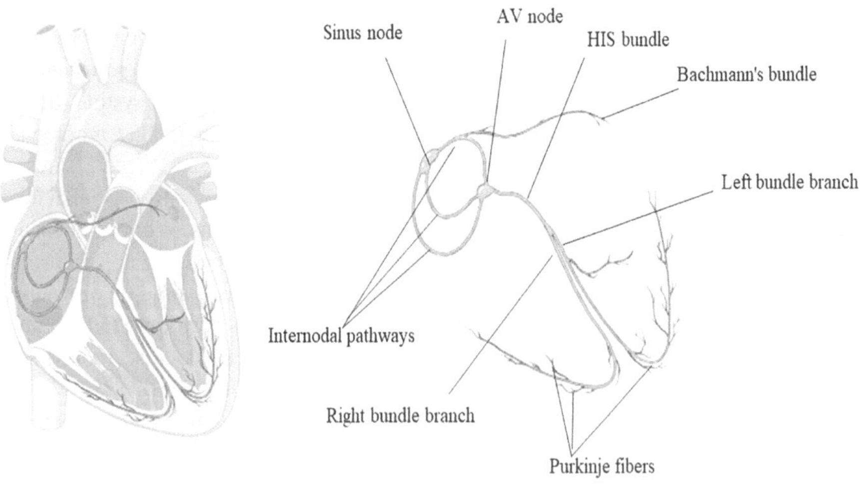

FIGURE 1.11 Human hearts conduction system with its simplified version.

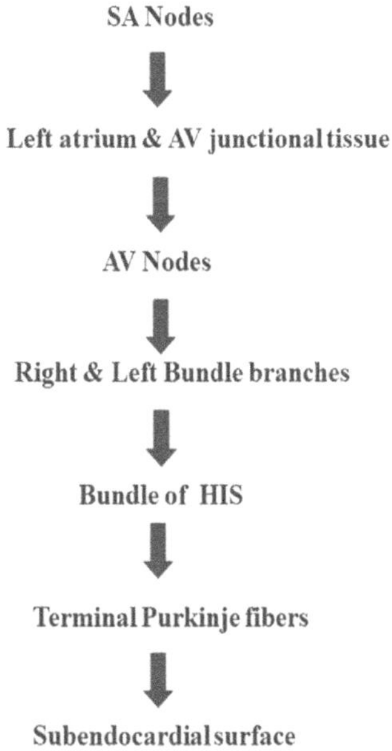

FIGURE 1.12 Flow chart of conduction system of human heart.

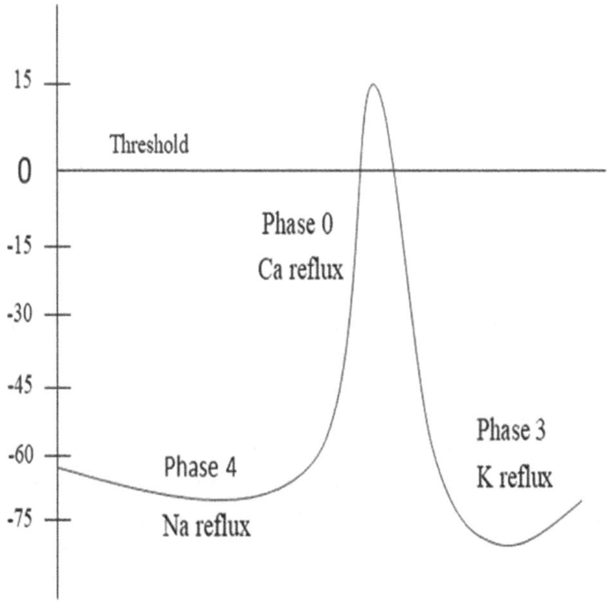

FIGURE 1.13 SA nodal potential graph.

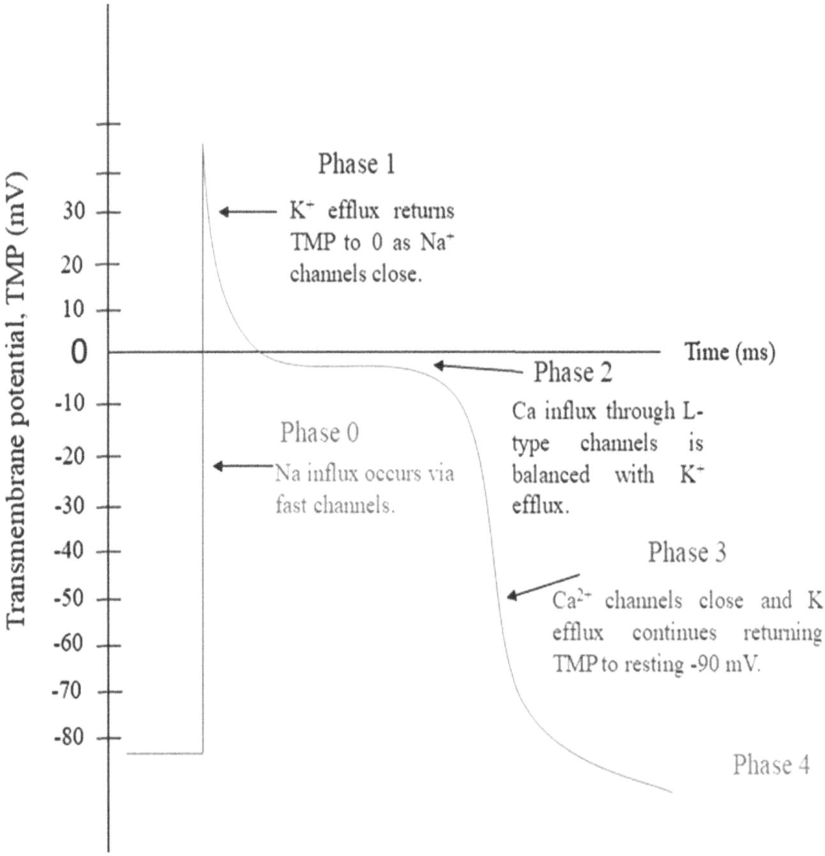

FIGURE 1.14 Cardiac action potential graph.

is the abrupt, brief rise in sodium (Na^{3+}) ion membrane conductance that occurs at the start of the action potential in cardiac cells, with the exception of the nodal tissue. The conductance of the potassium (K^{+}) ion membrane briefly increases after that, resulting in the first phase of repolarization [9, 16, 17].

Phase 1 of the action potential, which is the first repolarization phase, is also influenced by the reduction in sodium (Na^{3+}) ion conductance. The plateau phase, also known as phase 2, comes after this one. It is characterized by a brief rise in the inward conductance of calcium ions (Ca^{2+}) and an increase in the outward conductance of potassium ions (K^{+}). During the plateau period, the membrane potential is maintained by the balance between these inward and outward currents. Afterward, the action potential moves into phase 3, also known as the repolarization phase, which is defined by a rise in the conductance of outward K^{+} ion and a reduction in the inward Ca^{2+} ion conductance. Phase 4 of the repolarization phase occurs as a result of the membrane being hyperpolarized toward the K^{+} ion equilibrium due to the increased K^{+} conductance. The myocardium and the remainder of the conduction system have different action potentials than the SA node. Phase 4 of its characteristics includes an unstable resting membrane potential brought on by an inward Na^+ current and an enhanced Na^+ ion conductance. The previous action potential's repolarization initiates this inward Na^+ current. In the SA nodal potential graph, the action potential during phase 0 is driven by the inward refluxing of Ca^{2+} ion conductance instead of Na^+ ions, in contrast to surplus of the myocardium. Furthermore, the SA nodal action potential is devoid of the cardiac cell's phase 2, the plateau phase. Like the SA node, the AV node's action potential upstroke is caused by Ca^{2+} ion conductance. The Purkinje system has the quickest conduction velocity, whereas the AV node has the slowest.

1.9 CONCLUSION

The function of the anatomy of human heart is intricate, enthralling, and also essential. But in order to use this knowledge in clinical practice effectively, one must have a thorough comprehension of its underlying theories, workings, and functions. Understanding changes in cardiac architecture and physiology and having a firm grasp of these concepts helps in both diagnosing and forecasting prospective ailments as well as their symptoms. The HVMB model, put forth by G. Torrent, which provides a functional anatomical explanation for the observed twist as well as directional motions of the heart, is supported when comparing functional imaging with different structural models. Additional research is required to fully understand these notions of spatial anatomy. Keith's problem might be resolved, and a more precise knowledge of cardiac dynamics could result from the right validation of the coordination between heart structure and function.

DECLARATION OF CONFLICT OF INTEREST

The author declares that there is no competitive or financial interest known to influence the work reported in this chapter.

ACKNOWLEDGMENTS

The authors gratefully acknowledged HBTU Kanpur (SS) and UPCST, Uttar Pradesh for research project grant no. CST/D-831, Project id: 3993 (SK).

ABBREVIATIONS

AHL	Ascending helical limb
AL	Anterior leaflet
ALC	Anterolateral commissure
ATP	Adenosine Triphosphate
AV	node Atrioventricular node
CS	Coronary sinus

DHL	Descending helical limb
DIvPg	Diastolic intraventricular pressure gradient
HVMB	Helical ventricular myocardial band
IDHL	Inner descending helical limb
IVS	Interventricular septum
LA	Left atrium
LAD	Left anterior descending
LCf	Left circumflex
LV	Left ventricle
MVO	Mitral valve opening
OAHL	Outer ascending helical limb
PDA	Posterior descending artery
PMC	Posteromedial commissure
PL	Posterior leaflet
RA	Right atrium
RCA	Right coronary artery
RV	Right ventricle
TEE	Transesophageal echocardiography
TMR	Tagging magnetic resonance

REFERENCES

1. G. Heusch, P. Libby, B. Gersh, D. Yellon, M. Böhm, G. Lopaschuk, L. Opie, Cardiovascular remodelling in coronary artery disease and heart failure, The Lancet 383 (2014) 1933–1943. https://doi.org/10.1016/S0140-6736(14)60107-0
2. D.N. Ku, Blood flow in arteries, Annu Rev Fluid Mech 29 (1997) 399–434. https://doi.org/10.1146/annurev.fluid.29.1.399
3. G. Buckberg, J.I.E. Hoffman, A. Mahajan, S. Saleh, C. Coghlan, Cardiac mechanics revisited, Circulation 118 (2008) 2571–2587. https://doi.org/10.1161/CIRCULATIONAHA.107.754424
4. J. Zimmerman, pmc_2311951, 39 (1966) 348–366.
5. B. Gerald, N. Navin, N. Christopher, K. Mladen, What is the heart? Anatomy, function, pathophysiology, and misconceptions, J Cardiovasc Dev Dis 5 (2018). https://doi.org/10.3390/jcdd5020033
6. A. F, Early Science in Oxford, Nature 130 (1932) 946–947. https://doi.org/10.1038/130946a0
7. F. Torrent-Guasp, G.D. Buckberg, C. Clemente, J.L. Cox, H.C. Coghlan, M. Gharib, The structure and function of the helical heart and its buttress wrapping. I. The normal macroscopic structure of the heart, Semin Thorac Cardiovasc Surg 13 (2001) 301–319. https://doi.org/10.1053/stcs.2001.29953
8. R. Stoney, Gray's anatomy, 38th edition, J Vasc Surg 25 (1997) 964–965. https://doi.org/10.1016/S0741-5214(97)70243-X
9. S. Shah, G. Gnanasegaran, J. Sundberg-Cohon, J.R. Buscombe, The Heart: Anatomy, Physiology and Exercise Physiology, in: A. Movahed, G. Gnanasegaran, J. Buscombe, M. Hall (Eds.), Integrating Cardiology for Nuclear Medicine Physicians: A Guide to Nuclear Medicine Physicians, Springer Berlin Heidelberg, Berlin, Heidelberg, 2009: pp. 3–22. https://doi.org/10.1007/978-3-540-78674-0_1
10. E.L. Boulpaep, Organization of the Cardiovascular System, 2009. https://api.semanticscholar.org/CorpusID:78101857

11. J.F. Malouf, W. Edwards, J. Tajik, J.B. Seward, Functional Anatomy of the Heart, in: V. Fuster, R.A. Harrington, J. Narula, Z.J. Eapen, eds. Hurst's the Heart. McGraw-Hill Education, New York, USA, 2017: pp. 45–86.
12. Robert E. Shaddy, Daniel J Penny, Timothy F. Feltes, Frank Cetta, Seema Mital, Cardiac anatomy and Examination of Cardiac Specimens, in Moss and Adams' Heart Disease in Infants, Children, and Adolescents: Including the Fetus and Young Adult: Eighth Edition (Vol. 1-2). Wolters Kluwer Health Adis (ESP), 30 May 2013: USA, 2013.
13. S.Y. Ho, Anatomy of the mitral valve, Heart 88 (2002) iv5. https://doi.org/10.1136/heart.88.suppl_4.iv5
14. M. Castellá, G.D. Buckberg, S. Saleh, Diastolic dysfunction in stunned myocardium: A state of abnormal excitation–contraction coupling that is limited by Na+–H+ exchange inhibition, Eur J Cardiothorac Surg 29 (2006) S107–S114. https://doi.org/10.1016/j.ejcts.2006.02.042
15. C.H. Lee, F. Vancheri, M.S. Josen, D.G. Gibson, Discrepancies in the measurement of isovolumic relaxation time: A study comparing M mode and Doppler echocardiography, Heart 64 (1990) 214–218. https://doi.org/10.1136/hrt.64.3.214
16. W. Ganong, Lange Review of Medical Physiology, 21st ed., McGraw-Hill, New York, USA, 2003.
17. W. Ganong, Lange Review of Medical Physiology, 22nd ed., McGraw-Hill, New York, USA, 2005.
18. T.N. James, Anatomy of the coronary arteries in health and disease, Circulation 32 (1965) 1020–1033. https://doi.org/10.1161/01.cir.32.6.1020
19. Z. Vlodaver, H.N. Neufeld, J.E. Edwards, Coronary Arterial Variations in the Normal Heart and in Congenital Heart Disease, Academic Press, New York, 1975. https://api.semanticscholar.org/CorpusID:57553212
20. M. Loukas, C. Groat, R. Khangura, D.G. Owens, R.H. Anderson, The normal and abnormal anatomy of the coronary arteries, Clin Anat 22 (2009) 114–128. https://doi.org/10.1002/ca.20761
21. M.J. Schlesinger, P.M. Zoll, S. Wessler, The conus artery: A third coronary artery, Am Heart J 38 (1949) 823–836. https://doi.org/10.1016/0002-8703(49)90884-4
22. W. Edwards, Anatomy of the Cardiovascular System, Harper & Row, Philadelphia, 1984.
23. J. Bullock, J.I. Boyle, M. Wang, Physiology, The National Medical Series for Independent Study, 2nd ed., Williams and Wilkins, Maryland, 1991.
24. J.S. Robb, R.C. Robb, The normal heart: Anatomy and physiology of the structural units, Am Heart J 23 (1942) 455–467. https://doi.org/10.1016/S0002-8703(42)90291-6
25. D.H. MacIver, J.B. Partridge, P. Agger, R.S. Stephenson, B.J.D. Boukens, C. Omann, J.C. Jarvis, H. Zhang, The end of the unique myocardial band: Part II. Clinical and functional considerations, Eur J Cardiothorac Surg 53 (2018) 120–128. https://doi.org/10.1093/ejcts/ezx335
26. J.A. Armour, W.C. Randall, Electrical and mechanical activity of papillary muscle, Am J Physiol 218 (1970) 1710–1717. https://doi.org/10.1152/ajplegacy.1970.218.6.1710
27. G.D. Buckberg, J.I. Hoffman, H.C. Coghlan, N.C. Nanda, Ventricular structure-function relations in health and disease: Part I. The normal heart., Eur J Cardiothorac Surg. 47 (2015) 587–601. doi: 10.1093/ejcts/ezu278.
28. D.H. MacIver, R.S. Stephenson, B. Jensen, P. Agger, D. Sánchez-Quintana, J.C. Jarvis, J.B. Partridge, R.H. Anderson, The end of the unique myocardial band: Part I. Anatomical considerations, Eur J Cardiothorac Surg 53 (2018) 112–119. https://doi.org/10.1093/ejcts/ezx290
29. M. Castella, G.D. Buckberg, S. Saleh, M. Gharib, Structure function interface with sequential shortening of basal and apical components of the myocardial band, Eur J Cardiothorac Surg 27 (2005) 980–987. https://doi.org/10.1016/j.ejcts.2005.01.051

30. N.B. Ingels, D.E. Hansen, G.T. Daughters, E.B. Stinson, E.L. Alderman, D.C. Miller, Relation between longitudinal, circumferential, and oblique shortening and torsional deformation in the left ventricle of the transplanted human heart, Circ Res 64 (1989) 915–927. https://doi.org/10.1161/01.RES.64.5.915
31. R. Beyar, E.P. Shapiro, W.L. Graves, W.J. Rogers, W.H. Guier, G.A. Carey, R.L. Soulen, E.A. Zerhouni, M.L. Weisfeldt, J.L. Weiss, Quantification and validation of left ventricular wall thickening by a three-dimensional volume element magnetic resonance imaging approach, Circulation 81 (1990) 297–307. https://doi.org/10.1161/01.CIR.81.1.297
32. B. Jung, M. Markl, D. Föll, J. Hennig, Investigating myocardial motion by MRI using tissue phase mapping, Eur J Cardiothorac Surg 29 (2006) S150–S157. https://doi.org/10.1016/j.ejcts.2006.02.066
33. G.D. Buckberg, A. Mahajan, B. Jung, M. Markl, J. Hennig, M. Ballester-Rodes, MRI myocardial motion and fiber tracking: A confirmation of knowledge from different imaging modalities, Eur J Cardiothorac Surg 29 (2006) S165–S177. https://doi.org/10.1016/j.ejcts.2006.02.064
34. G.D. Buckberg, I.E. Hoffman, H.C. Coghlan, N.C. Nanda, Ventricular structure–function relations in health and disease: Part I. The normal heart, Eur J Cardiothorac Surg 47 (2015) 587–601. https://doi.org/10.1093/ejcts/ezu278
35. I. Starr, W.A. Jeffers, R.H. Meade, The absence of conspicuous increments of venous pressure after severe damage to the right ventricle of the dog, with a discussion of the relation between clinical congestive failure and heart disease, Am Heart J 26 (1943) 291–301. https://doi.org/10.1016/S0002-8703(43)90325-4
36. L.J. Dell'Italia, Anatomy and physiology of the right ventricle, Cardiol Clin 30 (2012) 167–187. https://doi.org/10.1016/j.ccl.2012.03.009
37. A.C.P. Bakos, The question of the function of the right ventricular myocardium: An experimental study, Circulation 1 (1950) 724–732. https://api.semanticscholar.org/CorpusID:30099641
38. A. Keith, Schorstein lecture on the fate of the bulbus cordis in the human heart: Given at the London Hospital Medical College on Dec. 17th, 1924, The Lancet 204 (1924) 1267–1273. https://doi.org/https://doi.org/10.1016/S0140-6736(01)23270-X
39. J.A. Armour, W.C. Randall, Structural basis for cardiac function, Am J Physiol 218 (1970) 1517–1523. https://doi.org/10.1152/ajplegacy.1970.218.6.1517
40. J.S. Rankin, P.A. McHale, C.E. Arentzen, D. Ling, J.C. Greenfield, R.W. Anderson, The three-dimensional dynamic geometry of the left ventricle in the conscious dog 39 (1976) 304–313. Circulation Research, doi: 10.1161/01.res.39.3.304.
41. C.C. Beladan, A. Călin, M. Roşca, C. Ginghină, B.A. Popescu, Left ventricular twist dynamics: Principles and applications, Heart 100 (2014) 731–740. https://doi.org/10.1136/heartjnl-2012-302064
42. P. Sengupta, J. Korinek, M. Belohlavek, J. Narula, M. Vannan, A. Jahangir, B. Khandheria, Left ventricular structure and function. Basic science for cardiac imaging, J Am Coll Cardiol 48 (2006) 1988–2001. https://doi.org/10.1016/j.jacc.2006.08.030
43. Y. Notomi, M.G. Martin-Miklovic, S.J. Oryszak, T. Shiota, D. Deserranno, Z.B. Popovic, M.J. Garcia, N.L. Greenberg, J.D. Thomas, Enhanced ventricular untwisting during exercise: A mechanistic manifestation of elastic recoil described by Doppler tissue imaging, Circulation 113 (2006) 2524–2533. doi: 10.1161/CIRCULATIONAHA.105.596502.
44. J. Bogaert, F.E. Rademakers, Regional nonuniformity of normal adult human left ventricle, Am J Physiol Heart Circ Physiol 280 (2001) H610–620. doi: 10.1152/ajpheart.2001.280.2.H610.
45. M.D. Arthur Selzer, W. Herbert, M.D. Bradley, M. Forrest, M.D. Willett, A critical appraisal of the concept of bernheim's syndrome, The American Journal of Medicine, 18 (1955) 567–576. https://doi.org/10.1016/0002-9343(55)90457-5.

46. Y. Henderson, A.L. Prince, The relative systolic discharges of the right and left ventricles and their bearing on pulmonary congestion and depletion, Heart 5 (1914) 217–226.
47. F. Triposkiadis, A. Xanthopoulos, K.D. Boudoulas, G. Giamouzis, H. Boudoulas, J. Skoularigis, The interventricular septum: Structure, function, dysfunction, and diseases, J Clin Med 11 (2022). https://doi.org/10.3390/jcm11113227
48. M. Nguyen-Truong, W. Liu, C. Doherty, K. LeBar, K.M. Labus, C.M. Puttlitz, J. Easley, E. Monnet, A. Chicco, Z. Wang, The interventricular septum is biomechanically distinct from the ventricular free walls, Bioengineering 8 (2021). https://doi.org/10.3390/bioengineering8120216
49. W.P. Santamore, L.J. Dell, Ventricular interdependence: Significant left ventricular contributions to right ventricular systolic function, Prog Cardiovasc Dis 40 (1998) 289–308. https://doi.org/10.1016/S0033-0620(98)80049-2

2 Cellular Sources and Biomechanical Conditioning for Cardiac Tissue Engineering

Shampa Ghosh, Krishna Kumar Singh, Surya Prakash Pandey, and Jitendra Kumar Sinha

2.1 INTRODUCTION

Cardiovascular disease (CVD) remains the leading cause of death worldwide, placing a significant burden on healthcare systems (Roth et al., 2020). Myocardial infarction (MI) presents challenges in treatment due to its restricted regenerative ability (Savoji et al., 2019). Conventional treatments for heart failure include pharmacotherapy, surgical intervention, and mechanical support devices (Ullah et al., 2023). They do not address the fundamental issue of lost or dysfunctional myocardial tissue. Cardiac tissue engineering (CTE) offers significant promise for repairing or preserving the damaged heart after MI and potentially regenerating the injured myocardium for long-term healing (Lai et al., 2023). This innovation opened up new research opportunities in CTE to bridge the gap between laboratory research and clinical application (Sharma et al., 2021). CTE aims to replicate the in vivo cardiac environment in vitro, with long-term objectives including the production of engineered tissues for cardiac repair and regeneration, preclinical models for drug toxicity assessment, and disease models to better understand heart-related illnesses (Echeverria Molina et al., 2021). With the global increase in CVD incidence improved treatment options are critical and overcome the limitations of donor tissue availability and immune rejection (Curtis and Russell, 2009). Various types of scaffolds (hydrogels, nanofibers, and decellularized tissues) may have the ability to replicate the environment of the heart (Roacho-Pérez et al., 2022). These scaffolds are appropriately porous, rigid, and biochemically active. The engineered scaffolds impersonate the mechanical and biochemical cues of the extracellular matrix (ECM) for promoting cell adhesion, proliferation, and differentiation in cardiac cells. This strategy also serves to deliver stem cells, CM mitogens, or drug carriers to the site of infarction. The ESCs, iPSCs, adult stem cells, MSCs, and cardiac progenitor cells (CPCs) are but a few of the cell lineages that have been explored for the purpose of CTE. These sources of cells each have distinct advantages and challenges related to their potential for differentiation, proliferation, and host tissue integration (Park et al., 2023; Zielińska et al., 2023). Therefore, the following requirements should be met by bioreactor-based frameworks for CTE application (Niu et al., 2023). There is assistance in uniform cell

DOI: 10.1201/9781003670995-2

transport, a controlled physiochemical environment, as well as oxygen levels, nutrition flow, and mechanical forces to imitate the physiological conditions of the human body in the bioreactors (Reina-Mahecha et al., 2023). This book chapter highlights recent progress in different types of cardiac stem cells with a particular focus on enhancing cardiomyocyte maturation for the fabrication of scaffolds.

2.2 CELLULAR SOURCES FOR CTE

Cardiac muscle cells (cardiomyocytes) are striated, branch, contain multiple mitochondria, and are under involuntary regulation. Each myocyte has a located core surrounded by a cell film known as the sarcolemma. The sarcolemma of cardiac muscle cells contains voltage-gated calcium channels, which have specialized particle channels that skeletal muscle lacks. Stem cells are undifferentiated cells that can self-renew and differentiate into various specialized cell types, allowing them to be used to cure several diseases that presently have no treatment. Stem cells can be found in both fetal and adult tissues. In an ideal scenario, stem cells and their sources should be available in sufficient quantities and capable of separating into beating CMs upon transplanting. They must be immune-compatible, allergy-free, and electro-physiologically compatible with the body's myocardium. The cardiac muscle generates electrical impulses from cardiomyocytes (Gittenberger-de Groot et al., 2012). The human heart muscle comprises a variety of cells, including CMs, pericytes, endothelial cells, and fibroblasts (Schwach and Passier, 2019). The CMs account for around 75% of the heart volume and 30–40% of the total cell number (Schwach and Passier, 2019). Variation in cellular composition and activity of expression in different cardiac regions reflects specialization in function. This section discusses the four primary cell types CPCs, iPSCs, MSCs, and ESCs in CTE (Augustine et al., 2021)

2.2.1 Cardiac Progenitor Cells (CPCs)

CPCs are a type of stem cell found in adult heart tissues. Their qualities support the healing of cardiac tissue repair. CPCs promote cardiomyocyte growth, angiogenesis, and blood flow. In addition, it is suggested that they inhibit apoptosis, reduce fibrosis and aggravation, resulting in a smaller scar. They can differentiate into several cell types, including cardiomyocytes, endothelium, and smooth muscle cells (Bryl et al., 2024). However, the regenerating capacity of cardiac tissue is confined because of the limited number of CPCs. Attempting to replicate the microenvironment of CPCs may help to enhance their ability for regeneration (Birket and Mummery, 2015). Cardiac tissue development aims to achieve this goal by mixing several microenvironmental components, such as cells, extracellular framework (ECM), and biochemical variables such as BMP2, VEGF, bFGF, DKK1, and IGF1(Ding et al., 2020). However, CPCs are no reliable CSC markers. It is difficult to identify them (Zhang et al., 2016). Few studies demonstrated that the CPCs derived from cardiac adipose tissue were successfully differentiated into cardiomyocytes, smooth muscle, and endothelial cells (Bryl et al., 2024). The therapeutic potential has also been highlighted in delivery systems with pericytes. They were able to restore vascular and muscle structures in infected mouse hearts (Barreto et al., 2019). CPCs are promising for CTE due to their proclivity to integrate and function inside cardiac tissue. In this regard, determining the optimal structure for assisting CPCs and their subordinates is critical. The scaffolds should be biodegradable, immune-privileged, provide electrical and/or mechanical qualities for cell connection and assembly, and promote back vascularization (Barreto et al., 2019). They have improved cardiac function when transplanted into wounded hearts (Pushp et al., 2021a). They can direct the differentiation of cardiac cells and stimulate epigenetic repair pathways (Mauretti et al., 2017). The use of CPCs is limited due to their rarity in the adult heart and difficulty in isolating and differentiation. There may be a need for an improved understanding of their regeneration mechanisms (Figure 2.1).

2.2.2 Induced Pluripotent Stem Cells

iPSCs are derived from adult somatic cells that have been genetically reprogrammed into cells similar to embryonic stem cells (ESCs). These cells can differentiate into cardiomyocytes (Clancy and Santana, 2024). iPSCs have pluripotency, self-tailored properties, and low immune rejection. iPSCs can generate enormous numbers of cardiomyocytes, which are necessary for the large-scale production of cardiac tissue

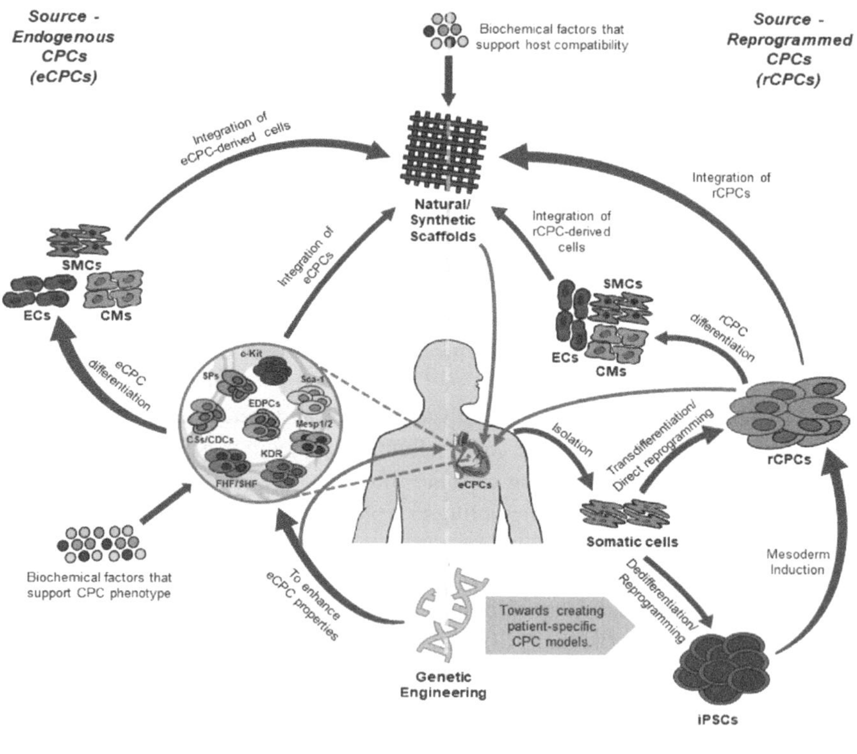

FIGURE 2.1 Different types of cardiac cells have regenerative applications (Barreto et al., 2019).

for therapeutic applications (Funakoshi and Yoshida, 2021). Significant progress has been made in optimizing methods for differentiating iPSCs into cardiomyocytes and other cardiac cells (Oikonomopoulos et al., 2018). These are generated by reprogramming patient-specific somatic cells with a variety of factors, including Oct4, Nanog, Sox2, Lin28 (ONSL), Klf4, and c-Myc (Cerneckis et al., 2024). These reprogramming methods have been improved through viral and nonviral delivery technologies. In addition, histone deacetylase inhibitors and growth factor modifications effectively induced human iPSCs to differentiate into cardiac cells (Xu et al., 2017). Comparative studies have shown that CMs generated from ESCs and iPSCs exhibit similar gene expression, beating patterns, and physiological responses. Recently, seeding on scaffolds/matrices helped differentiate them into functional cardiac cells (Prondzynski et al., 2024). PLGA-based scaffolds coated with polypyrrole were used to develop human iPSCs into beating cardiac cells (Gelmi et al., 2016). Furthermore, electrospun PCL-aligned nanofibers showed enhanced cell proliferation, adhesion (Pushp et al., 2021b). 3D culture of iPSCs improved electromechanical coupling into cardiac cells with characteristics similar to adult cardiomyocytes. The use of iPSCs is important in engineered cardiac tissue to treat cardiac damage (Cerneckis et al., 2024; Ye et al., 2013). A multifactorial approach successfully generated cardiac tissue sheets using temperature-responsive culture dishes, significantly restoring cardiac function (Kistamás et al., 2023). iPSCs have certain advantages, including minimizing the risk of immune rejection and the ethical and legal issues associated with ESCs.

2.2.3 Mesenchymal Stem Cells (MSCs)

These cells i.e. mesenchymal stem cells (MSCs) have been identified in the bone marrow, adipose tissue, placenta, and umbilical cord blood of adults. They contain some unique features, including multilineage differentiation potential, vascular and myocardial supportive capacity, and importantly, immunomodulatory properties. MSC therapies represent some of the most promising approaches for rejuvenation of the failing heart, especially their paracrine actions (Paul et al., 2009). Moreover, they have also been shown to adopt several of the phenotypic features and markers of cardiomyocytes (CMs) and to couple with residual CMs via Cx43 gap junctions, allowing the exchange of quasi-symmetrical junctional currents (Vasileios Karantalis, 2017). They have some advantages in tissue engineering compared to other sources of cells: anti-inflammation and immunomodulation, and differentiation into cardiomyocytes. Various studies performed the treatment of MI in rats using MSCs engrafted in 3D hydrogels (Guo et al., 2020).

The outcomes of such research have reported an improvement in the left ventricular function of injured cardiac animals (Wu et al., 2017). In addition, they enhanced the angiogenesis in the infracted region along with decreasing the damage of the tissue volume significantly as well as helped in hindering the death of muscular cells of the recipient heart four weeks after transplantation (Pittenger et al., 2019). These MSC layers help in myocardial tissue formation and paracrine signal. These effects help with promoting angiogenesis, protecting the heart, and enhancing left ventricular function (Fan et al., 2020; Ullah et al., 2015). Another study suggested that tissue-engineered vascular grafts (TEVGs) demonstrate to regulate the immune response, providing an additional advantage to vascular repair (Vasileios Karantalis, 2017). These findings have suggested that they may be laying the foundation for MSC-based therapies for heart conditions.

2.2.4 Embryonic Stem Cells (ESCs)

The ability of ESCs to differentiate into any one of the several hundred specialized cell types and their homogeneity makes them ideal to use in experimental studies. The latter capacity allows for the quantitative evaluation of begetter determination lineage fate-mapping and experimental manipulation of differentiation pathways. ESCs can generate an infinite number of progenies at defined formative phases useful in cellular therapy for heart infection. A major obstacle is the usually low efficiency of in vitro generation of cardiomyocytes from ESCs-1–3%. Due to their high degree of pluripotency, ESCs are a powerful tool for generating cardiac tissue; however, they also bear the risk of dangerous contaminants, including teratoma-forming cells (Csöbönyeiová et al., 2022). Further studies were then devoted to the refinement of methods for generating cardiac progenitors through guided differentiation and by forming embryoid bodies, procedures closely related to early developmental stages. It also finds applications in CTE (Zhao et al., 2021). More recently, cardiomyocytes differentiated from ESCs have been used in clinical trials to mature CMs themselves (Sacco et al., 2023). Developments like these have made the use of ESC-derived CMs in clinical trials questionable due to ethical concerns, possible immune responses, teratoma formation, and uncontrolled cell differentiation. Hence, their clinical usage in many parts of the world today is tightly restricted (Duelen and Sampaolesi, 2017; Min et al., 2024).

2.3 SCAFFOLD DESIGN AND FABRICATION TECHNIQUES IN CTE

CTE has focused on the development of scaffolds acting like a native environment niche of the heart. A properly designed scaffold besides enhancing cell attachment and proliferation will also facilitate the functional assembly of cardiac cells inside a tissue (Chiu and Radisic, 2013). The ideal scaffold will include numerous key features such as mechanical properties, anisotropy, elasticity, and contractility. Scaffolds may mimic the native cardiac microenvironment with fibrous anisotropic alignment and appropriate porosity (Carrier et al., 1999; Gálvez-Montón et al., 2013). It also helps to promote cardiac cell attachment, proliferation, and conductivity. Electrical stimulation has positively influenced the cell behavior of CMs (Wang and Guan Jianjun, 2010). The remaining portions of this chapter focused on the methodologies used to attain these required scaffold features. The development of cardiac tissue scaffold also depends on native CMs and impulsive and rhythmic contraction. The different stem cell sources show variations in contractile strength and tissue functionality (Maeda et al., 2017). Additionally, the protein composition within the cardiac ECM plays an important role in tissue maturation and functionality. The collagen type I (fibrous and structural) changes to type III collagen (spherical and elastic) during development, which affects the mechanical properties of the tissue (Eschenhagen et al., 2012). The presence of other ECM proteins (elastin) is important to provide elasticity to the continuous pumping action of the heart. The collagen type IV contributes to the structural integrity and functionality of the heart and influencing coronary artery stiffness. In addition, fibronectin and laminin are important for cell adhesion and migration, facilitating proper cell function within cardiac tissue. Connexin-43 plays roles in forming gap junctions necessary for electrical conductivity between cells for synchronized heart contractions (Radisic et al., 2007). Nevertheless, it becomes very important to explore various scaffold design and fabrication technologies with emphasis on their roles and also challenges. The findings indicate that intermediate stiffness levels (approximately 9 kPa) are most favorable for the formation of tissues with organized sarcomeres (Bouten et al., 2011). It increased the contractile strength and stiffness of native cardiac tissue (8–11 kPa). Scaffolds must be compatible with polymers and transplanted cells with minimal inflammatory responses (Huyer et al., 2015). Natural polymers such as collagen, fibrin, and polysaccharides have demonstrated the ability to promote effective cell differentiation of cardiac cells (Kieda et al., 2024). However, these natural biomaterials often lack appropriate mechanical strength. To address this, synthetic biocompatible polymers are used to provide mechanical strength (Bouten et al., 2011; Pomeroy et al., 2020). Cells are passively placed on scaffolds using traditional static seeding techniques. It may lead to insufficient cell penetration and low seeding effectiveness. To improve these results, alternative dynamic methods such as magnetic, vacuum, electrostatic, and centrifugal seeding have been developed for cell culture (Kieda et al., 2024; Patel and Patel, 2024). Different approaches offer distinct advantages and the seeding strategy should accord with both polymer properties and scaffold manufacturing processes (Figure 2.2).

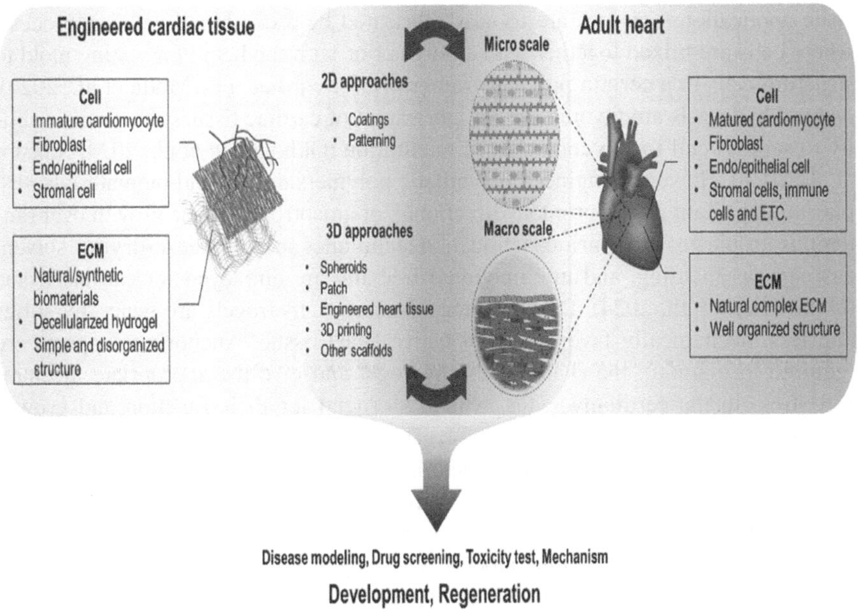

FIGURE 2.2 Different strategies to fabricate cardiac tissue by using cells and biomaterials (Sun and Nunes, 2017).

2.4 TECHNIQUES FOR SCAFFOLD FABRICATION

2.4.1 Hydrogels

MI, hypoxic conditions can cause tissue damage, cardiomyocyte loss, and alterations in the structure and function of the heart's ventricular wall and chambers (Mialet-Perez and Belaidi, 2024). Adult cardiomyocytes have limited regeneration capacity, making recovery of heart function after MI difficult (Mialet-Perez and Belaidi, 2024). There is an urgent need for therapies to heal the damaged heart particularly to address the long-term structural and functional damage reported following MI (Zheng et al., 2024a). The scarcity of donor hearts and the limited ability of CMs to regenerate have accelerated the development of hydrogel-based CVD treatments. These hydrogels are designed to mimic the ECM of native tissues. It also provides the necessary biophysical support and biochemical signals that promote the differentiation of stem cells into specific cardiac lineages.

Hydrogels are pivotal in tissue engineering for delivering bioactive agents like growth factors and proteins to mend damaged cardiac tissues (Ghosh et al., 2023, 2024a, 2024b; Nagayach et al., 2024; Narayanan et al., 2022; Patel and Patel, 2024; Sachdeva et al., 2023, 2024b). These polymers are particularly valued for their higher water content, which facilitates efficient gas and nutrient transfer (Choi and Kohane, 2024). This is important for oxygen and metabolite exchange (Motta et al., 2024). Their moldable nature allows them to be fabricated into various shapes. They can be easily modified or functionalized to include cellular adhesion sites such as RGD integrin-binding domains and ECM proteins (Choi and Kohane, 2024; Park et al., 2024). This flexibility in modification makes the hydrogel scalable for large-scale applications. Tissues are usually fabricated by a combined gelation process, where cells are mixed together with a polymer or with the help of a casting mold to structure cells in a certain polymer framework for cardiac TE (Motta et al., 2024). Natural hydrogels are favored for the fabrication of cardiac tissues due to their ability to support cell fusion and enhance maturation (Okhovatian et al., 2024; Rakshit et al., 2024). However, engineered synthetic polymers and hybrid biomaterials also play an important role to promote directional, or anisotropic, tissue growth over random, isotropic growth. Various fabrication techniques such as freeze-drying, solvent casting, gas foaming, and unidirectional freezing are employed for cardiac tissue (Okhovatian et al., 2024). Despite their advantages, hydrogels are generally softer and less mechanically favorable than native heart tissue. Anchoring supports are required to maintain the shape of the hydrogel and give the appropriate mechanical stress to the cardiomyocytes, which is crucial for their function and growth (Elkhoury et al., 2024; Guan et al., 2024). This configuration is additionally useful in measuring the force exerted by designed tissues, which can reach lengths of several millimeters, usually ranging from 7 to 9 mm.

Cabrerizo et al. found that injectable alginate-collagen hydrogel could retain heart function following MI in animal models. These hydrogels are injected into the heart of extracellular vesicles. It was indicating potential for heart repair based on studies that found an increase in scar thickness and an improvement in wall dimensions (Gil-Cabrerizo et al., 2022). Vuorenpää et al. were developed using gelatin gelin gum-based hydrogels with cardiomyocytes derived from iPSCs. The mechanical properties of these hydrogels were comparable to native rabbit heart tissue. The seeded cardiomyocytes were able to recover cardiac function (Vuorenpää et al., 2024). Hydrogels are also excellent carriers for drug delivery. They can be engineered to maximize the retention of therapeutic agents at targeted locations and their effectiveness in the body. Koivisto et al. (2019) developed dual-responsive hydrogel targeting inflammatory macrophages for atherosclerosis treatment (Koivisto et al., 2019). Also, the targeting studies using ApoE knockout mice and Cy7 as fluorescent tracers underlined specific signals in the heart region, which indicated precise delivery (Sachdeva et al., 2024a). These new formats provide for accurate regulation of drug release time and site, and even real-time monitoring of conditions, furthering diagnostic and therapeutic possibilities that hydrogels can bring to medical applications (Yi et al., 2024). All these innovations underline the importance of hydrogel technologies in solving complex problems of CVD therapy (Xu et al., 2024). The stimuli-responsive hydrogels are also known as "smart hydrogels," which exhibit a phase transition in response to external environmental stimuli such as pH, temperature, ultrasound, and reactive oxygen species. This phase change property makes the release of the drug encapsulated in the hydrogel matrix controlled. This feature increases the precision of therapeutic delivery, reducing side effects by making sure that medications are released only at specific sites (Elkhoury et al., 2024; Park et al., 2024).

Hybrid hydrogels combine the advantages of both natural and synthetic polymers offering cell recognition and mechanical properties for CTE. VEGF-loaded hybrid hydrogel was shown to improve neovascularization and cardiac recovery. While traditional hydrogels are typically applied directly to the heart or through epicardial coagulation, which requires significant surgical intervention than injectable hydrogels. These hydrogels use stimuli-responsive polymers that gel in response to environmental changes. A notable development is the thermo-responsive injectable polymer, which prevents adverse remodeling of the ventricular wall after ischemic events (Gao et al., 2024). These injectable hydrogels solidify after being injectable and providing support and potentially enhancing cardiac function. Furthermore, pH-responsive and self-healing supramolecular hydrogels have been used to effectively deliver growth factors in large animal MI models. It demonstrates the potential to reduce myocardial scarring. Other innovations include hydrogels with conductive, elastomeric, and oxygen-releasing properties, tailored to meet the specific mechanical and biological requirements of CTE (Elkhoury et al., 2024; Xu et al., 2024). Emphasis on CTE by hydrogel technology presents great promise for developing minimal invasive treatment options that can dramatically improve patient recovery after MI. These do point to the fact that further research needs to be done in optimizing properties in hydrogels, such as stiffness, gelation time, and physical stimuli response.

2.4.2 3D Printing

3D printing is considered an advanced tool for the fabrication of complicated tissue niches. This strategy has the potential for proper distribution and formation of tissues. It is possible to fabricate size, shape, and porosity by using 3D scaffolds. In addition, it is required to modify the geometry based on individual patients' medical imaging data. Extrusion, inkjet, laser-assisted printing, and stereolithography are some of the different bioprinting techniques that are commonly being employed in the fabrication of scaffolds. These methodologies have the potential to make a range of diverse tissues, including cartilage, brain tissue, and heart valves. It is challenging to bring adequate functional cardiomyocytes into a supportive scaffold to sustain its form and function at microscale during cardiac regeneration. The appropriate selection of cells with correct bioink is essential for the longevity and functional incorporation of tissue. This developing field is still growing within a frame from formulation of the bio-ink to functional testing of bio-printed cardiac tissues.

2.4.3 Electrospinning

Electrospinning represents a very effective method for the preparation of biomimetic non-woven scaffolds consisting of a great network of interconnected fibers and pores (Su et al., 2024). Electrospinning is based on the utilization of an electric field for the drawing of charged threads of polymer solutions or melts into fine fibers, capable of producing fibers in diameters ranging from nanometers up to micrometers (Huang et al., 2021). Electrospun scaffolds are morphologically similar to the fibrous structure of the ECM. The thin liquid jet of entangled polymer chains, ejected from the polymer reservoir towards the collection site due to electric field strength, determines the fiber orientation during passage through fast motion caused by instability in this jet (Ahmadi Bonakdar and Rodrigue, 2024; Gomes et al., 2022). Because of the physical similarities between micro-and nanofibers and protein fibrils in native ECM, micro and nanofibers hold high importance in tissue engineering (Huang et al., 2021).

These fibers have a high surface-area-to-volume ratio, which boosts substrate availability for cell adhesion and promotes tissue culture. Numerous studies have shown that electrospin fibers may promote cell attachment, proliferation, and ECM environment (Sekkarapatti Ramasamy et al., 2022; Singh et al., 2020, 2023a, 2023b). These scaffolds have been made from various polymers for a wide range of applications including nerve regeneration, bone, vascular, stem cell tissue, and skin tissue engineering. Many factors influence the electrospinning scaffolding process, including solution properties (such as viscosity and conductivity), controllable variables (such as flow rate and electric field strength), and ambient conditions (such as temperature and humidity). Traditional single-nozzle technology allows for the spinning of polymer mixtures. However, side-by-side or coaxial nozzles can produce fibers with distinct properties, which is useful for drug delivery applications (Ahmadi Bonakdar and Rodrigue, 2024; Su et al., 2024). The cell adhesion is strongly influenced on the hydrophilicity or hydrophobicity of synthetic polymers. The bio-composites have proven more successful in TE applications. Blending poly(1,8-octanediol-co-citrate) (POC) has been blended with poly(ε-caprolactone) (PCL) improves cell adherence and reduces degradation. It is suitable for use in cardiac patch (Vogt and Boccaccini, 2021).

In cardiac repair, the fibrous scaffolds seemed to minimize the immune responses and rejections. They allowed the cardiomyocytes to beat synchronously and maintained the anisotropic structure needed for heart function. Conductive polyaniline (PANI) was combined into the poly(glycerol acetate) (PGS) scaffolds tested in CTE application. (Wu et al., 2023). Combination of PGS and gelatin may also be used to develop clinically relevant constructs for CTE (Kharaziha et al., 2013).

This combination acts analogously to the architecture of the left ventricular myocardium and enhances the functionality of neonatal rat cardiac fibroblast cells. Cardiomyocytes are synthetic biodegradable patches repaired for a limited time. Polyester-based thermoplastic polymers such as PGA, PLA, and PCL have better elasticity and mechanical strength and hence preferred over patches. These patches are meant for biocompatibility and to bear continuous heartbeat during cardiac reconstruction (Broadwin et al., 2024). Smooth muscle cell growth was supported by electrospun PCL/PLA scaffolds. Besides, the scaffolds have been fabricated to promote entrance in SMCs and are blood-compatible (Shahverdi et al., 2022). The urgent need exists in the development of vascular structures similar to native blood vessels. Growth factors such as IGF-1 and HGF are transmitted through scaffolds that may stimulate angiogenesis, tissue regeneration at damaged sites. Scaffold embedding heparinized chitosan or poly ε-caprolactone (CS/PCL) nanofibers enhance rapid endothelialization. Its achievement of controlled degradation rates and enhancement of mechanical and electrical properties remains the main issues which electrospinning faces (Gomes et al., 2022). To overcome these challenges, research is being conducted to optimization the different combinations of synthetic and natural polymers.

2.5 DECELLULARIZATION TECHNIQUES

Decellularization and recellularization represent quite transformative approaches in the context of regenerative medicine, especially organ transplantation (Fu et al., 2014). This technology aims to transform donor heart organs into biocompatible scaffolds that can be subsequently re-cellularized with patient-specific cells to overcome some limitations in donor organ scarcity and immune rejection (Mendibil et al., 2020). Decellularization involves the removal of cells and maintaining ECM from the cardiac organ (Boccafoschi et al., 2017). The decellularization process needs to be maintained so that it does not affect the integrity and bioactivity of the ECM. It is similar to the cardiac tissue's natural microenvironment. Different types of proteins, glycoproteins, signaling molecules, and growth factors were within the ECM. They have also received some other important cell signaling, structural support, and tissue organization roles as well (Lu et al., 2012). Three kinds of methods were used such as physical treatment, chemical treatment, and enzymatic treatments for decellularization. Various types of detergents like SDS, Tween 20, and Triton X100 can remove the cellular material with a minimal amount of damage to ECM (Keane et al., 2015). These processes may, however, also interfere with protein conformation and remove inherent growth factors that play an active role in tissue growth (Bhaskar and Gupta, 2020; Bhaskar et al., 2022; Singh et al., 2021a, 2021b, 2022).

The subsequent step is recellularization, consisting of cell seeding an acellular scaffold with an appropriate population of cells capable of replacing functional properties. In the case of functional cardiac tissue, this step is critical because the tissue must be contractile and able to conduct electrical impulses (Tan et al., 2022). This will also ensure cell distribution and appropriate penetration throughout the scaffold. The most critical challenge is how to ensure the vascularization of the reseeded scaffold adequately to allow the survival and integration of the transplanted organ (Moroni and Mirabella, 2014). According to Barbulescu et al. (2022), the process of vascularization has been capable of providing nutrients and oxygen to the tissue (Barbulescu et al., 2022). Decellularization and recellularization techniques can be regarded as very promising for the fabrication of organ scaffolds meant for cardiac transplants. Such techniques have the potential to retain the structural and metabolic integrity of the ECM (Gilpin and Yang, 2017).

2.5.1 Microfabrication

Microfabrication of materials has newly rearranged the engineering to better simulate in vivo tissue environments. These methods allow one to stamp geometric patterns from masters onto the substrate in a rather precise manner, creating specified topographies that assist in the anisotropic organization of tissue structures (Ainslie and Desai, 2008; Brown and Khetani, 2018). Lithography permits the creation of substrates with microchannels and complicated microfluidic networks that mimic tissue vasculature. However, these manufacturing procedures can be labor-intensive, necessitating specialized equipment and facilities, and incur substantial production costs (Takeuchi et al., 2011). There are basic methods for creating material substrates that will help cardiomyocytes proliferate and sarcomeres align axially (Boudou et al., 2012). Alford et al. have developed biohybrid thin films composed of muscle cells micropatterned onto thin, flexible PDMS sheets (Alford et al., 2010).

The PDMS thin films with 20-μm-wide corrugated lines improved CM alignment and compliance during the cardiac cycle. Plasma design on polyethylene glycol substrates resulted in integrated spherical chambers with diameters ranging from 200 to 600 μm (Zeng et al., 2024; Zheng et al., 2024). These compartments contain iPSC colonies and direct the development of cardiac microchambers during differentiation (Liu et al., 2024). Patterned culture chambers help generate hydrogel-based cardiac tissues and promote long-term maturation by BioWireTM II. The Innovative applications of microfabrication have resulted in the creation of complex tissue architectures that resemble genuine myocardium (Takeuchi et al., 2011; Ugolini et al., 2018). Further advancements, the creation of accordion-like honeycomb scaffolds using laser microablation of poly(glycerol sebacate), are intended to improve CM alignment and optimize the mechano-microenvironment. Further studies have employed conductive biomaterials with nanoelectronics to create cardiac patches that are able to perform real-time electrophysiological recording and pacing. Such microfabrication techniques allow for outstanding intricacy and function at a tissue level, which can enable high-throughput studies (Elkhoury et al., 2021). This method opens up new frontiers in studying the complex structure and function of human heart tissue.

2.6 METHODS TO IMPROVE CARDIOMYOCYTE MATURATION IN CTE

Cardiomyocyte development may be a real obstacle to CTE; functional integration and long-term survival of bioengineered cardiac tissues depend largely on the development of cardiomyocytes within those tissues (Karbassi et al., 2020). Developed cardiomyocytes show certain functional, metabolic, and electrophysiological properties required for a healthy heart (Yang et al., 2023). This field of study encompasses numerous approaches that aim at the betterment of cardiomyocyte development, with a particular focus on further advances in this key area of CTE. Cardiomyocyte development encompasses a few significant changes, including improved sarcomeric organization, increased measurement, the formation of an adult-like metabolic profile, and advances in calcium signaling and electrical conductivity (Besser et al., 2018). Young cardiomyocytes frequently develop into tissue that is lacking in sufficient contractile property and unable to synchronize well with the surrounding myocardium; this therefore leads to problematic salutary results (Figure 2.3).

2.6.1 Electrical Stimulation

Electrical stimulation in the design of tissues is an active interventional strategy to enhance the formation of cardiomyocytes, which are critical to the successful incorporation of cardiac tissues (Tandon et al., 2009). The electrical stimulation significantly advances the cardiomyocytes of a phenotype that much more closely resembles the intrinsic electrical action of the heart (Serena et al., 2009). This bio-inspired methodology utilizes the electrophysiological experience within the heart to further cellular processes critical for utilitarian advancement. Electrical action is

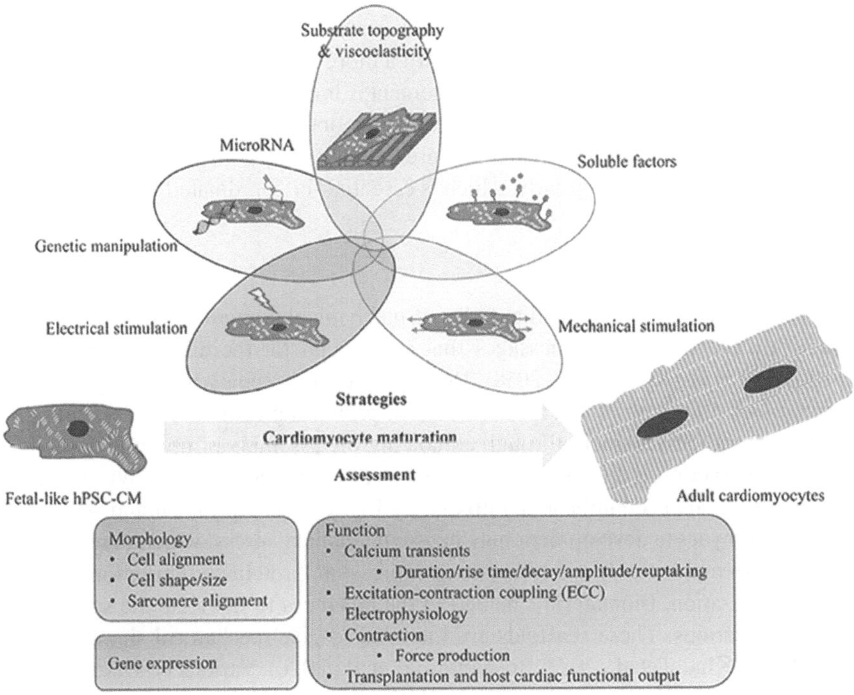

FIGURE 2.3 Schematic diagram showing the strategies to promote and the assessment of the maturation of cardiomyocytes (Sun and Nunes, 2017).

similarly fundamental to the general synchrony in muscle compression (Stoppel et al., 2016). Electrical stimulation supports the orientation of cardiomyocytes within the engineered cardiac tissue. Interconnected networks are a basic prerequisite of their structure for active contraction. More importantly, such stimulation increases the contractility of these cells, a vital feature that determines the beating efficiency of the muscle. The sarcomere is one of the most important basic components inside cardiomyocytes (Fomby et al., 2010; Love et al., 2018). They are made up of interdigitating actin and myosin fibers. Their intentional movement and basic keenness are essential for producing strong compression. It is altered by electrical excitation. Western blot and immunofluorescent staining revealed upregulation of cardio-progenitor markers (Nkx2.5, GATA-4, CTT, and C43) and enhanced cell communication after electrical stimulation, highlighting nanoscale biomimetic cues potential for electroactive tissue repair applications (Mooney et al., 2012). Integrating silicon nanowires into hiPSC cardiac spheroids significantly enhances cell–cell junctions and reduces spontaneous beat rate (Richards et al., 2016). Electrical stimulation promotes a greater assembly of sarcomeres within cardiomyocytes by mimicking the electrical impulses (Chan et al., 2013). Mechanical propellers in bioreactor designs have pushed the use of consistent and controlled electrical stimulus to generate heart tissues. Advanced bioreactors are designed with coordinate cathodes that provide continuous electrical stimulation to refined tissues, eliminating the variability that occurs with manual or less controlled stimulation procedures (Hernández et al., 2016). These include features that encode basic sarcomere proteins, particle channels, and other components critical to the cardiomyocyte's electrical and contractile capabilities. Upregulation of these characteristics indicates a formative shift toward a more developed cardiac phenotype, as observed in local heart tissue. This arrangement is important not only for the mechanical qualities of the tissue, but also for the generation of electrical signals inside the cardiac arrangement. Improved architecture increases the ability of the tissue to conduct electrical impulses regularly, which is essential for coordinated withdrawals.

2.6.2 Mechanical Stretch

The cardiac muscle performs the cycles of mechanical compression and relaxation. These are the mechanical messages that are crucial for the differentiation of the cardiomyocytes (Rysä et al., 2018). Recently, several studies have suggested that mechanical stretch plays a significant role in promoting cellular organization, prolongation, and development through enhancing the assembly of proteins needed for muscle contraction (Nguyen-Truong et al., 2020). The mechanical environment of the beating heart is complicated with energy by cyclic compression and relaxation. The cardiomyocyte development may cause mechanical stress, which may cause an alteration in molecular levels influencing expression, protein configuration, and cellular organization. Biomaterials helped in the advances to fabricate the scaffold for CTE applications. These scaffolds are intended to give mechanical signals to promote CMs (Khatat et al., 2023; Roshanbinfar et al., 2020). Various types of biomaterial are used to maintain rigidity and flexibility that support cellular communication and spatial framework for CMs. Electrospin fiber collagen (9.89%), hyaluronic acid (1.1%), and polyaniline (1.34%) had facilitate contraction periods, larger contractile amplitude, reduced beating rates, and increased connexin 43 expression postnatal rat cardiomyocytes. These findings indicate that such fibers are appropriate for human-induced pluripotent stem cell-derived CMs for CTE (Roshanbinfar et al., 2020). It can also influence the length of stretch-induced push channels with different compositions of materials. These promise to transform the production of functional cardiac tissues. It may be a better treatment option for cardiac diseases. Further, it helps to improve understanding of cardiac mechanics and pathogenesis.

2.6.3 Co-culture Systems

The human heart is composed of different cells such as fibroblasts, endothelial cells, smooth muscle cells, and cardiomyocytes. The CMs have around 30% to 40% of the total volume.

The heart has significant heterogeneity. The ventricles have different cellular signatures from atria (47.1% cardiomyocytes versus 31.1%, respectively) by single-cell sequencing research. The fraction of cFbs in the heart has been shown to range between 20% and 60% in rats and humans. Co-culture of different cardiac cells has emerged as a viable method for enhancing the development for constructed cardiac tissues (Gisone et al., 2022; Li et al., 2021). This strategy is based on the idea of replicating the complicated cellular environment of the heart. They will show more precise physiological to mimic the intuitive processes within the paracrine signaling and coordinated cell-cell interactions (Chu et al., 2020). They are essential for cellular separation, development, and function. Paracrine signals are produced by cells that affect nearby cells in the tissue microenvironment (Van Luyn et al., 2002). These signals stimulate cardiomyocyte growth, accelerate angiogenesis, and strengthen fibroblast and smooth muscle cell repair mechanisms (Ikeda et al., 2008).

The electrical coupling has to permit the physical and biochemical communications. They are necessary for the contraction and relaxation of the CMs (Li et al., 2024). While developing these co-culture systems, optimization is necessary concerning the culture medium and combination type of cells with several types of culture conditions media (Beauchamp et al., 2020). These ratios would mimic cardiac cellular morphology. The ratio between CMs and non-CMs dictates the structure of the tissue, the mechanical properties, and the electrical potential capacity (Kirkpatrick et al., 2011). Three-dimensional bioprinting and microfluidic devices have fundamentally expanded the ability to create complex co-culture environments. 3D printing enables printing different cell types that can mimic the 3D heart tissue architecture. This method allows the production of constructs with multiple cell types and bears a great resemblance to cardiac tissue (Battiston et al., 2014; Saini et al., 2015). It provides the study of cellular behavior under highly controlled conditions. It also provides effective tools in the design in vitro of cardiac models.

2.7 FUTURE PERSPECTIVES AND CONCLUSION

The landscape of CVD management is at a pivotal juncture with the integration of CTE into potential treatment paradigms. The persistent issue at the heart of CTE's promise lies in effectively addressing the irreversible loss and dysfunction of myocardial tissue post-MI. CTE represents a paradigm change from symptomatic treatment to restorative therapies by providing a bridge between acute mechanical intervention and true tissue repair using modern scaffold technologies and stem cell research. CTE represents the beginning of a new era in the treatment of cardiovascular medicine with overcoming the limitations of conventional treatment. The researchers are exploring to improve the potency of pluripotent stem cells (CMs, iPSCs, and ESCs) to generate cardiomyocytes in future developments in CTE. Furthermore, the emerging science of coordinate cell reconstruction or trans-differentiation points to a promising frontier in CTE applications.

The successful production of bioengineered cardiac tissues remains a significant problem. Future research will likely focus on applying electromechanical conditioning strategies for mimic the heart. These frameworks will advance to more accurately mimic the physiological settings in which cardiomyocytes participate in vivo, advancing the advancement of tissues with improved contractile quality and consistency.

Furthermore, biodegradable materials that mimic the mechanical and biochemical signals of the cardiac ECM would facilitate the integration of designer tissues with the existing heart, hence accelerating normal tissue regeneration following transplant. 3D bioprinting provides precise spatial distribution of various types of cells within bio-fabricated structures, better mimicking the heterogeneous structure of the heart. This could lead to more effective treatments for myocardial necrosis. As CTE approaches therapeutic applications, questions of resistive dismissal and integration with existing tissue will receive more attention. The use of stem cells will continue to drive debate to ensure that contemporary medications are safe and ethical. The long-term prospects for CTE are promising, with the potential to change the treatment of cardiac disease by addressing the critical limitations of present treatment. As the technology improves, it will certainly pose previously unanswered problems about the feasibility of retrieving human heart tissue.

FUNDING STATEMENT

No funding was received for the current work published in this chapter.

CONFLICT OF INTEREST

Authors declare no conflict of interest.

REFERENCES

Ahmadi Bonakdar, M., Rodrigue, D., 2024. Electrospinning: Processes, structures, and materials. Macromol 4, 58–103. https://doi.org/10.3390/macromol4010004

Ainslie, K.M., Desai, T.A., 2008. Microfabricated implants for applications in therapeutic delivery, tissue engineering, and biosensing. Lab Chip 8, 1864–1878. https://doi.org/10.1039/b806446f

Alford, P.W., Feinberg, A.W., Sheehy, S.P., Parker, K.K., 2010. Biohybrid thin films for measuring contractility in engineered cardiovascular muscle. Biomaterials 31, 3613–3621. https://doi.org/10.1016/j.biomaterials.2010.01.079

Augustine, R., Dan, P., Hasan, A., Khalaf, I.M., Prasad, P., Ghosal, K., Gentile, C., McClements, L., Maureira, P., 2021. Stem cell-based approaches in cardiac tissue engineering: Controlling the microenvironment for autologous cells. Biomed. Pharmacother. 138, 111425. https://doi.org/10.1016/j.biopha.2021.111425

Barbulescu, G.I., Bojin, F.M., Ordodi, V.L., Goje, I.D., Barbulescu, A.S., Paunescu, V., 2022. Decellularized extracellular matrix scaffolds for cardiovascular tissue engineering: Current techniques and challenges. Int. J. Mol. Sci. 23(21), 13040.

Barreto, S., Hamel, L., Schiatti, T., Yang, Y., George, V., 2019. Cardiac progenitor cells from stem cells: Learning from genetics and biomaterials. Cells 8, 1–55. https://doi.org/10.3390/cells8121536

Battiston, K.G., Cheung, J.W.C., Jain, D., Santerre, J.P., 2014. Biomaterials in co-culture systems: Towards optimizing tissue integration and cell signaling within scaffolds. Biomaterials 35, 4465–4476. https://doi.org/10.1016/j.biomaterials.2014.02.023

Beauchamp, P., Jackson, C.B., Ozhathil, L.C., Agarkova, I., Galindo, C.L., Sawyer, D.B., Suter, T.M., Zuppinger, C., 2020. 3D co-culture of hiPSC-derived cardiomyocytes with cardiac fibroblasts improves tissue-like features of cardiac spheroids. Front. Mol. Biosci. 7, 1–17. https://doi.org/10.3389/fmolb.2020.00014

Besser, R.R., Ishahak, M., Mayo, V., Carbonero, D., Claure, I., Agarwal, A., 2018. Engineered microenvironments for maturation of stem cell derived cardiac myocytes. Theranostics 8, 124–140. https://doi.org/10.7150/thno.19441

Bhaskar, R., Gupta, M.K., 2020. Testicular Tissue Engineering: An Emerging Solution for in Vitro Spermatogenesis, Biopolymer-Based Formulations: Biomedical and Food Applications. Elsevier Inc. https://doi.org/10.1016/B978-0-12-816897-4.00033-3

Bhaskar, R., Kumar Gupta, M., Soon Han, S., 2022. Tissue engineering approaches for the in vitro production of spermatids to treat male infertility: A review. Eur. Polym. J. 174, 111318. https://doi.org/10.1016/j.eurpolymj.2022.111318

Birket, M.J., Mummery, C.L., 2015. Pluripotent stem cell derived cardiovascular progenitors – A developmental perspective. Dev. Biol. 400, 169–179. https://doi.org/10.1016/j.ydbio.2015.01.012

Boccafoschi, F., Botta, M., Fusaro, L., Copes, F., Ramella, M., Cannas, M., 2017. Decellularized biological matrices: An interesting approach for cardiovascular tissue repair and regeneration. J. Tissue Eng. Regen. Med. 11, 1648–1657. https://doi.org/10.1002/term.2103

Boudou, T., Legant, W.R., Mu, A., Borochin, M.A., Thavandiran, N., Radisic, M., Zandstra, P.W., Epstein, J.A., Margulies, K.B., Chen, C.S., 2012. A microfabricated platform to measure and manipulate the mechanics of engineered cardiac microtissues. Tissue Eng. Part A 18, 910–919. https://doi.org/10.1089/ten.tea.2011.0341

Bouten, C.V.C., Dankers, P.Y.W., Driessen-Mol, A., Pedron, S., Brizard, A.M.A., Baaijens, F.P.T., 2011. Substrates for cardiovascular tissue engineering. Adv. Drug Deliv. Rev. 63, 221–241. https://doi.org/10.1016/j.addr.2011.01.007

Broadwin, M., Imarhia, F., Oh, A., Stone, C.R., Sellke, F.W., Bhowmick, S., Abid, M.R., 2024. Exploring electrospun scaffold innovations in cardiovascular therapy: A review of electrospinning in cardiovascular disease. Bioengineering 11. https://doi.org/10.3390/bioengineering11030218

Brown, G.E., Khetani, S.R., 2018. Microfabrication of liver and heart tissues for drug development. Philos. Trans. R. Soc. B Biol. Sci. 373. https://doi.org/10.1098/rstb.2017.0225

Bryl, R., Kulus, M., Bryja, A., Domagała, D., Mozdziak, P., Antosik, P., Bukowska, D., Zabel, M., Dzięgiel, P., Kempisty, B., 2024. Cardiac progenitor cell therapy: Mechanisms of action. Cell Biosci. 14, 1–15. https://doi.org/10.1186/s13578-024-01211-x

Carrier, R.L., Papadaki, M., Rupnick, M., Schoen, F.J., Bursac, N., Langer, R., Freed, L.E., Vunjak-Novakovic, G., 1999. Cardiac tissue engineering: Cell seeding, cultivation parameters, and tissue construct characterization. Biotechnol. Bioeng. 64, 580–589. https://doi.org/10.1002/(SICI)1097-0290(19990905)64:5<580::AID-BIT8>3.0.CO;2-X

Cerneckis, J., Cai, H., Shi, Y., 2024. Induced pluripotent stem cells (iPSCs): Molecular mechanisms of induction and applications. Signal Transduct. Target. Ther. 9, 1–26. https://doi.org/10.1038/s41392-024-01809-0

Chan, Y.C., Ting, S., Lee, Y.K., Ng, K.M., Zhang, J., Chen, Z., Siu, C.W., Oh, S.K.W., Tse, H.F., 2013. Electrical stimulation promotes maturation of cardiomyocytes derived from human embryonic stem cells. J. Cardiovasc. Transl. Res. 6, 989–999. https://doi.org/10.1007/s12265-013-9510-z

Chiu, L.L.Y., Radisic, M., 2013. Cardiac tissue engineering. Curr. Opin. Chem. Eng. 2, 41–52. https://doi.org/10.1016/j.coche.2013.01.002

Choi, W., Kohane, D.S., 2024. Hybrid nanoparticle-hydrogel systems for drug delivery depots and other biomedical applications. ACS Nano. https://doi.org/10.1021/acsnano.4c06888

Chu, A.J., Zhao, E.J., Chiao, M., Lim, C.J., 2020. Co-culture of induced pluripotent stem cells with cardiomyocytes is sufficient to promote their differentiation into cardiomyocytes. PLoS One 15, 1–15. https://doi.org/10.1371/journal.pone.0230966

Clancy, C.E., Santana, L.F., 2024. Advances in induced pluripotent stem cell-derived cardiac myocytes: Technological breakthroughs, key discoveries and new applications. J. Physiol. 16, 3871–3892. https://doi.org/10.1113/JP282562

Csöbönyeiová, M., Beerová, N., Klein, M., Debreová-Čeháková, M., Danišovič, Ľ, 2022. Cell-based and selected cell-free therapies for myocardial infarction: How do they compare to the current treatment options? Int. J. Mol. Sci. 23. https://doi.org/10.3390/ijms231810314

Curtis, M.W., Russell, B., 2009. Cardiac tissue engineering. J. Cardiovasc. Nurs. 24, 87–92. https://doi.org/10.1097/01.JCN.0000343562.06614.49

Ding, M., Andersson, H., Martinsson, S., Sabirsh, A., Jonebring, A., Wang, Q.D., Plowright, A.T., Drowley, L., 2020. Aligned nanofiber scaffolds improve functionality of cardiomyocytes differentiated from human induced pluripotent stem cell-derived cardiac progenitor cells. Sci. Rep. 10, 1–14. https://doi.org/10.1038/s41598-020-70547-4

Duelen, R., Sampaolesi, M., 2017. Stem cell technology in cardiac regeneration: A pluripotent stem cell promise. EBioMedicine 16, 30–40. https://doi.org/10.1016/j.ebiom.2017.01.029

Echeverria Molina, M.I., Malollari, K.G., Komvopoulos, K., 2021. Design challenges in polymeric scaffolds for tissue engineering. Front. Bioeng. Biotechnol. 9, 1–29. https://doi.org/10.3389/fbioe.2021.617141

Elkhoury, K., Kodeih, S., Enciso-Martínez, E., Maziz, A., Bergaud, C., 2024. Advancing cardiomyocyte maturation: Current strategies and promising conductive polymer-based approaches. Adv. Healthc. Mater. 13. https://doi.org/10.1002/adhm.202303288

Elkhoury, K., Morsink, M., Sanchez-Gonzalez, L., Kahn, C., Tamayol, A., Arab-Tehrany, E., 2021. Biofabrication of natural hydrogels for cardiac, neural, and bone tissue engineering applications. Bioact. Mater. 6, 3904–3923. https://doi.org/10.1016/j.bioactmat.2021.03.040

Eschenhagen, T., Eder, A., Vollert, I., Hansen, A., 2012. Physiological aspects of cardiac tissue engineering. Am. J. Physiol. Hear. Circ. Physiol. 303. https://doi.org/10.1152/ajpheart.00007.2012

Fan, X.L., Zhang, Y., Li, X., Fu, Q.L., 2020. Mechanisms underlying the protective effects of mesenchymal stem cell-based therapy. Cell. Mol. Life Sci. 77, 2771–2794. https://doi.org/10.1007/s00018-020-03454-6

Fomby, P., Cherlin, A.J., Hadjizadeh, A., Doillon, C.J., Sueblinvong, V., Weiss, D.J., Bates, J.H.T., Gilbert, T., Liles, W.C., Lutzko, C., Rajagopal, J., Prockop, D.J., Chambers, D., Giangreco, A., Keating, A., Kotton, D., Lelkes, P.I., Wagner, D.E., Prockop, D.J., 2010. Stem cells and cell therapies in lung biology and diseases: Conference report. Ann. Am. Thorac. Soc. 12, 181–204. https://doi.org/10.1002/term

Fu, R.H., Wang, Y.C., Liu, S.P., Shih, T.R., Lin, H.L., Chen, Y.M., Sung, J.H., Lu, C.H., Wei, J.R., Wang, Z.W., Huang, S.J., Tsai, C.H., Shyu, W.C., Lin, S.Z., 2014. Decellularization and recellularization technologies in tissue engineering. Cell Transplant. 23, 621–630. https://doi.org/10.3727/096368914X678382

Funakoshi, S., Yoshida, Y., 2021. Recent progress of iPSC technology in cardiac diseases. Arch. Toxicol. 95, 3633–3650. https://doi.org/10.1007/s00204-021-03172-3

Gálvez-Montón, C., Prat-Vidal, C., Roura, S., Soler-Botija, C., Bayes-Genis, A., 2013. Cardiac tissue engineering and the bioartificial heart. Rev. Española Cardiol. (English Ed) 66, 391–399. https://doi.org/10.1016/j.rec.2012.11.012

Gao, H., Liu, S., Qin, S., Yang, J., Yue, T., Ye, B., Tang, Y., Feng, J., Hou, J., Danzeng, D., 2024. Injectable hydrogel-based combination therapy for myocardial infarction: A systematic review and meta-analysis of preclinical trials. BMC Cardiovasc. Dis. https://doi.org/10.1186/s12872-024-03742-0

Gelmi, A., Cieslar-Pobuda, A., de Muinck, E., Los, M., Rafat, M., Jager, E.W.H., 2016. Direct mechanical stimulation of stem cells: A beating electromechanically active scaffold for cardiac tissue engineering. Adv. Healthc. Mater. 5, 1471–1480. https://doi.org/10.1002/adhm.201600307

Ghosh, S., Bhaskar, R., Mishra, R., Arockia Babu, M., Mohammad Abomughaid, M., Kumar Jha, N., Kumar Sinha, J., 2024a. Neurological insights into brain-targeted cancer therapy and bioinspired microrobots. Drug Discov. Today 29, 104105. https://doi.org/10.1016/j.drudis.2024.104105

Ghosh, S., Ghosh, S., Sharma, H., Bhaskar, R., Han, S.S., Sinha, J.K., 2024b. Harnessing the power of biological macromolecules in hydrogels for controlled drug release in the central nervous system: A review. Int. J. Biol. Macromol. 254, 127708. https://doi.org/10.1016/j.ijbiomac.2023.127708

Ghosh, S., Sinha, J.K., Ghosh, S., Sharma, H., Bhaskar, R., Narayanan, K.B., 2023. A comprehensive review of emerging trends and innovative therapies in epilepsy management. Brain Sci. 13. https://doi.org/10.3390/brainsci13091305

Gil-Cabrerizo, P., Saludas, L., Prósper, F., Abizanda, G., Echanove-González de Anleo, M., Ruiz-Villalba, A., Garbayo, E., Blanco-Prieto, M.J., 2022. Development of an injectable alginate-collagen hydrogel for cardiac delivery of extracellular vesicles. Int. J. Pharm. 629, 1–8. https://doi.org/10.1016/j.ijpharm.2022.122356

Gilpin, A., Yang, Y., 2017. Decellularization strategies for regenerative medicine: From processing techniques to applications. Biomed Res. Int. 2017. https://doi.org/10.1155/2017/9831534

Gisone, I., Cecchettini, A., Ceccherini, E., Persiani, E., Morales, M.A., Vozzi, F., 2022. Cardiac tissue engineering: Multiple approaches and potential applications. Front. Bioeng. Biotechnol. 10, 1–8. https://doi.org/10.3389/fbioe.2022.980393

Gittenberger-de Groot, A.C., Winter, E.M., Bartelings, M.M., Jose Goumans, M., DeRuiter, M.C., Poelmann, R.E., 2012. The arterial and cardiac epicardium in development, disease and repair. Differentiation 84, 41–53. https://doi.org/10.1016/j.diff.2012.05.002

Gomes, M.R., Castelo Ferreira, F., Sanjuan-Alberte, P., 2022. Electrospun piezoelectric scaffolds for cardiac tissue engineering. Biomater. Adv. 137, 212808. https://doi.org/10.1016/j.bioadv.2022.212808

Guan, H., Chen, Y., Liu, X., Huang, L., 2024. Research and application of hydrogel-encapsulated mesenchymal stem cells in the treatment of myocardial infarction. Colloids Surf. B Biointerfaces 239, 113942. https://doi.org/10.1016/j.colsurfb.2024.113942

Guo, Y., Yu, Y., Hu, S., Chen, Y., Shen, Z., 2020. The therapeutic potential of mesenchymal stem cells for cardiovascular diseases. Cell Death Dis. 11. https://doi.org/10.1038/s41419-020-2542-9

Hernández, D., Millard, R., Sivakumaran, P., Wong, R.C.B., Crombie, D.E., Hewitt, A.W., Liang, H., Hung, S.S.C., Pébay, A., Shepherd, R.K., Dusting, G.J., Lim, S.Y., 2016. Electrical stimulation promotes cardiac differentiation of human induced pluripotent stem cells. Stem Cells Int. 2016. https://doi.org/10.1155/2016/1718041

Huang, W., Huo, M., Cheng, N., Wang, R., 2021. New forms of electrospun nanofibers applied in cardiovascular field. Front. Cardiovasc. Med. 8, 1–8. https://doi.org/10.3389/fcvm.2021.801077

Huyer, L.D., Montgomery, M., Zhao, Y., Xiao, Y., Conant, G., Korolj, A., Radisic, M., 2015. Biomaterial based cardiac tissue engineering and its applications. Biomed. Mater. 10. https://doi.org/10.1088/1748-6041/10/3/034004

Ikeda, K., Tojo, K., Udagawa, T., Otsubo, C., Ishikawa, M., Tokudome, G., Hosoya, T., Tajima, N., Nakao, K., Kawamura, M., 2008. Cellular physiology of rat cardiac myocytes in cardiac fibrosis: In vitro simulation using the cardiac myocyte/cardiac non-myocyte co-culture system. Hypertens. Res. 31, 693–706. https://doi.org/10.1291/hypres.31.693

Karbassi, E., Fenix, A., Marchiano, S., Muraoka, N., Yang, X., Murry, C.E., 2020. Cardiomyocyte maturation: Advances in knowledge and implications for regenerative medicine. Nat. Rev. Cardiol. 17, 341–359. https://doi.org/10.1038/s41569-019-0331-x.

Keane, T.J., Swinehart, I.T., Badylak, S.F., 2015. Methods of tissue decellularization used for preparation of biologic scaffolds and in vivo relevance. Methods 84, 25–34. https://doi.org/10.1016/j.ymeth.2015.03.005

Kharaziha, M., Nikkhah, M., Shin, S.R., Annabi, N., Masoumi, N., Gaharwar, A.K., Camci-Unal, G., Khademhosseini, A., 2013. PGS:Gelatin nanofibrous scaffolds with tunable mechanical and structural properties for engineering cardiac tissues. Biomaterials 34, 6355–6366. https://doi.org/10.1016/j.biomaterials.2013.04.045

Khatat, M.M., Same, S., Moharamzadeh, K., Rad, J.S., Mehdipour, A., Roshangar, L., 2023. Mechanical properties of the rabbit and human decellularized patches for well-tolerated/reinforced organ in cardiac tissue engineering. J. Cardiovasc. Thorac. Res. 15, 244–249. https://doi.org/10.34172/jcvtr.2023.32926

Kieda, J., Shakeri, A., Landau, S., Wang, E.Y., Zhao, Y., Lai, B.F., Okhovatian, S., Wang, Y., Jiang, R., Radisic, M., 2024. Advances in cardiac tissue engineering and heart-on-a-chip. J. Biomed. Mater. Res. Part A 112, 492–511. https://doi.org/10.1002/jbm.a.37633

Kirkpatrick, C.J., Fuchs, S., Unger, R.E., 2011. Co-culture systems for vascularization - Learning from nature. Adv. Drug Deliv. Rev. 63, 291–299. https://doi.org/10.1016/j.addr.2011.01.009

Kistamás, K., Müller, A., Muenthaisong, S., Lamberto, F., Zana, M., Dulac, M., Leal, F., Maziz, A., Costa, P., Bernotiene, E., Bergaud, C., Dinnyés, A., 2023. Multifactorial approaches to enhance maturation of human iPSC-derived cardiomyocytes. J. Mol. Liq. 387. https://doi.org/10.1016/j.molliq.2023.122668

Koivisto, J.T., Gering, C., Karvinen, J., Maria Cherian, R., Belay, B., Hyttinen, J., Aalto-Setälä, K., Kellomäki, M., Parraga, J., 2019. Mechanically biomimetic gelatin-gellan gum hydrogels for 3D culture of beating human cardiomyocytes. ACS Appl. Mater. Interfaces 11, 20589–20602. https://doi.org/10.1021/acsami.8b22343

Lai, P., Sheng, M., Ye, J.H., Tang, Z.X., Hu, S., Wang, B., Yuan, J.L., Yang, Y.H., Zhong, Y.M., Liao, Y.L., 2023. Research trends in cardiovascular tissue engineering from 1992 to 2022: A bibliometric analysis. Front. Cardiovasc. Med. 10, 1–12. https://doi.org/10.3389/fcvm.2023.1208227

Li, Z., Hampton, M.J.W., Barajas, M.B., Riess, M.L., Riess, M.L., 2021. Development of a cell co-culture model to mimic cardiac ischemia/reperfusion in vitro. JoVE e62913. https://doi.org/doi:10.3791/62913

Li, Z., Hampton, M.J.W., Barajas, M.B., Riess, M.L., 2024. Development of a cell co-culture model to mimic cardiac ischemia/reperfusion in vitro. J. Vis. Exp (176), e62913. https://doi:10.3791/62913 (2021).

Liu, Y., Kamran, R., Han, X., Wang, M., Li, Q., Lai, D., Naruse, K., Takahashi, K., 2024. Human heart-on-a-chip microphysiological system comprising endothelial cells, fibroblasts, and iPSC-derived cardiomyocytes. Sci. Rep. 14, 1–14. https://doi.org/10.1038/s41598-024-68275-0

Love, M.R., Palee, S., Chattipakorn, S.C., Chattipakorn, N., 2018. Effects of electrical stimulation on cell proliferation and apoptosis. J. Cell. Physiol. 233, 1860–1876. https://doi.org/10.1002/jcp.25975

Lu, H., Hoshiba, T., Kawazoe, N., Chen, G., 2012. Comparison of decellularization techniques for preparation of extracellular matrix scaffolds derived from three-dimensional cell culture. J. Biomed. Mater. Res. Part A 100 A, 2507–2516. https://doi.org/10.1002/jbm.a.34150

Maeda, K., Suuronen, E.J., Ruel, M., 2017. Engineering Niches for Cardiovascular Tissue Regeneration, Biology and Engineering of Stem Cell Niches. Elsevier Inc. https://doi.org/10.1016/B978-0-12-802734-9.00029-9

Mauretti, A., Spaans, S., Bax, N.A.M., Sahlgren, C., Bouten, C.V.C., 2017. Cardiac progenitor cells and the interplay with their microenvironment. Stem Cells Int. 2017. https://doi.org/10.1155/2017/7471582

Mendibil, U., Ruiz-Hernandez, R., Retegi-Carrion, S., Garcia-Urquia, N., Olalde-Graells, B., Abarrategi, A., 2020. Tissue-specific decellularization methods: Rationale and strategies to achieve regenerative compounds. Int. J. Mol. Sci. 21, 1–29. https://doi.org/10.3390/ijms21155447

Mialet-Perez, J., Belaidi, E., 2024. Interplay between hypoxia inducible Factor-1 and mitochondria in cardiac diseases. Free Radic. Biol. Med. 221, 13–22. https://doi.org/10.1016/j.freeradbiomed.2024.04.239

Min, S., Kim, S., Sim, W.S., Choi, Y.S., Joo, H., Park, J.H., Lee, S.J., Kim, H., Lee, M.J., Jeong, I., Cui, B., Jo, S.H., Kim, J.J., Hong, S.B., Choi, Y.J., Ban, K., Kim, Y.G., Park, J.U., Lee, H.A., Park, H.J., Cho, S.W., 2024. Versatile human cardiac tissues engineered with perfusable heart extracellular microenvironment for biomedical applications. Nat. Commun. 15, 1–22. https://doi.org/10.1038/s41467-024-46928-y

Mooney, E., Mackle, J.N., Blond, D.J.P., O'Cearbhaill, E., Shaw, G., Blau, W.J., Barry, F.P., Barron, V., Murphy, J.M., 2012. The electrical stimulation of carbon nanotubes to provide a cardiomimetic cue to MSCs. Biomaterials 33, 6132–6139. https://doi.org/10.1016/j.biomaterials.2012.05.032

Moroni, F., Mirabella, T., 2014. Decellularized matrices for cardiovascular tissue engineering. Am. J. Stem Cells 3, 1–20.

Motta, I., Soccio, M., Guidotti, G., Lotti, N., Pasquinelli, G., 2024. Hydrogels for cardio and vascular tissue repair and regeneration. Gels 10, 1–17. https://doi.org/10.3390/gels10030196

Nagayach, A., Bhaskar, R., Ghosh, S., Kumar, K., Soo, S., Kumar, J., 2024. Advancing the understanding of diabetic encephalopathy through unravelling pathogenesis and exploring future treatment perspectives. Ageing Res. Rev. 100, 102450. https://doi.org/10.1016/j.arr.2024.102450

Narayanan, K.B., Bhaskar, R., Han, S.S., 2022. Recent advances in the biomedical applications of functionalized nanogels. Pharmaceutics 14. https://doi.org/10.3390/pharmaceutics14122832

Nguyen-Truong, M., Li, Y.V., Wang, Z., 2020. Mechanical considerations of electrospun scaffolds for myocardial tissue and regenerative engineering. Bioengineering 7, 1–24. https://doi.org/10.3390/bioengineering7040122

Niu, X., Xu, Z., Di, M., Huang, D., Li, X., 2023. Bioreactor strategies for tissue-engineered osteochondral constructs: Advantages, present situations and future trends. Compos. Part B Eng. 259, 110736. https://doi.org/10.1016/j.compositesb.2023.110736

Oikonomopoulos, A., Kitani, T., Wu, J.C., 2018. Pluripotent stem cell-derived cardiomyocytes as a platform for cell therapy applications: Progress and hurdles for clinical translation. Mol. Ther. 26, 1624–1634. https://doi.org/10.1016/j.ymthe.2018.02.026

Okhovatian, S., Khosravi, R., Wang, E.Y., Zhao, Y., Radisic, M., 2024. Biofabrication strategies for cardiac tissue engineering. Curr. Opin. Biotechnol. 88, 103166. https://doi.org/10.1016/j.copbio.2024.103166

Park, C.S., Kang, Y.W., Na, H., Sun, J.Y., 2024. Hydrogels for bioinspired soft robots. Prog. Polym. Sci. 150, 101791. https://doi.org/10.1016/j.progpolymsci.2024.101791

Park, S., Gwon, Y., Khan, S.A., Jang, K.J., Kim, J., 2023. Engineering considerations of iPSC-based personalized medicine. Biomater. Res. 27, 1–27. https://doi.org/10.1186/s40824-023-00382-x

Patel, R., Patel, D., 2024. Injectable hydrogels in cardiovascular tissue engineering. Polymers (Basel) 16, 1–27. https://doi.org/10.3390/polym16131878

Paul, D., Samuel, S.M., Maulik, N., 2009. Mesenchymal stem cell: Present challenges and prospective cellular cardiomyoplasty approaches for myocardial regeneration. Antioxid. Redox Signal. 11, 1841–1855. https://doi.org/10.1089/ars.2009.2455

Pittenger, M.F., Discher, D.E., Péault, B.M., Phinney, D.G., Hare, J.M., Caplan, A.I., 2019. Mesenchymal stem cell perspective: Cell biology to clinical progress. npj Regen. Med. 4. https://doi.org/10.1038/s41536-019-0083-6

Pomeroy, J.E., Helfer, A., Bursac, N., 2020. Biomaterializing the promise of cardiac tissue engineering. Biotechnol. Adv. 42, 107353. https://doi.org/10.1016/j.biotechadv.2019.02.009

Prondzynski, M., Berkson, P., Trembley, M.A., Tharani, Y., Shani, K., Bortolin, R.H., Sweat, M.E., Mayourian, J., Yucel, D., Cordoves, A.M., Gabbin, B., Hou, C., Anyanwu, N.J., Nawar, F., Cotton, J., Milosh, J., Walker, D., Zhang, Y., Lu, F., Liu, X., Parker, K.K., Bezzerides, V.J., Pu, W.T., 2024. Efficient and reproducible generation of human iPSC-derived cardiomyocytes and cardiac organoids in stirred suspension systems. Nat. Commun. 15, 1–17. https://doi.org/10.1038/s41467-024-50224-0

Pushp, P., Bhaskar, R., Kelkar, S., Sharma, N., Pathak, D., Gupta, M.K., 2021a. Plasticized poly(vinylalcohol) and poly(vinylpyrrolidone) based patches with tunable mechanical properties for cardiac tissue engineering applications. Biotechnol. Bioeng. 118, 2312–2325. https://doi.org/10.1002/bit.27743

Pushp, P., Nogueira, D.E.S., Rodrigues, C.A.V., Ferreira, F.C., Cabral, J.M.S., Gupta, M.K., 2021b. A concise review on induced pluripotent stem cell-derived cardiomyocytes for personalized regenerative medicine. Stem Cell Rev. Rep. 17, 748–776. https://doi.org/10.1007/s12015-020-10061-2

Radisic, M., Park, H., Gerecht, S., Cannizzaro, C., Langer, R., Vunjak-Novakovic, G., 2007. Biomimetic approach to cardiac tissue engineering. Philos. Trans. R. Soc. B Biol. Sci. 362, 1357–1368. https://doi.org/10.1098/rstb.2007.2121

Rakshit, P., Giri, T.K., Mukherjee, K., 2024. Progresses and perspectives on natural polysaccharide based hydrogels for repair of infarcted myocardium. Int. J. Biol. Macromol. 269, 132213. https://doi.org/10.1016/j.ijbiomac.2024.132213

Reina-Mahecha, A., Beers, M.J., van der Veen, H.C., Zuhorn, I.S., van Kooten, T.G., Sharma, P.K., 2023. A review of the role of bioreactors for iPSCs-based tissue-engineered articular cartilage. Tissue Eng. Regen. Med. 20, 1041–1052. https://doi.org/10.1007/s13770-023-00573-6

Richards, D.J., Tan, Y., Coyle, R., Li, Y., Xu, R., Yeung, N., Parker, A., Menick, D.R., Tian, B., Mei, Y., 2016. Nanowires and electrical stimulation synergistically improve functions of hiPSC cardiac spheroids. Nano Lett. 16, 4670–4678. https://doi.org/10.1021/acs.nanolett.6b02093

Roacho-Pérez, J.A., Garza-Treviño, E.N., Moncada-Saucedo, N.K., Carriquiry-Chequer, P.A., Valencia-Gómez, L.E., Matthews, E.R., Gómez-Flores, V., Simental-Mendía, M., Delgado-Gonzalez, P., Delgado-Gallegos, J.L., Padilla-Rivas, G.R., Islas, J.F., 2022. Artificial scaffolds in cardiac tissue engineering. Life 12, 1–21. https://doi.org/10.3390/life12081117

Roshanbinfar, K., Vogt, L., Ruther, F., Roether, J.A., Boccaccini, A.R., Engel, F.B., 2020. Nanofibrous composite with tailorable electrical and mechanical properties for cardiac tissue engineering. Adv. Funct. Mater. 30. https://doi.org/10.1002/adfm.201908612

Roth, G.A., Mensah, G.A., Johnson, C.O., Addolorato, G., Ammirati, E., Baddour, L.M., Barengo, N.C., Beaton, A.Z., Benjamin, E.J., Benziger, C.P., 2020. Global burden of cardiovascular diseases and risk factors, 1990–2019: Update from the GBD 2019 study. J. Am. Coll. Cardiol. 76, 2982–3021. https://doi.org/10.1016/j.jacc.2020.11.010

Rysä, J., Tokola, H., Ruskoaho, H., 2018. Mechanical stretch induced transcriptomic profiles in cardiac myocytes. Sci. Rep. 8, 1–14. https://doi.org/10.1038/s41598-018-23042-w

Sacco, A.M., Castaldo, C., Di Meglio, F., Nurzynska, D., Palermi, S., Spera, R., Gnasso, R., Zinno, G., Romano, V., Belviso, I., 2023. The long and winding road to cardiac regeneration. Appl. Sci. 13, 1–41. https://doi.org/10.3390/app13169432

Sachdeva, P., Badri, K., Kumar, J., Gupta, S., 2024a. Recent advances in drug delivery systems targeting insulin signalling for the treatment of Alzheimer's disease. J. Alzheimer's Dis. 98, 1169–1179. https://doi.org/10.3233/JAD-231181

Sachdeva, P., Ji, S., Ghosh, S., Ghosh, S., Raghunath, M., 2023. Plausible role of stem cell types for treating and understanding the pathophysiology of depression. Pharmaceutics 15, 814, 1–15. https://doi.org/10.3390/pharmaceutics15030814

Sachdeva, P., Narayanan, K.B., Sinha, J.K., Gupta, S., Ghosh, S., Singh, K.K., Bhaskar, R., Almutary, A.G., Zothantluanga, J.H., Kotta, K.K., Nelson, V.K., Paiva-Santos, A.C., Abomughaid, M.M., Kamal, M., Iqbal, D., Alharbi, M.H., Almutairi, A.A., Dewanjee, S., Nuli, M.V., Vippamakula, S., Jha, S.K., Ojha, S., Jha, N.K., 2024b. Recent advances in drug delivery systems targeting insulin signalling for the treatment of Alzheimer's disease. J. Alzheimer's Dis. 98, 1169–1179. https://doi.org/10.3233/JAD-231181

Saini, H., Navaei, A., Van Putten, A., Nikkhah, M., 2015. 3D cardiac microtissues encapsulated with the co-culture of cardiomyocytes and cardiac fibroblasts. Adv. Healthc. Mater. 4, 1961–1971. https://doi.org/10.1002/adhm.201500331

Savoji, H., Mohammadi, M.H., Rafatian, N., Toroghi, M.K., Wang, E.Y., Zhao, Y., Korolj, A., Ahadian, S., Radisic, M., 2019. Cardiovascular disease models: A game changing paradigm in drug discovery and screening. Biomaterials 198, 3–26. https://doi.org/10.1016/j.biomaterials.2018.09.036

Schwach, V., Passier, R., 2019. Native cardiac environment and its impact on engineering cardiac tissue. Biomater. Sci. 7, 3566–3580. https://doi.org/10.1039/c8bm01348a

Sekkarapatti Ramasamy, M., Bhaskar, R., Narayanan, K.B., Purohit, S.D., Park, S.S., Manikkavel, A., Kim, B., Han, S.S., 2022. Combination of polydopamine and carbon nanomaterials coating enhances the piezoelectric responses and cytocompatibility of biodegradable PLLA nanofiber scaffolds for tissue engineering applications. Mater. Today Commun. 33, 104659. https://doi.org/10.1016/j.mtcomm.2022.104659

Serena, E., Figallo, E., Tandon, N., Cannizzaro, C., Gerecht, S., Elvassore, N., Vunjak-Novakovic, G., 2009. Electrical stimulation of human embryonic stem cells: Cardiac differentiation and the generation of reactive oxygen species. Exp. Cell Res. 315, 3611–3619. https://doi.org/10.1016/j.yexcr.2009.08.015

Shahverdi, M., Seifi, S., Akbari, A., Mohammadi, K., Shamloo, A., Movahhedy, M.R., 2022. Melt electrowriting of PLA, PCL, and composite PLA/PCL scaffolds for tissue engineering application. Sci. Rep. 12, 1–16. https://doi.org/10.1038/s41598-022-24275-6

Sharma, V., Dash, S.K., Govarthanan, K., Gahtori, R., Negi, N., Barani, M., Tomar, R., Chakraborty, S., Mathapati, S., Bishi, D.K., Negi, P., Dua, K., Singh, S.K., Gundamaraju, R., Dey, A., Ruokolainen, J., Thakur, V.K., Kesari, K.K., Jha, N.K., Gupta, P.K., Ojha, S., 2021. Recent advances in cardiac tissue engineering for the management of myocardium infarction. Cells. https://doi.org/10.3390/cells10102538

Singh, H., Purohit, S.D., Bhaskar, R., Yadav, I., Bhushan, S., Gupta, M.K., Gautam, S., Showkeen, M., Mishra, N.C., 2021a. Biomatrix from goat-waste in sponge/gel/powder form for tissue engineering and synergistic effect of nanoceria. Biomed. Mater. 16. https://doi.org/10.1088/1748-605X/abdb74

Singh, H., Purohit, S.D., Bhaskar, R., Yadav, I., Gupta, M.K., Mishra, N.C., 2021b. Development of decellularization protocol for caprine small intestine submucosa as a biomaterial. Biomater. Biosyst. 100035. https://doi.org/10.1016/j.bbiosy.2021.100035

Singh, H., Purohit, S.D., Bhaskar, R., Yadav, I., Bhushan, S., Gupta, M.K., Mishra, N.C., 2022. Curcumin in decellularized goat small intestine submucosa for wound healing and skin tissue engineering. J. Biomed. Mater. Res. Part B Appl. Biomater. 110, 210–219. https://doi.org/10.1002/jbm.b.34903

Singh, Y.P., Dasgupta, S., Nayar, S., Bhaskar, R., 2020. Optimization of electrospinning process & parameters for producing defect-free chitosan/polyethylene oxide nanofibers for bone tissue engineering. J. Biomater. Sci. Polym. Ed. 31, 781–803. https://doi.org/10.1080/09205063.2020.1718824

Singh, Y.P., Mishra, B., Gupta, M.K., Bhaskar, R., Han, S.S., Mishra, N.C., Dasgupta, S., 2023a. Gelatin/monetite electrospun scaffolds to regenerate bone tissue: Fabrication, characterization, and in-vitro evaluation. J. Mech. Behav. Biomed. Mater. 137, 105524. https://doi.org/10.1016/j.jmbbm.2022.105524

Singh, Y.P., Purohit, S.D., Gupta, M.K., Bhaskar, R., Han, S.S., Dasgupta, S., 2023b. Preparation, characterization, and bioactivity of reinforced monetite with chitosan-gelatin electrospun composite scaffold for bone tissue engineering. Biomed. Mater. 18. https://doi.org/10.1088/1748-605X/ace7a3

Stoppel, W.L., Kaplan, D.L., Black, L.D., 2016. Electrical and mechanical stimulation of cardiac cells and tissue constructs. Adv. Drug Deliv. Rev. 96, 135–155. https://doi.org/10.1016/j.addr.2015.07.009

Su, R., Ai, Y., Wang, J., Wu, L., Sun, H., Ding, M., Xie, R., Liang, Q., 2024. Engineered microfibers for tissue engineering. ACS Appl. Bio Mater. https://doi.org/10.1021/acsabm.4c00615

Sun, X., Nunes, S.S., 2017. Bioengineering approaches to mature human pluripotent stem cell-derived cardiomyocytes. Front. Cell Dev. Biol. 5, 1–8. https://doi.org/10.3389/fcell.2017.00019

Takeuchi, A., Nakafutami, S., Tani, H., Mori, M., Takayama, Y., Moriguchi, H., Kotani, K., Miwa, K., Lee, J.K., Noshiro, M., Jimbo, Y., 2011. Device for co-culture of sympathetic neurons and cardiomyocytes using microfabrication. Lab Chip 11, 2268–2275. https://doi.org/10.1039/c0lc00327a

Tan, Y.H., Helms, H.R., Nakayama, K.H., 2022. Decellularization strategies for regenerating cardiac and skeletal muscle tissues. Front. Bioeng. Biotechnol. 10, 1–23. https://doi.org/10.3389/fbioe.2022.831300

Tandon, N., Cannizzaro, C., Chao, P.H.G., Maidhof, R., Marsano, A., Au, H.T.H., Radisic, M., Vunjak-Novakovic, G., 2009. Electrical stimulation systems for cardiac tissue engineering. Nat. Protoc. 4, 155–173. https://doi.org/10.1038/nprot.2008.183

Ugolini, G.S., Visone, R., Cruz-Moreira, D., Mainardi, A., Rasponi, M., 2018. Generation of Functional Cardiac Microtissues in a Beating Heart-on-a-Chip, 1st ed, Methods in Cell Biology. Elsevier Inc. https://doi.org/10.1016/bs.mcb.2018.05.005

Ullah, A., Kumar, M., Sayyar, M., Sapna, F., John, C., Memon, S., Qureshi, K., Agbo, E.C., Ariri, H.I., Chukwu, E.J., Varrassi, G., Khatri, M., Kumar, S., Elder, N.M., Mohamad, T., 2023. Revolutionizing cardiac care: A comprehensive narrative review of cardiac rehabilitation and the evolution of cardiovascular medicine. Cureus 15. https://doi.org/10.7759/cureus.46469

Ullah, I., Subbarao, R.B., Rho, G.J., 2015. Human mesenchymal stem cells - current trends and future prospective. Biosci. Rep. 35. https://doi.org/10.1042/BSR20150025

Van Luyn, M.J.A., Tio, R.A., Gallego, Y., Van Seijen, X.J., Plantinga, J.A., De Leij, L.F.M.H., DeJongste, M.J.L., Van Wachem, P.B., 2002. Cardiac tissue engineering: Characteristics of in unison contracting two- and three-dimensional neonatal rat ventricle cell (co)-cultures. Biomaterials 23, 4793–4801. https://doi.org/10.1016/S0142-9612(02)00230-2

Vasileios Karantalis, J.M.H., 2017. Use of mesenchymal stem cells for therapy of cardiac disease. Physiol. Behav. 176, 139–148. https://doi.org/10.1161/CIRCRESAHA.116.303614.

Vogt, L., Boccaccini, A.R., 2021. Random and aligned electrospun poly(ε-caprolactone) (PCL)/poly(1,8-octanediol-co-citrate) (POC) fiber mats for cardiac tissue engineering using benign solvents. Eur. Polym. J. 160, 110772. https://doi.org/10.1016/j.eurpolymj.2021.110772

Vuorenpää, H., Valtonen, J., Penttinen, K., Koskimäki, S., Hovinen, E., Ahola, A., Gering, C., Parraga, J., Kelloniemi, M., Hyttinen, J., Kellomäki, M., Aalto-Setälä, K., Miettinen, S., Pekkanen-Mattila, M., 2024. Gellan gum-gelatin based cardiac models support formation of cellular networks and functional cardiomyocytes. Cytotechnology 76, 483–502. https://doi.org/10.1007/s10616-024-00630-5

Wang, F., Guan Jianjun, J., 2010. Cellular cardiomyoplasty and cardiac tissue engineering for myocardial therapy. Adv. Drug Deliv. Rev. 62, 784–797. https://doi.org/10.1016/j.addr.2010.03.001

Wu, Z., Chen, G., Zhang, J., Hua, Y., Li, J., Liu, B., Huang, A., Li, H., Chen, M., Ou, C., 2017. Treatment of myocardial infarction with gene-modified mesenchymal stem cells in a small molecular hydrogel. Sci. Rep. 7, 1–11. https://doi.org/10.1038/s41598-017-15870-z

Wu, Z., Li, Q., Wang, L., Zhang, Y., Liu, W., Zhao, S., Geng, X., Fan, Y., 2023. A novel biomimetic nanofibrous cardiac tissue engineering scaffold with adjustable mechanical and electrical properties based on poly(glycerol sebacate) and polyaniline. Mater. Today Bio. 23, 100798. https://doi.org/10.1016/j.mtbio.2023.100798

Xu, J., Lian, W., Li, L., Huang, Z., 2017. Generation of induced cardiac progenitor cells via somatic reprogramming. Oncotarget 8, 29442–29457. https://doi.org/10.18632/oncotarget.15272

Xu, Q., Xiao, Z., Yang, Q., Yu, T., Deng, X., Chen, N., Huang, Y., Wang, L., Guo, J., Wang, J., 2024. Hydrogel-based cardiac repair and regeneration function in the treatment of myocardial infarction. Mater. Today Bio. 25, 100978. https://doi.org/10.1016/j.mtbio.2024.100978

Yang, H., Yang, Y., Kiskin, F.N., Shen, M., Zhang, J.Z., 2023. Recent advances in regulating the proliferation or maturation of human-induced pluripotent stem cell-derived cardiomyocytes. Stem Cell Res. Ther. 14, 1–17. https://doi.org/10.1186/s13287-023-03470-w

Ye, L., Swingen, C., Zhang, J., 2013. Induced pluripotent stem cells and their potential for basic and clinical sciences. Curr. Cardiol. Rev. 9, 63–72.

Yi, B., Xu, Y., Wang, X., Wang, G., Li, S., Xu, R., Liu, X., Zhou, Q., 2024. Overview of injectable hydrogels for the treatment of myocardial infarction. Cardiovasc. Innov. Appl. 9, 960. https://doi.org/10.15212/CVIA.2024.0019

Zeng, Z., Li, H., Li, Q., Sun, R., Zhang, X., Zhang, D., Zhu, Q., Chen, C., 2024. Quantitative measurement of acute myocardial infarction cardiac biomarkers by "All-in-One" immune microfluidic chip for early diagnosis of myocardial infarction. Spectrochim. Acta Part A Mol. Biomol. Spectrosc. 315. https://doi.org/10.1016/j.saa.2024.124256

Zhang, Y., Cao, N., Huang, Y., Spencer, C.I., Fu, J.D., Yu, C., Liu, K., Nie, B., Xu, T., Li, K., Xu, S., Bruneau, B.G., Srivastava, D., Ding, S., 2016. Expandable cardiovascular progenitor cells reprogrammed from fibroblasts. Cell Stem Cell 18, 368–381. https://doi.org/10.1016/j.stem.2016.02.001

Zhao, D., Lei, W., Hu, S., 2021. Cardiac organoid — A promising perspective of preclinical model. Stem Cell Res. Ther. 12, 1–10. https://doi.org/10.1186/s13287-021-02340-7

Zheng, K., Hao, Y., Xia, C., Cheng, S., Yu, J., Chen, Z., Li, Y., Niu, Y., Ran, S., Wang, S., Ye, W., Luo, Z., Li, X., Zhao, J., Li, R., Zong, J., Zhang, H., Lai, L., Huang, P., Zhou, C., Xia, J., Zhang, X., Wu, J., 2024a. Effects and mechanisms of the myocardial microenvironment on cardiomyocyte proliferation and regeneration. Front. Cell Dev. Biol. 12, 1–22. https://doi.org/10.3389/fcell.2024.1429020

Zheng, H., Tai, L., Xu, C., Wang, W., Ma, Q., Sun, W., 2024b. Microfluidic-based cardiovascular systems for advanced study of atherosclerosis. J. Mater. Chem. B 7225–7245. https://doi.org/10.1039/d4tb00756e

Zielińska, A., Karczewski, J., Eder, P., Kolanowski, T., Szalata, M., Wielgus, K., Szalata, M., Kim, D., Shin, S.R., Słomski, R., Souto, E.B., 2023. Scaffolds for drug delivery and tissue engineering: The role of genetics. J. Control. Release 359, 207–223. https://doi.org/10.1016/j.jconrel.2023.05.042

3 Biomaterials for Cardiac Tissue Engineering

Ira Singh and Santosh Kumar

3.1 INTRODUCTION

The biomaterials employed in tissue engineering have seen a significant transformation in the past ten years [1]. Heart tissue engineering has led to the development of medical technologies such as gene delivery methods, stem cell treatments, and diagnostic systems based on nanotechnology [1–4]. Traditionally used materials in these technologies comprise ceramics, metals, and man-made polymers [1]. The creation of 3D structures that closely replicate the original tissue's chemical and biological characteristics is one of the biggest challenges in the creation of tissue constructions using these standard materials [5, 6]. Progress in biomimetic materials has exhibited the assimilation of advantageous characteristics including mechanical strength, porosity, swelling, biocompatibility, and biodegradability [6, 7]. However, in order to make typical materials friendly, such as polymers, metals, ceramics, and composites, they must undergo costly production procedures, lengthy processing, and chemical treatments [8, 9]. Because of their structural properties and inertness, Biomedical structures and equipment have been made using metals including cobalt, titanium, and stainless steel [10]. Commercially available pure titanium is one of the most used alloys based on titanium. It is highly renowned for having outstanding corrosion resistance and tensile strength, which make it perfect for use in the heart [11]. Nevertheless, the production of bare metal stents is expensive, and their drawbacks include thrombosis of the stent and sizing errors with respect to the target arterial [11]. Moreover, iron stents can cause blood arteries to swell and block branches [11]. Creating drug-eluting stents (DESs) with a polymer that absorbs biologically to address the issues brought on by bare metal stents [11, 12]. These DESs are further divided into metallic, polymer-carrying, and without polymer stents. Subsequently, DES advancements were linked to late and subacute thrombosis, from which polymers may arise in persistent vascular hypersensitivity, endothelial dysfunction, and irritation around the stent [11]. Due to these obstacles, research is now focusing on more innovative approaches to create biocompatible materials for cardiovascular tissue engineering with the added benefit of sustainability, using uncomplicated, naturally occurring ingredients and straightforward production processes. Figure 3.1 summarizes the advantages of employing biomaterials and provides a quick explanation of the characteristics that make them such important instruments in the area.

In this regard, current research has made great use of the diversity and adaptability of biomaterials to create novel patches, hydrogels, scaffolds, and delivery systems with enormous potential for clinical application in the future. The use of

DOI: 10.1201/9781003670995-3

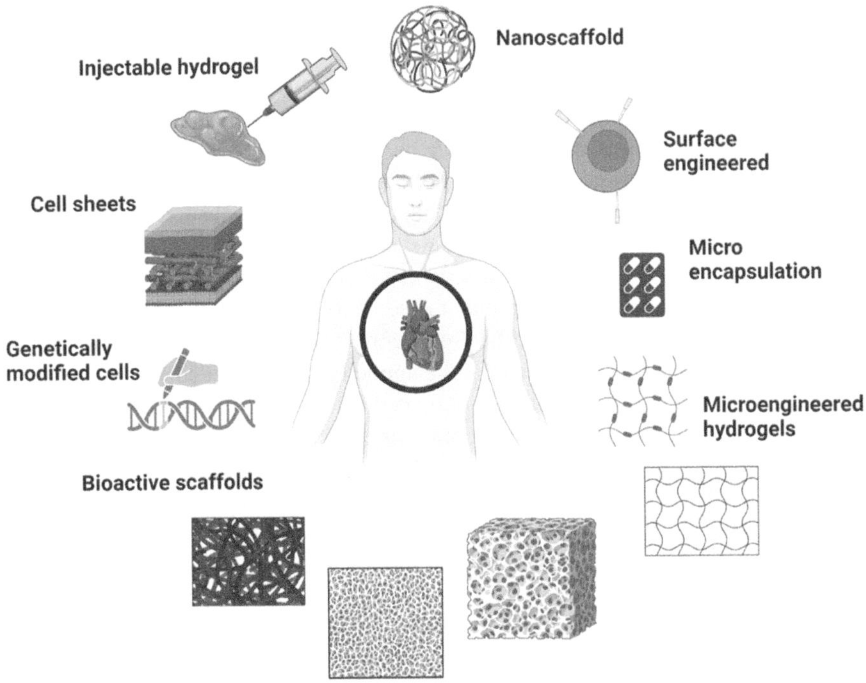

FIGURE 3.1 Engineered biomaterial for the restoration of heart tissue. Adapted from [2] with some modifications.

non-traditional biomaterials in cardiovascular tissue engineering is examined in this book chapter, along with how they might influence the creation of cardiac and circulatory tissue structures.

3.2 MODERN TISSUE ENGINEERING

The mismatch between the availability and demand of appropriate organ donors leads to the engineering of tissues for transplantation. Over 113,000 men, women, and children are on the national transplant list, according to US Government Information on Organ Donation and Transplantation [13]. According to estimates from the International Society of Heart and Lung Transplantation's xenotransplantation advisory committee, the number of Americans waiting for heart transplants is believed to be ten times greater than the country's transplantation need [14]. The worries regarding public health difficulties are significantly increased by the unfulfilled need for organs for transplantation [15]. According to Roger et al., 2333 heart transplants were carried out in the United States in 2010; however, in 2011, over 3000 individuals were waiting for a heart transplant and were consequently suffering from end-stage heart failure [16]. Creating tissue structures and functional organs for implantation can contribute to changing healthcare and assist patient handling. A tissue construct's engineering requires consideration of certain factors. Consists of biodegradability to dissolve in the body's natural environment and biocompatibility to prevent an immunological reaction—the cellular microenvironment without resulting in cytotoxicity, as well as cost-effectiveness to have affordable creation. Stents for biological applications are made of materials like metals and polymers, which have the drawbacks of causing inflammation, hypersensitivity, and vascular irritation at the implantation location [11]. Due to these difficulties, scientists are now looking at unconventional sources of naturally occurring biomaterials to produce off-the-shelf cardiovascular tissue constructions that are clinically viable. Biomaterials, which can be broadly categorized into two approaches to induce functional repair to the heart muscle after injury, have been used extensively in the field of cardiac regenerative therapy. (a) The development of viable cardiac patches in vitro that can be applied to the wounded region and used to replace the non-viable section of a damaged heart; and (b) injectable biomaterials like hydrogels that aid in the prevention of cardiac remodeling, provide cells to replace the damaged tissue, and draw in endogenous cell types in an effort to restore functionality [17]. Figure 3.2 illustrates an overview of the last ten years' advancements in tissue engineering. Along with genetic editing techniques that allow for more extensive cell modification, Additional cell sources such as adult stem cells and induced pluripotent stem cells are now accessible. Improvements in chemistries, growth factor delivery systems, and tissue design technologies have made it possible to engineer tissues that greatly resemble their native counterparts in terms of structure, content, and function.

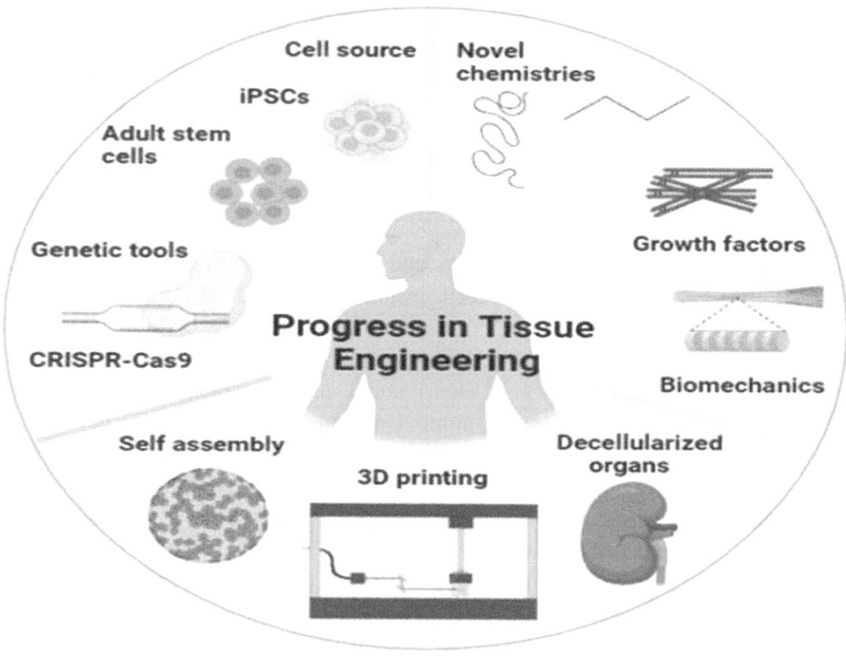

FIGURE 3.2 An overview of the last ten years' advancements in tissue engineering. Adapted from [6] with some modifications.

3.2.1 Advances in Tissue Engineering

Over the past ten years, there have been more approaches to reprogramming cells due to significant advancements in our comprehension of the reprogramming of cells. Since the discovery of PSCs, the stem cell field has seen significant changes in its terrain. To reprogram adult cells into iPSCs, four distinct genes (Oct4 and Sox2 with either c-Myc and Klf4 or Nanog and Lin28) that encode the required reprogramming factors were first added [18, 19]. Because many different types of somatic cells can be induced to become pluripotent, autologous cell sources are a promising option for various uses for tissue engineering. Because iPSCs are readily obtained from the patients, they may open up new possibilities for personalized therapy, such as the engineering and repair of tissues using the patient's cells. Additionally, combining allogeneic iPSCs and immunoisolation capsules has promise as a flexible means of treating conditions like diabetes. Numerous significant advancements in adult stem cell research have been made possible. For instance, mesenchymal stem cells' (MSCs') capacity to migrate is a potent means of stimulating tissue rejuvenation. It is possible to modify these cells to create a variety of desirable cytokines and growth factors that support the treatment of illnesses and the repair of minor wounds [18–21]. Novel techniques for modifying a cell's genetic makeup have also been created; the most well-known of these is the technology known as clustered regularly interspaced short palindromic repeats, or CRISPR [22–25]. CRISPR technology makes it possible to precisely target DNA and then cut at that precise position to modify mammalian cells' genomes with previously unheard-of ease and accuracy. In the future, we see the field of personalized tissue engineering be revolutionized by CRISPR technology and its derivatives, which also promote tissue modulation and cell engineering's flexibility. Attempts to genetically modify pig organs for possible human transplantation are among the examples [26–28]. Figure 3.3 offers an

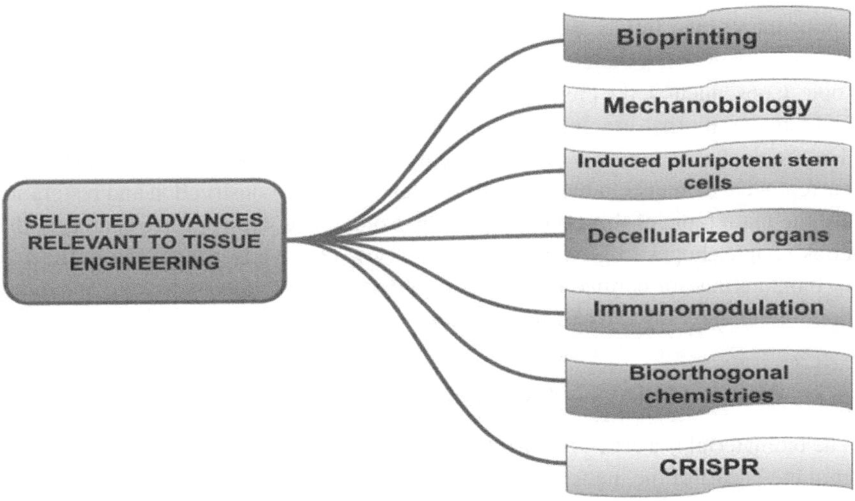

FIGURE 3.3 Significant developments in tissue engineering. Adapted from [17] with some modifications.

illustration of how tissue engineering has come a long way in the past ten years in overcoming these challenges, thanks to advancements in the fields of biology, chemistry, materials science, and engineering tactics, as well as the integration of these fields.

Pharmacological therapy aims to decrease workload (with nitrates and diuretics) and protect against the overactivity of toxic humoral elements in heart failure [29]. These include aldosterone (spironolactone), ACE inhibitors, and catecholamines (b-blockers). The prevention of these humoral variables is the Presently recommended conservative level of care for those with mild heart failure symptoms and little limitations during daily activities [29]. Interventional therapy is becoming increasingly widely used, especially for individuals with noticeable symptoms and severe limitations in their activities. It involves surgery or the insertion of pacing devices to regulate electrical/mechanical asynchrony [29–34]. However, medication and interventional therapy together are unable to effectively stop the disease from progressing to its final stage [35]. Eventually, a heart transplant is the only treatment available for end-stage heart failure. However, because of the scarcity of organ donors and side effects from immune-suppressive medications, researchers and doctors are always searching for fresh approaches to mend the damaged heart [36]. More effective and efficient care generation measures need to be pursued in this situation. Extensive research endeavors have been focused on integrating bioengineering principles into enhanced cardiovascular medications to address the limitations of existing treatments [37, 38]. Heart tissue engineering is one particularly intriguing multidisciplinary strategy that has gained popularity recently. To repair and restore heart tissue, various biomaterials, cells, and bioactive substances are integrated [39–42]. In particular, a variety of man-made and natural biomaterials can serve as delivery systems and scaffolds to allow cells to divide and become healthy. In this regard, novel patches, hydrogels, scaffolds, and delivery systems have been made possible by recent research, which has taken advantage of the diversity and adaptability of biomaterials to create materials with great potential for clinical application in the future. While some of these subjects have been covered in earlier reviews [38, 43–47], the goal of this work is to present a modern perspective on the topic. Consequently, the present review focuses primarily on the latest developments in biomaterials that are employed in cardiac tissue engineering and regeneration. This book chapter seeks to offer a contemporary perspective on the topic. The most current advancements in biomaterials for cardiac tissue construction and restoration are the main topic of this book chapter. By using this comprehensive approach, this book chapter hopes to give readers an overview of the advances made in the area of biomaterials for cardiac repair, act as a catalyst for further research, and aid in developing more effective treatment plans.

3.3 BIOMATERIALS—AN OVERVIEW

The biomaterial is a crucial element in tissue engineering; in fact, it could be considered the "heart of the matter." Biomaterials are a diverse range of materials that can be scaled up or down to replace or restore damaged tissues. These materials include metals, ceramics, nano- and micro-sized polymers, composites, and ceramics [48].

In tissue engineering, they can take on several shapes such as scaffolds, hydrogels, and carriers. They are essential for stabilizing cells and providing support for their continued growth and development [49]. Biomaterial form and function should closely resemble the natural characteristics of extracellular matrix (ECM) in order to facilitate cardiac tissue engineering. It should also provide an appropriate micro-environment to improve cell viability [50, 51]. Because of their structural properties and inertness, metals like titanium, cobalt, and stainless steel have been utilized to build biomedical structures and equipment [10]. In particular, biocompatible and biodegradable materials with mechanical and biological characteristics akin to the native myocardium support cell integration, lessen the antagonistic nature of the surrounding environment, guarantee a gradual release of bioactive molecules, and possess the proper electrical conductivity are essential for biomaterials intended for cardiac repair [48, 50, 52]. Furthermore, the incorporation of antioxidant compounds into biomaterials may act as a mediator between fibrosis and inflammation. Antioxidant structures can lessen oxidative damage, pro-inflammatory polarization of macrophages, and the fibrotic response to heart repair by scavenging reactive oxygen species [53]. Many natural (fibrin, gelatin alginate, chitosan, collagen, hyaluronic acids, silk) and synthetic polymers (PGA, PLA, PLGA, PU, and their derivatives) have been reported to resemble (to varying degrees) several important ECM properties, despite the complex requirements for an appropriate biomaterial [48–50, 54]. Its advantageous qualities include biocompatibility, suitable mechanical capabilities, hydrogel formation ability, proper chemistry, and a satisfactory degradation rate [41, 50, 55]. Furthermore, target progenitor and/or stem cells can be grown on biomaterials or in combination with them [48]. As a result, biomaterials and cells work in concert to enable tissue regeneration and repair while providing the support required for cell-to-tissue activities like adhesion, proliferation, and differentiation [49, 55]. In the last ten years, sophisticated chemicals that employ conjugation techniques for bioactive molecules have been put out to increase the biomaterials' activity and compatibility. For example, bioorthogonal click chemistry has greatly boosted the variety and intricacy of biomaterial compositions because of its exceptionally high yield, simplicity, adaptability, and selectivity [56, 57]. Biomaterials can also be paired with pro-survival factors, which shield transplanted cells from the harsh environment of post-MI damaged tissues, and regeneration factors, which promote reparative processes in the infarcted heart, to optimize restorative potential [50]. Furthermore, because of their customized 3D structure, which encourages the secretion of ECM, revascularization, and paracrine functions, biomaterials facilitate the development of blood vessels that support vascular substructures as well as the passage of gasses and nutrients [49]. Due to the contractile nature of the heart, various mechanical stresses occur on the cardiac tissues, causing irregular 3D deformations [58]. To replicate the normal stretching and compression of the myocardium, the biomaterials used in cardiac regeneration must be able to tolerate stresses such as mechanical strain, tensile forces, and shearing forces. Additionally, electrical conductivity should be stimulated by biomaterial implants in order to support dynamic heart tissue functions [52, 59]. To make things more understandable, Figure 3.4 was made to list the precise qualities of the biomaterials needed for heart tissue regeneration.

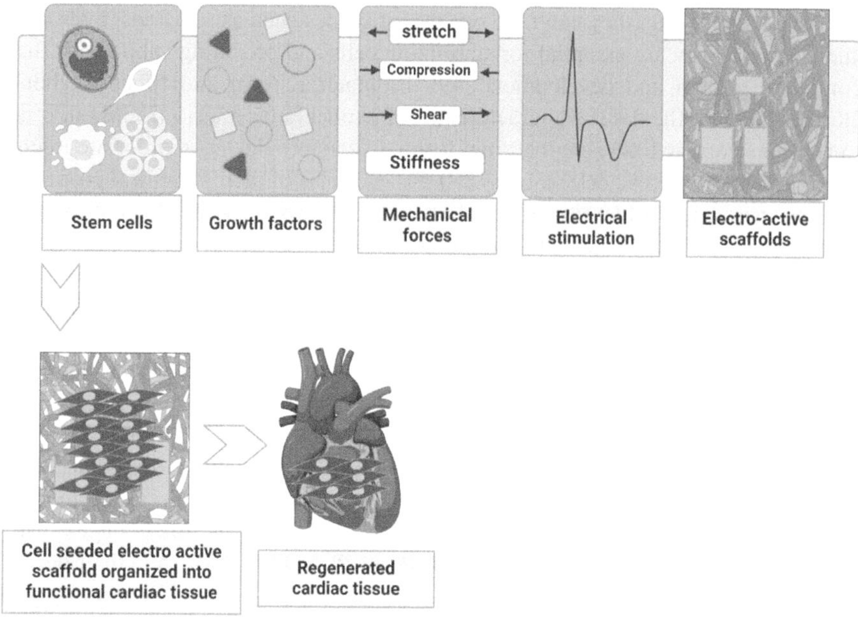

FIGURE 3.4 Summarizes the essential elements for heart tissue regeneration. Adapted from [39, 58, 60] with some modifications.

3.3.1 Design Standards for Cardiac Tissue Engineering Biomaterials

The development of biomaterial treatment and design solutions is hampered by the complexity of the natural heart environment. Taking the biomaterial application's goal into account is a crucial part of the biomaterial design process. Depending on whether the biomaterial is a functionalized substance used to artificially preserve normal ventricular shape or a scaffold for creating tissue patches, or a vehicle for the delivery of cells, different design criteria will apply. But before anything else, a few standard design requirements need to be addressed [17, 61–64].

3.3.1.1 Biocompatibility

The accepted meaning of "biocompatibility" in modern times is the "ability of a material to perform with an appropriate host response in a specific application" [65]. This includes the need for the material to maintain the contractile function of the heart and cardiomyocyte survival without cytotoxicity both in vivo and in vitro in the context of cardiac tissue engineering, without eliciting a significant foreign-body response in vivo [61–63]. This concentrates on reducing and managing the kind of reaction to avoid further harm to the heart and not impair its function rather than preventing the host's inflammatory and immunological response from being activated. A biocompatible substance should, in particular, be immunogenic and resistant to bacterial colonization and blood coagulation. It should also avoid attracting cell types that might speed up the remodeling process.

3.3.1.2 Biodegradability

"Biodegradability" describes the natural lifespan of an implanted material as well as the process by which it degrades. The several mechanisms and their ensuing definitions are thoroughly discussed elsewhere [66]. The breakdown of material through hydrolytic mechanisms, such as bulk and surface erosion, is referred to as bioerosion. Degradation through cellular activity is referred to as bioresorption. Enzymatic activity is referred to as biodegradation. These are the three modes of degradation that need to be considered. A biomaterial in cardiac tissue engineering is said to be biodegradable. If it degrades in vivo through disintegration, hydrolysis, or enzymatic activity, and if the breakdown products also satisfy the requirements for biocompatibility and biodegradability [61–64]. Table 3.1 provides a comprehensive overview of all the biomaterials and different approaches covered in this Book chapter, which covers material, design aspects, scaffold (Natural, Synthetic), hydrogel (Natural, Semi-synthetic, Synthetic), and use of each.

Although biocompatibility and biodegradability are two different concepts, they are frequently taken into account simultaneously when creating biomaterials because it makes little sense to create a biocompatible material that breaks down into hazardous constituents. The subject has seen a shift in recent years toward the study and creation of novel materials that satisfy the particular performance requirements of materials intended for use in tissue engineering.

3.3.2 Types of Biomaterials

3.3.2.1 Synthetic Biomaterials

Precise control over characteristics including the polymer's molecular weight, rate of degradation, mechanical attributes, and hydrophobicity is possible with synthetic materials. Nevertheless, unlike biologically generated materials, they might not engage in any beneficial interactions with cells. The most widely used synthetic scrim materials are the biodegradable polyesters made of glycolide (PLG) and lactide (PLA), as well as the copolymers of these two molecules (PLGA). Depending on the co-monomer ratio and molecular weight, the polymers degrade over a period of days to years. The FDA has approved the polymers, which are simple to make and have an excellent safety profile. Tissue engineering products using these polymers include DERMAGRAFT®, a treatment for skin regeneration [86]. These identical polymers, however, did not perform well when combined to generate thick porous structures for use in tissue engineering applications such as cardiac applications. The scaffolds tended to collapse and quickly lost their mechanical strength as the materials deteriorated [87, 88]. Additionally, the cell seeding procedure onto the scaffold formed of this polymer was ineffective, and the bulk of the cells gathered close to the scaffold boundaries because the majority of these polymers are hydrophobic in nature (particularly those having greater ratios of the co-monomer LA) [89]. Following the scaffolds' implantation, there was little tissue ingrowth or vascularization, and the majority of the interior volume of the scaffold remained empty [90]. Additionally, as polyester scaffolds deteriorate, an accumulation of acidic breakdown products occurs, which impacts cell viability and results in unfavorable tissue reactivity upon implantation [91]. Krupnick et al. have

TABLE 3.1
Biomaterial Techniques for Heart Tissue Restoration [67]

Scaffold	Material	Design	Utilize	References
Natural	Alignate	Scaffold that has been prevascularized	Whole replacement of the LV wall tissue	[68, 69]
	Sheets of cells	Prevascularized multilayer cell sheets in vitro	Patch made of tissue engineering	[70–72]
	Collagen	Proangiogenic biodegradable framework	Patch made of tissue engineering	[73]
Synthetic	strengthened with a fabric made of knitted poly-L-lactide (ε-Caprolactone-L-lactide)	seeded in a scaffold with vSMCs	Whole replacement of the LV wall tissue	[74]
	Poly (2-hydroxyethyl methacrylate-comethacrylic acid)	Engineered (spatially controlled) scaffold	Tissue-engineered patch	[75]
	Polylactic glycolic acid and poly-L-lactic acid	Multi-cell seeding for scaffolding and vascularization promotion	Tissue patch	[76]
Hydrogel	**Material**	**Design**	**Use**	**References**
Natural	Alginate	Hydrogel with chemical cross-linking	Bulking material	[77, 78]
	Chitosan–collagen	Thermogelling bioactive hydrogel	Internalized Repair	[79]
	Glycerol phosphate–chitosan	Chemically cross-linked hydrogel that is thermoresponsive	Cell transplantation	[80]
Semi-synthetic	fibrinogen–PEG	Hydrogel that can be photocrosslinked or polymerized by UV light	Bulking material, transplanting cells, and endogenous repair	[81, 82]
Synthetic	Methacrylated hyaluronic acid	Hydrogel with chemical cross-linking	hefty substance	[83]
	NIPAAm-co-AAc-co-HEMAPTMC	Thermoresponsive hydrogel	hefty substance	[84]
	Polyester	Bioactive thermoresponsive hydrogel	Natural mending and filling materials	[85]

demonstrated that the use of PGA mesh in the heart causes strong inflammatory reactions [92]. The manufacture of hydrogels, such as those based on polyethylene glycol, can address a number of the shortcomings of synthetic polyesters. Although these hydrophilic materials lack the biological characteristics of natural polymers like collagen, they nevertheless resemble the original ECM in many respects.

3.3.2.2 Natural Biomaterials

Natural polymers include substances produced from plants and seaweed as well as ECM proteins and derivatives such as collagen. Certain sticky sequences, like RGD, on the surfaces of natural polymers formed from ECM, such as Type I collagen and fibronectin, offer advantages for tissue engineering applications by promoting cell adherence and preserving cell differentiation. Unfortunately, if these materials are not chemically cross-linked, they will break down in the body quite quickly due to their lack of mechanical strength [93, 94]. Concerns are also raised by batch-to-batch variability in material characteristics and possible contaminations when extracted from animal tissues. To avoid utilizing animal products, recombinant human collagen, and other components are being created by expressing them in cell lines, including yeast. Apart from molecules based on proteins, natural polysaccharides are of tremendous interest. Alginate is a negatively charged polysaccharide from seaweed that forms hydrogels in the presence of calcium ions. Both native and modified versions of alginate are being created for use in tissue engineering [95, 96].

3.3.2.3 Conductive Biomaterials

Hydrogel networks that contain conductive biomaterials have made it possible to produce electrically conductive hydrogels. By using a straightforward ultraviolet-assisted capillary molding approach, reliable PEG nanopillar hydrogels featuring a distinct three-dimensional guiding structure made of PEG-DMA may promote the growth of CMs while preserving their conductive qualities [97]. GelMA hydrogel based on CNTs may be able to address several advantageous aspects of organic porous scaffolds at once, including high porosity, biodegradability, and electrical conductivity. The CNTs facilitated cell spreading and elongation and led to extensive nanofiber crisscrossing in the porous GelMA scaffold. Heart-protective scaffolds made of a photocrosslinkable derivative GelMA could lessen or prevent damage to the heart's tissues [98]. After an MI, damaged hearts could be combined with conductive biomaterials were used to construct cardiac tissues, which effectively prevented the infarcted heart from worsening. PPy-chitosan hydrogel is created when PPy is linked conductive PPy onto chitosan side chains [99].

When injected into rat hearts after myocardial infarction, this hydrogel was able to drastically enhance heart function and synchronize myocyte function ex vivo [100]. It was discovered that the elastic and conductive Hybrid hydrogels MeTro/GO made from graphene oxide (GO) nanoparticles could withstand stronger cyclic tensile and torsional pressures. A highly elastic, light-sensitive injectable scaffold with uniform GO spreading was created in two stages. These MeTro/GO hybrid hydrogels may promote the development and functionality of CMs [101]. Because of its carboxyl groups in the backbone (PTAA), one type of derivative of conductive polythiophene, forms a cross-linked network hydrogel with ease. Through the addition of Irgacure 2959 to facilitate conductive PTAA photocrosslinking with MAAG, and exposure to UV light for fifteen minutes, a well-proportioned hydrogel with high biocompatibility in vitro and in vivo was produced. This hydrogel satisfies the prerequisites for heart repair [102]. Using a similar synthesis method, a biocompatible cardiac patch might be formed by photosynthesis-based incorporation of GNR into GelMA hydrogels [103]. Wu et al.

[104] encased electrospun conductive nanofiber yarns (NFYs-NET) in a hydrogel shell to create endothelialized, anisotropic, three-dimensional multilayer cardiac tissues.

3.3.2.4 Extracellular Matrix-Based Biomaterials

The components of natural ECMs have been used in numerous research [105, 106] as a hydrogel to provide tissue-like water content and enable efficient encapsulation. The mechanical properties of hydrogels based on ECM have been altered by a variety of physical and chemical cross-linking methods. Numerous physical and chemical cross-linking methods have been employed, such as photopolymerization, hydrogen bonding, heat-induction-mediated solid-to-gel phase change, and enzyme cross-linking (i.e., cross-linking between two molecules with opposite charges) [107]. Conditions related to light exposure, including exposure times, locations, and intensities, can alter how ECM-based hydrogels behave mechanically [108, 109]. Seaweed-derived alginate is a polymer that is commonly utilized as an (ECM) for encasing living cells since it can be cross-linked at both room temperature and physiological pH [110]. Hydrophobic interactions have been exploited to create hydrogels from polysaccharides like chitosan and dextran [111].

3.3.2.5 Biomaterials Made of Silk

According to research, SF is the silk-based biomaterial that is most frequently employed in cardiac patch applications. Chung et al. made several breakthroughs in the cardiac patch field and were the first to use SF into CTE. By pressing SF, CS, and HA microparticles and creating an SF/CS/HA hybrid matrix of natural biomaterials by cross-linking them using genipin, a naturally occurring, mildly cytotoxic agent for cross-linking [112]. They demonstrated how the SF matrix encouraged MSC adherence and proliferation and that the existence of 5-azacytidine (5-aza) could slightly induce the attached MSCs to differentiate into CMs. However, the incorporation of polysaccharides like CS and HA greatly enhanced the MSCs' capacity for growth and differentiation [113]. Chung et al.'s research proved that it is possible to restore injured cardiac tissue with natural hybrid materials. Chen and colleagues have presented materials made of cellulose that had better mechanical qualities. By adding CS/SF multilayers to electrospun cellulose nanofibers, the CS/SF/cellulose nanofibrous cardiac patch was produced by them. In addition to providing biomimetic ECM support for the engrafted MSCs made from adipose tissue to adhere to and survive, the patch also blocked unfavorable remodeling of the left ventricle (LV) and stopped the heart failure from progressing [114]. Additionally, a pure SF scaffold was created and put to the test for study on cardiac patches. By lyophilizing B. mori SF solution, SF porous matrices with the right mechanical and physical characteristics may be easily created for myocardial restoration [115, 116]. Because of its repeated RGD sequences in vitro, AMSF matrices attached more rat neonatal CMs than B. mori. Additionally, they discovered that AMSF matrices promoted increased connexin 43 (Cx43) expression and CM development, leading to the intercellular coupling of CMs and tractable patches [117]. Figure 3.5 shows how biomaterials can be made from unconventional materials like paper, silk, and plant leaves. These materials are readily obtained and found in nature and can be imaginatively used to create inexpensive, long-lasting, and functional cardiovascular tissue constructs.

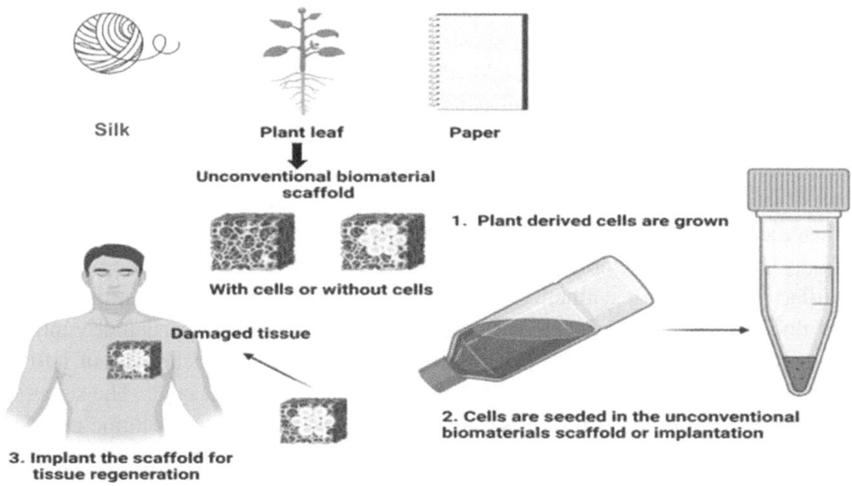

FIGURE 3.5 Application of novel biomaterials in tissue regeneration and repair. Unconventional biomaterials can be engineered to create novel biomaterials for the creation of affordable and functional cardiovascular tissue constructs. These materials can come from readily accessible, naturally occurring sources including silk, plant leaves, and paper. Adapted from [118] with some modifications.

3.4 METHODS FOR ENGINEERING AND REGENERATING HEART TISSUE

Since recent advancements showed promising results in enhancing heart function, encouraging angiogenesis, and reducing adverse immunological responses in animal tests and human trials, biomaterial-based approaches have drawn more attention to cardiac tissue engineering and regeneration [119, 120]. The following subsections provide an overview of the state of the art in heart regeneration therapies by describing the latest advancements in the administration of therapeutics using scaffolds, extracellular vesicles, injectable hydrogels, and cardiac patches.

3.4.1 Cardiac Patches

As long as the right cells adhere to and proliferate on the injured heart, cardiac patches can restore its functionality. Improved compatibility can be achieved by adjusting cardiac patches to the right dimensions, form, and mechanical tensile strength. Additionally, cardiac patches with cell strength can be planted, which improves compatibility. Additionally, before being implanted in biological reactors or in culture, it is possible to seed cardiac patches with cells to promote their development and maturation [121]. By distributing different bioactive substances or cells to the infarction site on the heart surface, these biomaterial constructs can enhance cardiac function [122]. The utilization of decellularized swine biological resources [123, 124], polymers derived from nature (such as cellulose [114, 125], CS [114, 126,127], SF [114], collagen [128, 129], and GelMA [130]), and synthetic polymers (such as PEGDA [130], PCL [131], PVA [132], and PVP [132]) are the main topics of recent studies regarding substrate materials. The benefit of utilizing native tissues' decellularized natural ECM is found in its intricate protein composition, which is interwoven with proteoglycans to give cells the support they need to orient and interact through signaling pathways. However, these biological materials offer a number of problems when transferring from in vitro and in vivo testing to human investigations. These challenges include pathogen translocation when employing allogenic and xenogenic tissues, host responses, and the lack of autologous tissue or organs [133]. Consequently, There's a growing body of research focused on creating cardiac patches using synthetic materials that are biocompatible or natural sources that do not include animals. He and associates have suggested a particularly intriguing recent study avenue [125]. The authors created cardiac patches out of leftover biomass and sea squirts in an attempt to address two issues at once. The scientists demonstrated how the naturally self-conductive structures made of tunic cellulose functioned as effective cardiac patches, encouraging the growth of cardiomyocytes and their spontaneous contraction. Thus, in addition to improving the available treatment choices for MI, their solution may also help reduce biopollution in maritime environments.

3.4.2 Injectable Hydrogels

Biomaterials of the hydrogel type can be used to distribute biological components that are acellular as well as cellular. As effective injectable carrier materials for active components, natural polymers such as hyaluronic acid, keratin, fucoidan, collagen, fibrin, chitosan, and alginate have been used [41].

The use of injectable hydrogels that have self-healing properties is one particularly intriguing heart repair technique. These hydrogels have the ability to rebuild their own structure and regain original properties after damage, all while physically supporting infarcted tissue and preventing pathological ventricular remodeling [134–136]. An intramyocardial injection of an ECM-mimicking hydrogel was suggested as an alternative by Contessotto et al. [137]. The injectable hydrogel consisting of elastin-related recombinamers resulted in complete functional recovery of the ejection fraction 21 days following the intervention in an ovine model. In the infarct border zone, there was also enhanced protection for GATA4+ cardiomyocytes, reduced fibrosis, and more angiogenesis. Alternatively, Bai et al. [138] have developed an injectable, temperature-sensitive hydrogel based on ECM derived from decellularized rat hearts that were seeded with brown adipose tissue-derived cardiomyogenic cells. The ECM hydrogel retained heart function and chamber form because it encouraged myocardial regeneration and cell engraftment. A dibenzaldehyde-terminated poly(ethylene glycol) and chitosan-graft-aniline tetramer-based self-healing conductive hydrogel have been created by Dong et al. [139] and injected into hearts that have been infarcted. The hydrogels that are injected are biocompatible, biodegradable, and have a release rate that can be adjusted. Their conductivity is comparable to natural heart tissue at about 10^{-3} S·cm^{-1}. An injectable hydrogel with mechanical resilience has been developed by Navaei et al. [140] for the delivery of cardiac cells for tissue engineering. Gelatin cross-linked to temperature-responsive polymer (PNIPA) makes up the hydrogel. The hybrid material provided increased water content and bioactivity, which led to optimal cell adhesion, spreading, and survival. It also helped organize markers particular to the heart and cytoskeleton. The injectable matrix enhanced the cell-embedded hydrogel's performance by providing a space for cardiac fibroblasts.

3.4.3 Extracellular Vesicles

Extracellular vesicles or spheres made from diverse cell types have shown promise as a treatment for heart regeneration when used alone or in different combinations [80]. When hydrogels or cardiac patches are utilized as delivery vehicles instead of injecting parent cells, which produce a variable release, extracellular vesicles can be delivered in a personalized manner [119].

Therefore, the majority of recent research has focused on employing different biomaterials in conjunction with extracellular vesicle-based treatments as feasible, biocompatible carriers to create therapeutic platforms that serve several purposes [141]. For example, Lv et al. [142] discussed the possibility of using tiny extracellular vesicles produced from MSCs to treat MI. To optimize their retention in the cardiac tissue and improve the therapeutic results, they have included them in alginate hydrogel. Overall cardiac function and infarct size were reported to be enhanced by the as-designed treatment, which also significantly reduced cardiac cell apoptosis, encouraged macrophage polarization on day three following MI, and four weeks following the incident, thicker scar tissue and enhanced angiogenesis. Exosomes produced from MSCs in the human umbilical cord have been shown to be useful in heart regeneration, according to studies by Han et al. [143]. To increase the exosomes' stability and retention, the authors encased them in useful peptide hydrogels. The hybrid formulation was found to produce better results in terms of increasing angiogenesis and lowering apoptosis, fibrosis, and inflammation when compared to exosome therapy alone. This improvement in outcomes ultimately resulted in an improvement in myocardial function. Shear-thinning gel that was injected was created by Chen and colleagues [144] using extracellular vesicles that were extracted from endothelial progenitor cells (EPCs). It was found that the new formulation improved the hemodynamic function following myocardial infarction, allowed for the preservation of ventricular shape, and increased peri-infarct vascular proliferation. On the other hand, Liu and colleagues [145] have opted to utilize extracellular vesicles released by cardiomyocytes that are produced from induced pluripotent stem cells. These vesicles were able to decrease cell apoptosis 24 hours after MI, decrease arrhythmic load, encourage ejection fraction recovery and four weeks following MI, diminish the extent of the infarct and the hypertrophy of the cells when they were enclosed in a synthetic hydrogel patch.

3.4.4 Scaffolds

For cardiac applications, it has been observed that certain parameters—such as substrate form, stiffness, matrix topography, and electrical stimulation—are crucial. Given their established impact on cellular behavior, motility regulation, proliferation, and differentiation responses, these parameters need to be precisely adjusted in order to facilitate the process by which planted cells differentiate to become highly functioning [49, 52, 146]. In this context, numerous studies have looked at different scaffolds based on substrate materials, embedded nanostructures, and seeded cells; a few of these are discussed in more detail below. Liang et al. [147] recently developed a conductive scaffold by combining solutions of SF and PPy. The researchers experimented with different SF concentrations and ratios for polymer blending, finding that a 7% SF solution had mechanical properties that were most similar to those of native heart tissues and that a PPy-to-SF 15:85 is the ratio provided cardiomyocytes with sufficient electrical conductivity. As an alternative, Li and associates [148] have produced biomaterial scaffolds with improved mechanical and electrical conductivity by combining high-aspect-ratio GNWs with GelMA hydrogels. Because cardiomyocytes grown on their scaffold showed increased spontaneous beating rate and increased synchronous beating activity on nanocomposite hydrogels, as well as increased cell viability and maturation status when compared to those grown on plain GelMA hydrogels, their scaffold served as an appropriate medium for the construction of functional cardiac tissue. Gold has also been used by Saravanan et al. [149] in an effort to create a better heart restoration scaffold. The scientists combined GO gold nanosheets with a chitosan matrix to form a conductive, biodegradable structure. The synthetic frameworks supported cell adhesion and proliferation without exhibiting any harmful effects because of its well-controlled porosity design, swelling, and degradation features. The scaffold increased cardiac contractility and restored ventricular function after implantation. Feiner and colleagues [60] have developed a different electronic wherein the substrate and passivation layer for the evaporated gold electrodes are electrospun albumin fibers. The highly effective frameworks facilitated the organization of cardiomyocytes into functioning cardiac tissue, acted as a means of actuating the designed tissue, and initiated the release of medication. The electronic scaffolds also deteriorated after implantation, which makes them a desirable option for temporary in vivo use.

3.5 CURRENT CHALLENGES

The search for efficient biomaterials for cardiac tissue engineering faces a variety of difficulties, including those related to mechanical integration, electrical functionality, biocompatibility, and the intricacy of cardiac physiology. One major challenge is making sure materials not only blend in with human biology but also break down safely. It is crucial to match the strength and flexibility of the heart's particular mechanical characteristics in order to support and improve cardiac function. Furthermore, the requirement for materials that promote electrical conduction echoes the heart's inherent ability to pace, highlighting the difficulty in developing technical solutions that can be easily incorporated into the cardiac system. The complexity of cardiac tissue necessitates novel techniques that can replicate these complex environments because of its unique requirements for cellular adhesion, proliferation, and differentiation in a three-dimensional setting. Moreover, problems with repeatability and scalability make it difficult to convert clinical breakthroughs from the lab into broadly accessible treatments, calling for developments that can reliably generate high-quality materials at scale. To overcome these challenges, interdisciplinary teams must work together to push the limits of heart regeneration and repair by utilizing the most recent developments in tissue engineering, biomaterial science, and clinical insights.

3.6 CONCLUSION

The investigation of Biomaterials for tissue engineering of the heart is a new area of study in medicine with the potential to completely change how heart disease is treated. The path toward fully functional, integrated cardiac repair solutions emphasizes the necessity for ongoing creativity and persistence, despite the notable advancements accomplished. The intricate process of simulating the cardiac environment, along with the difficulties of mechanical and electrical integration and biocompatibility, necessitates a multidisciplinary strategy that connects research and clinical application. The creation of biomaterials that support the dynamic cellular processes necessary for tissue regeneration in addition to imitating the structural and functional characteristics of the heart should be the primary focus of future research. In addition, these solutions' scalability, long-term sustainability, and ethical considerations continue to be critical. Collaboration between scientific fields, technological developments, and a better comprehension of cardiac biology will all contribute to our progress and open the door to discoveries that will provide patients with more efficient, individualized treatment options. With manufactured tissues and materials, it may soon be possible to totally restore cardiac function, ushering in a new age in cardiovascular care.

ACKNOWLEDGMENTS

The authors gratefully acknowledged HBTU Kanpur (IS) and UPCST, Uttar Pradesh for research project grant no. CST/D-831, Project id: 3993 (SK).

ABBREVIATIONS

5-aza	5-azacytidine
ACE	angiotensin-converting enzyme
CM	cytomembrane
CNTs	carbon nanotubes
CRISPR	clustered regularly interspaced short palindromic repeats
CS	chitosan
ECM	extracellular matrix
EPCs	endothelial progenitor cells
FDA	Food and Drug Administration
GelMA	gelatin methacrylate
GNRs	gold nanorods
GNWs	gold nanowires
GO	graphene oxide
HA	hyaluronic acid

iPSCs generate induced pluripotent stem cells
iPSCs pluripotent stem cells
MAAG methacrylated aminated gelatin
MSCs mesenchymal stem cells
NFYs-NET nanofiber yarns network
PCL polycaprolactone
PEGDA polyethylene glycol diacrylate
PEG polyethylene glycol
PEG-DMA poly(ethylene glycol)-dimethacrylate
PGA polyglycolic acid
PLA polylactic acid
PLG polyglycolide
PLGA poly(lactic-co-glycolic acid)
PPy polypyrrole
PTAA poly(thiophene-3-acetic acid)
PU polyurethane
PVA polyvinyl alcohol
PVP polyvinyl pyrrolidone
ROS reactive oxygen species
SF silk fibroin
VEGF vascular endothelial growth factor
PIPA Poly (N-isopropylacrylamide)

REFERENCES

1. D.F. Williams, On the nature of biomaterials, Biomaterials 30 (2009) 5897–5909.
2. A. Hasan et al., Engineered biomaterials to enhance stem cell-based cardiac tissue engineering and therapy, Macromol Biosci 16 (2016) 958–977.
3. J.M. Dang, K.W. Leong, Natural polymers for gene delivery and tissue engineering, Adv Drug Deliv Rev 58 (2006) 487–499.
4. A.S.T. Smith et al., Micro- and nano-patterned conductive graphene-PEG hybrid scaffolds for cardiac tissue engineering, Chem Commun (Cambridge, England) 53 (2017) 7412–7415.
5. M.A. Nguyen, G. Camci-Unal, Unconventional tissue engineering materials in disguise, Trends Biotechnol 38 (2020) 178–190.
6. A. Khademhosseini, R. Langer, A decade of progress in tissue engineering, Nat Protoc 11 (2016) 1775–1781.
7. F.-M. Chen, X. Liu, Advancing biomaterials of human origin for tissue engineering, Prog Polym Sci 53 (2016) 86–168.
8. R. Song et al., Current development of biodegradable polymeric materials for biomedical applications, Drug Des Dev Ther 12 (2018) 3117–3145.
9. W. Xiao et al., Fabrication and assembly of porous micropatterned scaffolds for modular tissue engineering, Mater Lett 228 (2018) 360–364.
10. A. Mahapatro, Metals for biomedical applications and devices, J Biomater Tissue Eng 2 (2012) 259–268.
11. S.K. Jaganathan et al., Biomaterials in cardiovascular research: Applications and clinical implications, BioMed Res Int 2014 (2014) 459465.
12. R. Waksman, Biodegradable stents: They do their job and disappear, J Invasive Cardiol 18 (2006) 70–74.

13. B. Desschans, P. Evrard, Coordinator transplant section of the Belgian transplant society. Organ donation and transplantation statistics in Belgium for 2012 and 2013, Transplant Proc 46 (2014) 3124–3126.
14. D.K.C. Cooper et al., Report of the xenotransplantation advisory committee of the international society for heart and lung transplantation: The present status of xenotransplantation and its potential role in the treatment of end-stage cardiac and pulmonary diseases, J Heart Lung Transplant 19 (2000) 1125–1165.
15. S. Giwa et al., The promise of organ and tissue preservation to transform medicine, Nat Biotechnol 35 (2017) 530–542.
16. V.L. Roger, A.S. Go, D.M. Lloyd-Jones et al., Heart disease and stroke statistics – 2012 update: A report from the American Heart Association, Circulation, 125 (2012) e2–e220.
17. P. Menasché, Current status and future prospects for cell transplantation to prevent congestive heart failure, Semin Thorac Cardiovasc Surg 20 (2008) 131–137.
18. J.M. Karp, G.S. Leng Teo, Mesenchymal stem cell homing: The devil is in the details, Cell Stem Cell 4 (2009) 206–216.
19. S.H. Ranganath, O. Levy, M.S. Inamdar, J.M. Karp, Harnessing the mesenchymal stem cell secretome for the treatment of cardiovascular disease, Cell Stem Cell 10 (2012) 244–258.
20. D. Sarkar et al., Engineered cell homing, Blood 118 (2011) e184–e191.
21. O. Levy et al., mRNA-engineered mesenchymal stem cells for targeted delivery of interleukin-10 to sites of inflammation, Blood 122 (2013) e23–e32.
22. M. Jinek et al., A programmable dual-RNA-guided DNA endonuclease in adaptive bacterial immunity, Science 337 (2012) 816–821.
23. L. Cong et al., Multiplex genome engineering using CRISPR/Cas systems, Science 339 (2013) 819–823.
24. F.A. Ran et al., Genome engineering using the CRISPR-Cas9 system, Nat Protoc 8 (2013) 2281–2308.
25. H. Wang et al., One-step generation of mice carrying mutations in multiple genes by CRISPR/Cas-mediated genome engineering, Cell 153 (2013) 910–918.
26. K. Servick, Gene-editing method revives hopes for transplanting pig organs into people, Science, 10 (2015) doi:10.1126/science.aad4700.
27. S. Reardon, New life for pig-to-human transplants, Nature 527 (2015) 152–154.
28. S. Reardon, Gene-editing record smashed in pigs, Nature News, (2015) 6.
29. J.B. Young, R.M. Mills, Clinical Management of Heart Failure, Professional Communications, Caddo, OK, 2004.
30. F.Y. Chen, L.H. Cohn, The surgical treatment of heart failure. A new frontier: nontransplant surgical alternatives in heart failure, Cardiol Rev 10 (2002) 326–333.
31. M. Loebe, E. Soltero, V. Thohan, J.A. Lafuente, G.P. Noon, New surgical therapies for heart failure, Curr Opin Cardiol 18 (2003) 194–198.
32. N.M. Hawkins, M.C. Petrie, M.R. MacDonald, K.J. Hogg, J.J.V. McMurray, Selecting patients for cardiac resynchronization therapy: electrical or mechanical dyssynchrony?, Eur Heart J 27 (2006) 1270–1281.
33. C. Martinez, A. Tzur, H. Hrachian, J. Zebede, G.A. Lamas, Pacemakers and defibrillators: recent and ongoing studies that impact the elderly, Am J Geriat Cardiol 15 (2006) 82–87.
34. S.K. Kohli, P. Elliott, Cardiac resynchronization therapy: the procedure and progress so far, Br J Hosp Med 66 (2005) 469–473.
35. M. Packer, The impossible task of developing a new treatment for heart failure, J Card Fail 8 (2002) 193–196.
36. P. Zammaretti, M. Jaconi, Cardiac tissue engineering: regeneration of the wounded heart, Curr Opin Biotechnol 15 (2004) 430–434.

37. S. Pascual-Gil, E. Garbayo, P. Díaz-Herráez, F. Prosper, M.J. Blanco-Prieto, Heart regeneration after myocardial infarction using synthetic biomaterials, J Control Release 203 (2015) 23–38.
38. Y. Zhao, N.T. Feric, N. Thavandiran, S.S. Nunes, M. Radisic, The role of tissue engineering and biomaterials in cardiac regenerative medicine, Can J Cardiol 30 (2014) 1307–1322.
39. K. Ashtari, H. Nazari, H. Ko, P. Tebon, M. Akhshik, M. Akbari, S.N. Alhosseini, M. Mozafari, B. Mehravi, M. Soleimani et al., Electrically conductive nanomaterials for cardiac tissue engineering, Adv Drug Deliv Rev 144 (2019) 162–179.
40. M. Tamimi, S. Rajabi, M. Pezeshki-Modaress, Cardiac ECM/chitosan/alginate ternary scaffolds for cardiac tissue engineering application, Int J Biol Macromol 164 (2020) 389–402.
41. Q.A. Majid, A.T.R. Fricker, D.A. Gregory, N. Davidenko, O. Hernandez Cruz, R.J. Jabbour, T.J. Owen, P. Basnett, B. Lukasiewicz, M. Stevens, Natural biomaterials for cardiac tissue engineering: A highly biocompatible solution, Front Cardiovasc Med 7 (2020) 554597.
42. H. Esmaeili, A. Patino-Guerrero, M. Hasany, M.O. Ansari, A. Memic, A. Dolatshahi-Pirouz, M. Nikkhah, Electroconductive biomaterials for cardiac tissue engineering, Acta Biomater 139 (2022) 118–140.
43. Z. Cui, B. Yang, R.-K. Li, Application of biomaterials in cardiac repair and regeneration, Engineering 2 (2016) 141–148.
44. L. Reis, L.L.Y. Chiu, N. Feric, L. Fu, M. Radisic, 3–Injectable biomaterials for cardiac regeneration and repair, in: R.-K. Li, R.D. Weisel, Eds., Cardiac Regeneration and Repair, Woodhead Publishing, Sawston, UK, 2014, pp. 49–81.
45. V. Vasanthan, A. Fatehi Hassanabad, S. Pattar, P. Niklewski, K. Wagner, P.W.M. Fedak, Promoting cardiac regeneration and repair using acellular biomaterials, Front Bioeng Biotechnol 8 (2020) 291.
46. Q.-Z. Chen, S.E. Harding, N.N. Ali, A.R. Lyon, A.R. Boccaccini, Biomaterials in cardiac tissue engineering: Ten years of research survey, Mater Sci Eng R Rep 59 (2008) 1–37.
47. L.D. Huyer, M. Montgomery, Y. Zhao, Y. Xiao, G. Conant, A. Korolj, M. Radisic, Biomaterial based cardiac tissue engineering and its applications, Biomed Mater 10 (2015) 034004.
48. C. Gokce, C. Gurcan, L.G. Delogu, A. Yilmazer, 2D materials for cardiac tissue repair and regeneration, Front Cardiovasc Med 9 (2022) 802551.
49. A.H. Nguyen, P. Marsh, L. Schmiess-Heine, P.J. Burke, A. Lee, J. Lee, H. Cao, Cardiac tissue engineering: State-of-the-art methods and outlook, J Biol Eng 13 (2019) 57.
50. B. Pournemati, H. Tabesh, A. Jenabi, R. Mehdinavaz Aghdam, A. Hossein Rezayan, A. Poorkhalil, S.H. Ahmadi Tafti, K. Mottaghy, Injectable conductive nanocomposite hydrogels for cardiac tissue engineering: Focusing on carbon and metal-based nanostructures, Eur Polym J 174 (2022) 111336.
51. E. Ruvinov, S. Cohen, Biomaterials for cardiac tissue engineering and regeneration, in: J. Hescheler, E. Hofer, Eds., Adult and Pluripotent Stem Cells: Potential for Regenerative Medicine of the Cardiovascular System, Springer, Dordrecht, The Netherlands, 2014, pp. 83–111.
52. F. Ibrahim, A. Thiha, W.S. Wan Kamarul Zaman, Y. Kamarulzaman, N.A. Dahlan, N.F. Jamaluddin, M.J. Madou, Cardiac tissue engineering: A comparative analysis on microscaffold patterning, Mater Today Commun 33 (2022) 104285.
53. Y. Yao, A. Li, S. Wang, Y. Lu, J. Xie, H. Zhang, D. Zhang, J. Ding, Z. Wang, C. Tu et al., Multifunctional elastomer cardiac patches for preventing left ventricle remodeling after myocardial infarction in vivo, Biomaterials 282 (2022) 121382.
54. S. Farzamfar, M. Aleahmad, S.K. Gholamreza, S. Majid, N. Niloofar, Polycaprolactone/gelatin nanofibrous scaffolds for tissue engineering, Biointerface Res Appl Chem 11 (2021) 11104–11115.

55. B. Shadman, A. Marzban, A. Asadi, S. Zahri, A. Barzegar, Design of PLGA-based scaffolds for developing and differentiating mesenchymal stem cells (MSCs), Biointerface Res Appl Chem 11 (2021) 12732–12742.
56. C.A. DeForest, B.D. Polizzotti, K.S. Anseth, Sequential click reactions for synthesizing and patterning three-dimensional cell microenvironments, Nat Mater 8 (2009) 659–664.
57. C.A. DeForest, K.S. Anseth, Cytocompatible click-based hydrogels with dynamically tunable properties through orthogonal photoconjugation and photocleavage reactions, Nat Chem 3 (2011) 925–931.
58. L. Stewart, N.A. Turner, Channelling the force to reprogram the matrix: Mechanosensitive ion channels in cardiac fibroblasts, Cells 10 (2021) 990.
59. P. Chansoria, E.L. Etter, J. Nguyen, Regenerating dynamic organs using biomimetic patches, Trends Biotechnol 40 (2022) 338–353.
60. R. Feiner, S. Fleischer, A. Shapira, O. Kalish, T. Dvir, Multifunctional degradable electronic scaffolds for cardiac tissue engineering, J Control Release 281 (2018) 189–195.
61. J. Leor, N. Landa, S. Cohen, Renovation of the injured heart with myocardial tissue engineering, Expert Rev Cardiovasc Ther 4 (2006) 239–252.
62. Q.Z. Chen, S.E. Harding, N.N. Ali et al., Biomaterials in cardiac tissue engineering: Ten years of research survey, Mat Sci Eng R 59 (2008) 1–37.
63. G. Vunjak-Novakovic, N. Tandon, A. Godier et al., Challenges in cardiac tissue engineering, Tissue Eng B Rev 16 (2010) 169–187.
64. C.V. Bouten, P.Y. Dankers, A. Driessen-Mol et al., Substrates for cardiovascular tissue engineering, Adv Drug Deliv Rev 63 (2011) 221–241.
65. D.F. Williams, European Society for Biomaterials, "Definitions in biomaterials," Proceedings of a Consensus Conference of the European Society for Biomaterials, Chester, UK, 3–5 March 1986, Elsevier: New York, 1987.
66. M. Treiser, S. Abramson, R. Langer, et al., Degradable and resorbable biomaterials, in Biomaterials Science, 3rd ed., B.D. Ratner, A.S. Hoffman, F.J. Schoen, J.E. Lemons (eds), Academic Press, New York, 2013, 179–195.
67. L. Reis, L.L. Chiu, N. Feric, L. Fu, M. Radisic, Biomaterials in myocardial tissue engineering, J Tissue Eng Regen Med, 10(1) (2016) 11–28.
68. G. Amir, L. Miller, M. Shachar et al., Evaluation of a peritoneal-generated cardiac patch in a rat model of heterotopic heart transplantation, Cell Transpl 18 (2009) 275–282.
69. Y. Sapir, O. Kryukov, S. Cohen, Integration of multiple cell–matrix interactions into alginate scaffolds for promoting cardiac tissue regeneration, Biomaterials 32 (2011) 1838–1847.
70. T. Shimizu, M. Yamato, Y. Isoi et al., Fabrication of pulsatile cardiac tissue grafts using a novel three-dimensional cell sheet manipulation technique and temperature-model of chronic ischemic cardiomyopathy, J Thorac Cardiovasc Surg 137 (2002) 180–187.
71. S. Masuda, T. Shimizu, M. Yamato et al., Cell sheet engineering for heart tissue repair, Adv Drug Deliv Rev 60 (2008) 277–285.
72. H. Sekine, T. Shimizu, K. Sakaguchi et al., In vitro fabrication of functional three-dimensional tissues with perfusable blood vessels, Nat Commun 4 (2013) 1399.
73. L.L. Chiu, M. Radisic, Scaffolds with covalently immobilized VEGF and Angiopoietin1 for vascularization of engineered tissues, Biomaterials 31 (2010) 226–241.
74. K. Matsubayashi, P.W. Fedak, D.A. Mickle, et al., Improved left ventricular aneurysm repair with bioengineered vascular smooth muscle grafts, Circulation, 108(suppl 1) (2003) II219–II225.
75. L.R. Madden, D.J. Mortisen, E.M. Sussman et al., Proangiogenic scaffolds as functional templates for cardiac tissue engineering, Proc Natl Acad Sci U S A 107 (2010) 15211–15216.
76. A. Lesman, M. Habib, O. Caspi et al., Transplantation of a tissue-engineered human vascularized cardiac muscle, Tissue Eng A 16 (2010) 115–125.

77. J. Leor, S. Tuvia, V. Guetta et al., Intracoronary injection of in situ forming alginate hydrogel reverses left ventricular remodelling after myocardial infarction in swine, J Am Coll Cardiol 54 (2009) 1014–1023.
78. K.Y. Lee, D.J. Mooney, Alginate: Properties and biomedical applications, Progr Polym Sci 37 (2012) 106–126.
79. L.A. Reis, L.L.Y. Chiu, Y. Liang et al., A peptide-modified chitosan-collagen hydrogel for cardiac cell culture and delivery, Acta Biomater 8 (2012) 1022–1036.
80. W.N. Lu, S.H. Lü, H.B. Wang et al., Functional improvement of infarcted heart by co-injection of embryonic stem cells with temperature-responsive chitosan hydrogel, Tissue Eng A 15 (2009) 1437–1447.
81. M. Habib, K. Shapira-Schweitzer, O. Caspi et al., A combined cell therapy and in-situ tissue-engineering approach for myocardial repair, Biomaterials 32 (2011) 7514–7523.
82. A.J. Rufaihah, S.R. Vaibavi, M. Plotkin et al., Enhanced infarct stabilisation and neovascularization mediated by VEGFloaded PEGylated fibrinogen hydrogel in a rodent myocardial infarction model, Biomaterials 34 (2013) 8195–8202.
83. J.L. Ifkovits, E. Tous, M. Minakawa et al., Injectable hydrogel properties influence infarct expansion and extent of postinfarction left ventricular remodelling in an ovine model, Proc Natl Acad Sci USA, 107 (2010) 11507–11512.
84. K.L. Fujimoto, Z. Ma, D.M. Nelson et al., Synthesis, characterization and therapeutic efficacy of a biodegradable, thermoresponsive hydrogel designed for application in chronic infarcted myocardium, Biomaterials 30 (2009) 4357–4368.
85. J. Wu, F. Zeng, X.P. Huang et al., Infarct stabilisation and cardiac repair with a VEGF-conjugated, injectable hydrogel, Biomaterials 32 (2011) 579–586.
86. M. Shachar, S. Cohen, Cardiac tissue engineering, ex-vivo: Design principles in biomaterials and bioreactors, Heart Fail Rev 8 (2003) 271–276.
87. J.M. Pachence, J. Kohn, Biodegradable polymers for tissue engineering, in: R.P. Lanza, R. Langer, W.L. Chick, Eds., Principles of Tissue Engineering, Landes Biosciences Academic Press, 1997, pp. 273–293.
88. B.S. Kim, D.J. Mooney, Engineering smooth muscle tissue with a predefined structure, J Biomed Mater Res 41 (1998) 322–332.
89. R.L. Carrier, M. Papadaki, M. Rupnick, F.J. Schoen, N. Bursac, R. Langer, L.E. Freed, G. Vunjak-Novakovic, Cardiac tissue engineering: Cell seeding, cultivation parameters, and tissue construct characterization, Biotech Bioeng 64 (1999) 580–589.
90. A.G. Mikos, G. Sarakinos, M.D. Lyman, D.E. Ingber, J.P. Vacanti, R. Langer, Prevascularization of porous biodegradable polymers, Biotechnol Bioeng 42 (1993) 716–723.
91. O.E. Bostman, E. Hirvensalo, J. Makinen, P. Rokkanen, Foreign-body reactions to fracture fixation implants of biodegradable synthetic polymers, J Bone Joint Surg 72-B (1990) 592–596.
92. A.S. Krupnick, A. Shabaan, A. Radu, A.W. Flake, Bone marrow tissue engineering, Tissue Eng 8 (2002) 145–155.
93. A. Ben-Yishay, D.A. Grande, R.E. Schwartz, D. Mneche, M.S. Pitman, Repair of articular cartilage defects with collagen-chondrocytes allografts, Tissue Eng 1 (1995) 119–132.
94. L.H.H. Olde Damink, P.J. Dijkstra, M.J.A. Van Luyn, P.B. Van Wachem, P. Nieuwenhuis, J. Feijen, Changes in the mechanical properties of dermal sheep collagen during in vitro degradation, J Biomed Mater Res 20 (1995) 139–145.
95. L. Shapiro, S. Cohen, Novel alginate sponges for cell culture and transplantation, Biomaterials 18 (1997) 583–590.
96. J.A. Rowley, G. Madlambayan, D.J. Mooney, Alginate hydrogels as synthetic extracellular matrix materials, Biomaterials 20 (1999) 45–53.
97. D.H. Kim, P. Kim, I. Song et al., Guided three-dimensional growth of functional cardiomyocytes on polyethylene glycol nanostructures, Langmuir 22 (2006) 5419–26.

98. S.R. Shin, S.M. Jung, M. Zalabany et al., Carbon-nanotube-embedded hydrogel sheets for engineering cardiac constructs and bioactuators, ACS Nano 7 (2013) 2369–2380.
99. J. Zhou, J. Chen, H. Sun et al., Engineering the heart: Evaluation of conductive nanomaterials for improving implant integration and cardiac function, Sci Rep 4 (2014) 3733.
100. A. Mihic, Z. Cui, J. Wu et al., A conductive polymer hydrogel supports cell electrical signalling and improves cardiac function after implantation into myocardial infarct, Circulation 132 (2015) 772–784.
101. N. Annabi, S.R. Shin, A. Tamayol et al., Highly elastic and conductive human-based protein hybrid hydrogels, Adv Mater 28 (2016) 40–49.
102. B. Yang, F. Yao, T. Hao et al., Development of electrically conductive double-network hydrogels via one-step facile strategy for cardiac tissue engineering, Adv Healthc Mater 5 (2016) 474–488.
103. A. Navaei, H. Saini, W. Christenson et al., Gold nanorod incorporated gelatin-based conductive hydrogels for engineering cardiac tissue constructs, Acta Biomater 41 (2016) 133–146.
104. Y. Wu, L. Wang, B. Guo et al., Interwoven aligned conductive nanofiber Yarn/Hydrogel composite scaffolds for engineered 3D cardiac anisotropy, ACS Nano 11 (2017) 5646–5659.
105. G.S. Hussey, J.L. Dziki, S.F. Badylak, Extracellular matrix-based materials for regenerative medicine, Nat Rev Mater 3 (2018) 159–173.
106. N.A. Peppas, J.J. Sahlin, Hydrogels as mucoadhesive and bioadhesive materials: A review, Biomaterials 17 (1996) 1553–1561.
107. W. Hu, Z. Wang, Y. Xiao, S. Zhang, J. Wang, Advances in crosslinking strategies of biomedical hydrogels, Biomater. Sci 7 (2019) 843–855.
108. K.T. Nguyen, J.L. West, Photopolymerizable hydrogels for tissue engineering applications, Biomaterials 23 (2002) 4307–4314.
109. S. Wu, S. Peng, C.H. Wang, Multifunctional polymer nanocomposites reinforced by aligned carbon nanomaterials, Polymers, 10(5) (2018) 542.
110. F. Yokoyama, I. Masada, K. Shimamura, T. Ikawa, K. Monobe, Morphology and structure of highly elastic poly (vinyl alcohol) hydrogel prepared by repeated freezing-and-melting, Colloid Polym Sci 264 (1986) 595–601.
111. W.E. Hennink, C.F. van Nostrum, Novel crosslinking methods to design hydrogels, Adv Drug Deliv Rev 64 (2012) 223–236.
112. H.J. Koo, Y.S. Song, H.J. Kim, Y.H. Lee, S.M. Hong, S.J. Kim, B.C. Kim, C.J. Lim, E.H. Park, Antiinflammatory effects of genipin, an active principle of gardenia, Eur J Pharmacol, 495 (2004) 201.
113. M.C. Yang, S.S. Wang, N.K. Chou, N.H. Chi, Y.Y. Huang, Y.L. Chang, M.J. Shieh, T.W. Chung, The cardiomyogenic differentiation of rat mesenchymal stem cells on silk fibroin-polysaccharide cardiac patches in vitro, Biomaterials, 30 (2009) 3757.
114. J. Chen, Y. Zhan, Y. Wang, D. Han, B. Tao, Z. Luo, S. Ma, Q. Wang, X. Li, L. Fan, C. Li, H. Deng, F. Cao, Chitosan/silk fibroin modified nanofibrous patches with mesenchymal stem cells prevent heart remodeling post-myocardial infarction in rats, Acta Biomater, 80 (2018) 154.
115. M. Rahimi, H. Mohseni-Kouchesfehani, A.H. Zarnani, S. Mobini, S. Nikoo, S. Kazemnejad, Evaluation of menstrual blood stem cells seeded in biocompatible Bombyx mori silk fibroin scaffold for cardiac tissue engineering, J Biomater Appl, 29 (2014) 199.
116. M. Rahimi, A.H. Zarnani, S. Mobini, S. Khorasani, M. Darzi, S. Kazemnejad, Comparative effectiveness of three-dimensional scaffold, differentiation media and co-culture with native cardiomyocytes to trigger in vitro cardiogenic differentiation of menstrual blood and bone marrow stem cells Biologicals, 54 (2018) 13.
117. C. Patra, S. Talukdar, T. Novoyatleva, S.R. Velagala, C. Muhlfeld, B. Kundu, S.C. Kundu, F.B. Engel, Silk protein fibroin from Antheraea mylitta for cardiac tissue engineering, Biomaterials, 33 (2012) 2673.

118. E. Morrison, S. Suvarnapathaki, L. Blake, G. Camci-Unal, Unconventional biomaterials for cardiovascular tissue engineering, Curr Opin Biomed Eng, 17 (2021) 100263.
119. S. Vasu, J. Zhou, J. Chen, P.V. Johnston, D.H. Kim, Biomaterials-based approaches for cardiac regeneration, Korean Circ J, 51 (2021) 943–960.
120. Y. Li, L. Wei, L. Lan, Y. Gao, Q. Zhang, H. Dawit, J. Mao, L. Guo, L. Shen, L. Wang, Conductive biomaterials for cardiac repair, Acta Biomater, 139 (2022) 157–178.
121. A. Ghofrani, L. Taghavi, B. Khalilivavdareh, A. Rohani Shirvan, A. Nouri, Additive manufacturing and advanced functionalities of cardiac patches: A review, Eur Polym J, 174 (2022) 111332.
122. T. Chang, C. Liu, K. Lu, Y. Wu, M. Xu, Q. Yu, Z. Shen, T. Jiang, Y. Zhang, Biomaterials based cardiac patches for the treatment of myocardial infarction, J Mater Sci Technol, 94 (2021) 77–89.
123. K. Huang, E.W. Ozpinar, T. Su, J. Tang, D. Shen, L. Qiao, S. Hu, Z. Li, H. Liang, K. Mathews, et al., An off-the-shelf artificial cardiac patch improves cardiac repair after myocardial infarction in rats and pigs, Sci Transl Med, 12 (2020) eaat9683.
124. M. Shah, P. Kc, G. Zhang, In vivo assessment of decellularized porcine myocardial slice as an acellular cardiac patch, ACS Appl Mater Interfaces, 11 (2019) 23893–23900.
125. Y. He, H. Hou, S. Wang, R. Lin, L. Wang, L. Yu, X. Qiu, From waste of marine culture to natural patch in cardiac tissue engineering, Bioact Mater, 6 (2021) 2000–2010.
126. M. Kapnisi, C. Mansfield, C. Marijon, A.G. Guex, F. Perbellini, I. Bardi, E.J. Humphrey, J.L. Puetzer, D. Mawad, D.C. Koutsogeorgis, et al., Auxetic cardiac patches with tunable mechanical and conductive properties toward treating myocardial infarction, Adv Funct Mater, 28 (2018) 1800618.
127. S. Kazemi Asl, M. Rahimzadegan, R. Ostadrahimi The recent advancement in the chitosan hybrid-based scaffolds for cardiac regeneration after myocardial infarction, Carbohydr Polym, 300 (2023) 120266.
128. K. Hosoyama, M. Ahumada, C.D. McTiernan, D.R. Davis, F. Variola, M. Ruel, W. Liang, E.J. Suuronen, E.I. Alarcon, Nanoengineered Electroconductive Collagen-Based Cardiac Patch for Infarcted Myocardium Repair ACS Appl Mater Interfaces, 10 (2018) 44668–44677.
129. H.S. O'Neill, J. O'Sullivan, N. Porteous, E. Ruiz-Hernandez, H.M. Kelly, F.J. O'Brien, G.P. Duffy, A collagen cardiac patch incorporating alginate microparticles permits the controlled release of hepatocyte growth factor and insulin-like growth factor-1 to enhance cardiac stem cell migration and proliferation, J Tissue Eng Regen Med, 12 (2018) e384–e394.
130. H. Cui, C. Liu, T. Esworthy, Y. Huang, Z.-x Yu, X. Zhou, H. San, S.-j Lee, S.Y. Hann, M. Boehm, et al., 4D physiologically adaptable cardiac patch: A 4-month in vivo study for the treatment of myocardial infarction, Sci Adv, 6 (2020) eabb5067.
131. W.L. Chen, C.D. Kan, In Proceedings of the 40th Annual International Conference of the IEEE Engineering in Medicine and Biology Society (EMBC), Honolulu, HI, USA, 18–21 July 2018; pp. 5338–5341.
132. P. Pushp, R. Bhaskar, S. Kelkar, N. Sharma, D. Pathak, M.K. Gupta, Plasticized poly (vinylalcohol) and poly (vinylpyrrolidone) based patches with tunable mechanical properties for cardiac tissue engineering applications, Biotechnol Bioeng, 118 (2021) 2312–2325.
133. Z. Qian, D. Sharma, W. Jia, D. Radke, T. Kamp, F. Zhao, Engineering stem cell cardiac patch with microvascular features representative of native myocardium, Theranostics, 9 (2019) 2143–2157.
134. J. Karvinen, M. Kellomäki, Characterization of self-healing hydrogels for biomedical applications, Eur Polym J, 181 (2022) 111641.
135. N.C. Sanoh, G.M. Salazar, D.P. Penaloza, Magnetic biopolymeric hydrogel composite material with self-healing attribute, Biointerface Res Appl Chem, 11 (2021) 14881–14888.

136. N. Weerawan, J. Chalitangkoon, P. Monvisade, Self-healing hydrogels based on sodium carboxymethyl cellulose/poly (vinyl alcohol) reinforced with montmorillonite, Biointerface Res Appl Chem, 12 (2022) 4770–4779.
137. P. Contessotto, D. Orbanić, M. Da Costa, C. Jin, P. Owens, S. Chantepie, C. Chinello, J. Newell, F. Magni, D. Papy-Garcia, et al., Elastin-like recombinamers-based hydrogel modulates post-ischemic remodeling in a non-transmural myocardial infarction in sheep, Sci Transl Med, 13 (2021) eaaz5380.
138. R. Bai, L. Tian, Y. Li, J. Zhang, Y. Wei, Z. Jin, Z. Liu, H. Liu, Combining ECM hydrogels of cardiac bioactivity with stem cells of high cardiomyogenic potential for myocardial repair, Stem Cells Int, 2019 (2019) 6708435.
139. R. Dong, X. Zhao, B. Guo, P.X. Ma, Self-healing conductive injectable hydrogels with antibacterial activity as cell delivery carrier for cardiac cell therapy, ACS Appl Mater Interfaces, 8 (2016) 17138–17150.
140. A. Navaei, D. Truong, J. Heffernan, J. Cutts, D. Brafman, R.W. Sirianni, B. Vernon, M. Nikkhah, PNIPAAm-based biohybrid injectable hydrogel for cardiac tissue engineering, Acta Biomater, 32 (2016) 10–23.
141. E.S.H. Cheow, W.C. Cheng, C.N. Lee, D. De Kleijn, V. Sorokin, S.K. Sze, Plasma-derived extracellular vesicles contain predictive biomarkers and potential therapeutic targets for myocardial ischemic (MI) injury, Mol Cell Proteom, 15 (2016) 2628–2640.
142. K. Lv, Q. Li, L. Zhang, Y. Wang, Z. Zhong, J. Zhao, X. Lin, J. Wang, K. Zhu, C. Xiao, et al., Incorporation of small extracellular vesicles in sodium alginate hydrogel as a novel therapeutic strategy for myocardial infarction, Theranostics, 9 (2019) 7403–7416.
143. C. Han, J. Zhou, C. Liang, B. Liu, X. Pan, Y. Zhang, Y. Wang, B. Yan, W. Xie, F. Liu, et al., Human umbilical cord mesenchymal stem cell derived exosomes encapsulated in functional peptide hydrogels promote cardiac repair, Biomater Sci, 7 (2019) 2920–2933.
144. C.W. Chen, L.L. Wang, S. Zaman, J. Gordon, M.F. Arisi, C.M. Venkataraman, J.J. Chung, G. Hung, A.C. Gaffey, L.A. Spruce, et al., Sustained release of endothelial progenitor cell-derived extracellular vesicles from shear-thinning hydrogels improves angiogenesis and promotes function after myocardial infarction, Cardiovasc Res, 114 (2018) 1029–1040.
145. B. Liu, B.W. Lee, K. Nakanishi, A. Villasante, R. Williamson, J. Metz, J. Kim, M. Kanai, L. Bi, K. Brown, et al., Cardiac recovery via extended cell-free delivery of extracellular vesicles secreted by cardiomyocytes derived from induced pluripotent stem cells, Nat Biomed Eng, 2 (2018) 293–303.
146. D. Kalhori, N. Zakeri, M. Zafar-Jafarzadeh, L. Moroni, M. Solati-Hashjin, Cardiovascular 3D bioprinting: A review on cardiac tissue development, Bioprinting, 28 (2022) e00221.
147. Y. Liang, A. Mitriashkin, T.T. Lim, J.C.-H. Goh, Conductive polypyrrole-encapsulated silk fibroin fibers for cardiac tissue engineering, Biomaterials, 276 (2021) 121008.
148. X.-P. Li, K.-Y. Qu, F. Zhang, H.-N. Jiang, N. Zhang, C. Nihad, C.-M. Liu, K.-H. Wu, X.-W. Wang, N.-P. Huang, High-aspect-ratio water-dispersed gold nanowires incorporated within gelatin methacrylate hydrogels for constructing cardiac tissues in vitro, J Mater Chem B, 8 (2020) 7213–7224.
149. S. Saravanan, N. Sareen, E. Abu-El-Rub, H. Ashour, G.L. Sequiera, H.I. Ammar, V. Gopinath, A.A. Shamaa, S.E. Sayed, M. Moudgil, et al., Graphene oxide-gold nanosheets containing chitosan scaffold improves ventricular contractility and function after implantation into infarcted heart, Sci Rep, 8 (2018) 15069.

4 Electroconductive Biomaterials for Cardiac Tissue Engineering

U.S.K. Madduma-Bandarage, H.G. Jayasinghe, and S.V. Madihally

4.1 INTRODUCTION

The heart and blood vessels (arteries, veins, and capillaries) are collectively called the cardiovascular system. The cardiovascular system ensures sufficient blood flow throughout the body and is regulated by many stimuli, such as hormones, changes in blood volume, and drugs [1, 2].

Cardiovascular diseases (CVDs) are the leading cause of death globally. CVD is a general term for conditions that include disorders of the heart and blood vessels. Types of CVDs are coronary heart disease, cerebrovascular disease, peripheral arterial disease, rheumatic heart disease, congenital heart disease, deep vein thrombosis, and pulmonary embolism. Coronary heart diseases include angina, heart attacks, and heart failure. Strokes and transient ischemic attacks are examples of cerebrovascular diseases. More common CVD deaths are due to heart attacks and strokes [2].

It is a great challenge to regain the original condition of the heart once the cardiac cells get damaged due to cardiovascular disease. This chapter briefly discusses different strategies currently practiced and proposed to treat damaged heart tissues and emphasizes electroconductive biomaterials as an alternative therapeutic approach.

4.1.1 Myocardial Infarction (MI)

Myocardial infarction (MI) is the most common cause of heart failure. The heart wall comprises three layers: endocardium, myocardium, and epicardium. The middle layer of the heart wall is the myocardium. The myocardium consists of cardiac muscle cells known as cardiomyocytes – striated, branched cells containing many mitochondria. These cells are under involuntary control. Cardiomyocytes contain branched fibers connecting via intercalated discs with gap junctions and desmosomes. These interconnections allow the cells to contract together. Gap junctions permit the electrical coupling between adjacent cells – propagation of coordinated action potentials between adjacent cells [3]. Myocardium has a direct current conductivity of 0.1 S/m and Young's modulus of 10–20 kPa at the start of the diastole and 200–500 kPa at the end of the diastole [4]. Figure 4.1 shows the anatomy of the human heart and the MI-affected heart.

The swirling pattern of the cardiac muscle is responsible for the effective blood pumping of the heart. The interruption or complete stop of blood flow to a part of the myocardium can lead to an MI, which is commonly known as a "heart attack." In

DOI: 10.1201/9781003670995-4

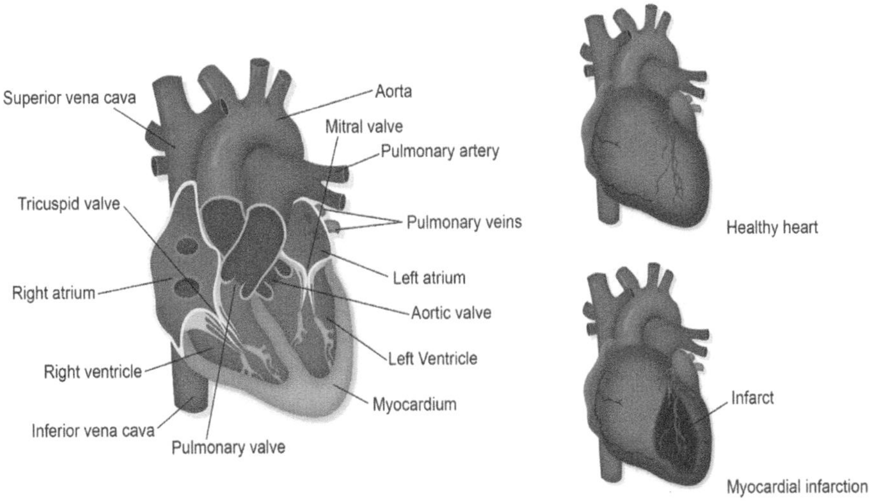

FIGURE 4.1 Anatomy of the human heart (left), healthy heart (top right), and a heart after a myocardial infarction (bottom right).

some cases, an MI passes away undetectably; however, in some cases, this condition can lead to sudden death [5–7]. The interruption of blood flow to the myocardium is typically caused by coronary artery occlusion.

After an MI, patients develop a high risk for heart failure in the future. Therefore, screening and prevention are essential for those patients to avoid heart failure in the future [7]. Clinical factors that may lead to heart failure after an MI are age, gender, number and location of infarct-related artery, history of previous MI, arterial hypertension, higher heart rate (increase by 10 b.p.m.), atrial fibrillation, diabetes, and chronic kidney disease. Biomarkers can detect the condition of the heart after an MI. For example, cardiac troponins can be used to determine infarct size, as these proteins are released when the heart muscle is damaged. Furthermore, natriuretic peptides give information on cardiac dysfunction [7].

4.1.2 Therapeutic Approaches for the Treatment of MI

MI can damage a large number of cardiac muscle cells. For example, a single MI can destroy 2–4 billion cardiomyocytes in the left ventricle (LV) [8]. The function of the LV is to force oxygenated blood through the aortic valve (Figure 4.1) and force the distribution in the entire body. Left ventricle ejection fraction (LVEF) measures the heart's mechanical contraction loss. The percentage ratio between the fraction of chamber volume ejected in systole, *stroke volume*, to blood volume at the end of diastole, *end-diastolic volume*, is known as LVEF, where stroke volume is the difference between end-diastolic volume and end-systolic volume [9].

$$\text{LVEF} = \frac{\text{Stroke volume}}{\text{End-diastolic volume}} \times 100\%$$

An LVEF between 50% and 70% is considered normal, and less than 30% is a severe dysfunction [9].

Since cardiomyocytes have an extremely low renewal rate, the adult human heart has a limited regenerative capacity. After MI, the myocardium undergoes the healing process through a series of events before developing the fibrotic scar tissue. These changes include initiating inflammation, transitioning to anti-inflammation before the tissue repair, and ending with scar formation [10]. However, the low regenerative capability of cardiomyocytes makes it difficult for the heart to regain its normal function promptly, which may even lead to the expansion of the damaged tissue [11].

The drugs currently used to treat an MI-damaged heart come in three classes: angiotensin-converting enzyme inhibitors/angiotensin II receptor blockers, aldosterone antagonists, and β-adrenergic blockers. These drugs relieve the hemodynamic burden by reducing the stress on the myocardium, and neurohormonal pathways balance the reduced myocardial functions. Two other approaches used in MI treatment are the implantation of an internal cardioverter-defibrillator and cardiac resynchronization therapy. These therapies do not reconstruct the damaged tissues and might even lead to the slowdown of the remodeling process of the myocardium. If the above therapeutic strategies fail, the next approach is the implantation of a mechanical left ventricular assist device (LVAD), and ultimately heart transplant based on severity of injury [11].

Regenerative medicine has been a novel, promising approach to treat MI-damaged hearts. In this approach, the focus is to regain the functions by repairing the heart; therefore, it would eliminate the majority of side effects or complications of current treatment techniques. Typically, stem cells, progenitor cells, or terminally differentiated cells are introduced to the damaged site of the myocardium by a bolus injection. Cells to be injected are harvested from various sources and expanded in vitro before being introduced to the targeted site. Newly introduced cells are selected based on their proliferation capacity, differentiation capacity, availability, and abundance [12]. Clinical trials have shown modest improvement in cardiac function for cell-based therapies. However, cell-based therapies have several drawbacks, such as attrition of cells (only 10–15% of cells remain) and no control over the cell fate and organization of the remaining cells [12, 13]. Hence, there is a concern about tumor formation by direct injection of stem cells [14].

Tissue engineering is another regenerative medicine-based approach that can potentially treat damaged heart tissues. Functional tissue is grown in vitro and implanted on the targeted site in this approach. Cardiac microtissues, engineered 3D cardiac tissue in the micrometer range, have a precise cellular organization and architecture with modulated electromechanical cues. These can produce synchronized unidirectional contractions and eliminate disruption of tissue homeostasis and emergence linked to some CVDs. Therefore, tissue engineering techniques are more advantageous than cell-based ones as they can modulate cellular and tissue-level structure and function [11]. Also, this method has shown that it could reduce infarct size and lead to angiogenesis and the formation of new blood vessels [15]. However, introducing the new tissue has to be done via invasive surgical procedures. Determining the implant's size, geometry, or location is challenging. Another challenge is to find scaffolding materials with the optimal degradation rate. Too fast degradation will lead to poor cell interaction with other cells and the extracellular matrix, and slow degradation will lead to a foreign body reaction and fibrotic encapsulation [11].

Scaffold-free cardiac tissue engineering is another approach that eliminates the use of scaffolding materials, and it has advantages of both cell-based methods and tissue engineering techniques. Here, the microtissues can be engineered in a range of self-assembled cell spheroid aggregates to complex organoid structures composed of different cell types, such as cardiomyocytes and cardiac fibroblasts; this technique can precisely control the microtissue's cell organization, architecture, and geometry [11]. However, this technology is still developing, and more studies need to be conducted to evaluate its full potential to use as a method to treat infarcts.

As mentioned, scaffolding biomaterial is vital in scaffold-based cardiac tissue engineering. Even though regenerative medicine is rapidly evolving, this study area faces many challenges. Some significant issues are loss or low survival rate of implant cells, poor engraftment of the engineered tissue with the host myocardium, and weak electrochemical coupling of engineered tissue with the native tissue [11]. However, engineered biomaterials can improve cell retention, survival, and proper engraftment. The common scaffolding materials used for cardiac tissue engineering are polymers, hydrogels, electrospun fibers, and composite biomaterials [11]. Since the myocardium has the characteristic feature of electrical conductivity, introducing non-conductive biomaterials may inhibit the electrical signal transmission and block the contracting synchronization of cardiomyocytes [16]. Therefore, an electroconductive biomaterial is more suitable to facilitate electrical signal transmission across the non-conductive fibrotic tissue and better suited for the scaffold-based tissue engineering techniques used to regenerate injured myocardium.

Exogenous materials are used in some scaffold-free tissue engineering techniques as well. Cell aggregation, a key feature in scaffold-free techniques, needs ultra-low adhesion surfaces. Therefore, cell culture plates coated with agarose or hydrogels with low adhesion of cells, such as methylcellulose hydrogel, induce cell aggregation. Some techniques in scaffold-free cardiac tissue engineering use electrically conductive nanomaterials, such as graphene and graphene oxide flakes, silicon nanoparticles and nanowires, polymeric nanofibers, and iron-based magnetic nanoparticles to promote differentiation and cell fate of stem cells in vitro conditions [11].

Overall, conductive biomaterials have shown promising results in regulating cell maturation and functionalizing cardiomyocytes, and they can induce differentiation and determine the cell fate of stem cells or progenitor cells. Moreover, conductive biomaterials are studied as conductive patches to promote in vivo myocardial repair [17].

4.2 CONDUCTIVE BIOMATERIALS FOR TISSUE ENGINEERING

Conductive biomaterials are materials that interact with biological systems and can conduct electricity. These materials have potential tissue engineering applications on cardiac, neural, bone, and muscle tissue. Also, conductive biomaterials may exhibit antibacterial properties, on-demand drug release, and biosensing [18,19].

Scaffolds should have an analogous function to the extracellular matrix. Therefore, the architecture of the scaffold should facilitate vascularization, new tissue formation, and host tissue integration. The scaffold should facilitate efficient nutrient and metabolite transport while maintaining mechanical stability while degrading at a rate that allows sufficient time for the implanted tissue to produce a new matrix and integrate with the native tissue. Tissue compatibility and active engagement of cellular components of the engineered tissues to facilitate and regulate their activities are also essential features of a scaffold [20]. Scaffolds should match tissue properties such as stiffness and biosignals as they determine cellular activities such as adhesion, proliferation, differentiation, and growth. As cell-scaffold interactions govern cellular fate, the scaffold's topography, 3D geometry, and chemical composition are essential in achieving the desired cell type in a tissue. Also, some external factors can influence cell-scaffold interactions. These include physical, biochemical, mechanical, and electrical stimulations [18].

In 1964, Bassett et al. showed that the formation of bone in adult dogs could be induced by applying low-intense direct electrical currents [21]. This finding led to more investigations and showed a significant influence of electrical stimulations on cellular activities and growth. The migration of cells guided by an applied electric field is called electrotaxis or galvanotaxis, and it has been widely tested for multiple types of cells [22]. In many in vitro experiments, cells show directional migration as a response to an external electric field. In response to electrical stimulation, cells can migrate into deeper scaffold regions and improve their differentiation [23]. It is evident that electrical stimulations influence cell migrations and affect stem cells' regenerative potential. However, the biophysical mechanism behind this phenomenon is still unclear [22].

4.2.1 Electroconductive Biomaterials for MI Treatment

4.2.1.1 Polymers

Small molecules called "monomers" can covalently bond to form large molecules with higher molecular weight, usually 10^3 to 10^6 g/mol, called polymers. In most cases, polymer molecules are long chains. Crosslinking polymer chains with each other results in more complex three-dimensional structures. The most exciting feature of polymers is that we can tweak their properties by modifications. For example, surface modifications, making crosslinks, changing the number of crosslinks, and making composites change the properties of polymers. Polymers can be natural or synthetic. Some examples of natural polymers are silk, latex, protein, starch, cellulose, and DNA. Polyvinyl chloride, polystyrene, polyester, nylon, polyethylene, Teflon, and epoxy are synthetic polymers, to name a few. Polymers can be reinforced by adding composite materials.

Natural, synthetic, or combinations of both have garnered special interest in tissue engineering applications due to their vast range of physical and chemical properties. Biological applications, especially tissue engineering, require designed polymeric materials to be biocompatible. Since biocompatibility is not an intrinsic material property, the fabricated polymer should match the properties of the native tissue. Also, knowing the cytotoxicity of the material and the toxicity of the breakdown products is essential [24]. Moreover, polymers must be purified thoroughly before the actual biological application to avoid leaching any starting materials, including unreacted monomers, which may be harmful to cells.

The next level of polymers includes network polymers. Interconnections between polymer chains, known as crosslinks, lead to the formation of network polymers. The crosslinks can be physical or chemical. These network structures are designed to hold large quantities of solvents, and the solvent-absorbed polymers are called gels. The polymers with large water retention capacity are known as hydrogels. Hydrogels mimic the extracellular matrix and can be adjusted to fit the physical and chemical properties of the native tissue. Therefore, hydrogels are ideal scaffolding materials for tissue engineering applications. With hydrogels, tissue engineering can be conducted in vitro or in vivo. Polymer gels can be designed to be injected as low viscous liquids, which can gelate inside the body [24]. Generally, a scaffolding material used in tissue engineering applications should have mechanical, chemical, and biological properties compatible with the native tissue for its optimum functionality. Thus, a polymer gel should integrate with the host cardiac tissue without causing complications for successful applications in cardiac tissue engineering. Both natural and synthetic polymers have been extensively studied to design scaffolds for cardiac tissue engineering, as each type has pros and cons. Some naturally degradable polymers investigated in cardiac tissue engineering are chitosan, fibrin gel, collagen, alginate, gelatin, and Matrigel [25]. However, blending these polymers with other materials may be necessary because these polymers alone may not comprise all the properties required for cardiac tissue growth [25, 26].

4.2.1.2 Electroconductive Polymers

Polymers that can conduct electricity are electroconductive polymers. These materials can be fabricated as smart materials with controllable electrical properties. Synthesis, properties, and application of electroconductive polymers have been discussed elsewhere [27–30].

Electroconductive polymers can be synthesized by chemical or electrochemical synthesis methods [31]. Chemical synthesis methods include oxidative polymerization, addition polymerization, condensation polymerization, etc [27, 31, 32]. Examples of electrochemical synthesis methods include electrochemical spinning and electrodeposition [33, 34]. Generally, chemical methods require chemical initiators and oxidizing agents for the polymerization reaction [35, 36]. In contrast, electrochemical methods use electric current, and the synthesis takes place in an electrochemical cell containing monomers, solvents, and dopants. The polymerization reaction begins with the oxidation of monomers by the electric current. These oxidized species can further react with other monomers in the medium, forming polymer chains [28, 35]. Chemical polymerization methods yield bulk polymers as powders or thick films, whereas electrochemical methods produce thin films of electroconductive polymers [28, 37]. However, the chemical polymerization methods are advantageous because they can produce polymers starting from any monomer. Unlike chemical methods, electrochemical methods can polymerize only monomers that an applied potential can oxidize [28].

4.2.1.2.1 Electrical Conductivity in Polymers

A material can conduct electricity if it has electrons that can move freely. In electroconductive solids, electrons move within and between energy levels known as bands. Each band has a specific energy and can hold a finite number of electrons. A band can be empty, partially filled, or full. A material can conduct electricity only if it has partially filled bands. For instance, metals are conductors because they have partially filled bands. The highest band or energy level that holds electrons is known as the valence band. The empty band immediately above the valence band is the conduction band. In a semiconductor, the valence band and conduction band are separated by a small energy gap, whereas in an insulator, the energy gap between the two bands is large. The early explanations of the conductivity of polymers used the band theory. According to the band theory, polymers have full valence bands and empty conduction bands separated by a considerable energy gap and, therefore, are non-conductive [38]. Nevertheless, the band theory could not explain the low conductivity of polymers in their pristine state [39]. The low electrical conductivity of polymers arises from their chemical structures. A characteristic feature of electroconductive polymers is the conjugated backbone that mainly contributes to their electrical conductivity (Figure 4.2). The conjugated backbone contains alternative

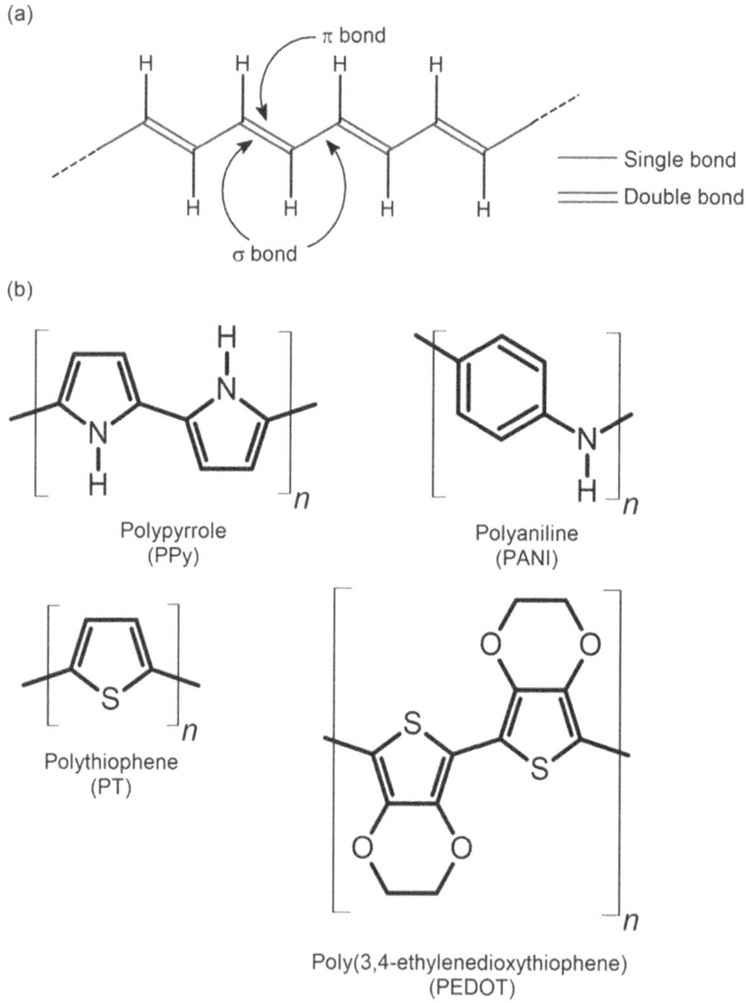

FIGURE 4.2 (A) Conjugated backbone of an electroconductive polymer and (B) chemical structures of common electroconductive polymers studied in cardiac tissue engineering.

single bonds and double bonds. The strong σ bonds in both single and double bonds tightly hold the atoms in the polymer backbone to provide mechanical strength, whereas the π bonds in the double bond facilitate the movement of electrons [27, 29, 31]. The p orbitals in the π bond overlap continuously allowing the electrons to move along the carbon backbone [39]. However, the conjugated backbone alone cannot make the polymer highly conductive. A process known as doping is used to change the electronic structure of a pristine polymer to enhance its electroconductivity.

4.2.1.2.2 Doping in Polymers

Doping in polymers is a process that introduces a molecule or ions known as a dopant. The dopant removes or contributes electrons from or to the polymer. Aromatic sulphonates such as polystyrene sulfonate (PSS), para-toluenesulphonate (pTS), and sodium benzene sulphonate (BS) are a group of widely used dopants [40, 41]. Other common dopants include hyaluronic acid (HA) chloride (Cl^-) ions, tetrafluoroborate (BF_4^-) ions, perchlorate (ClO_4^-) ions, and iodine, etc. [28, 42]. Doping can be either positive (p-doping) or negative (n-doping) based on the activity of the dopant. In p-doping, the dopant oxidizes the polymer by taking electrons from the polymer's valence band, so the polymer acquires a positive charge. In contrast, in n-doping, the dopant adds electrons to the conduction band of the polymer or reduces the polymer, thus making a negatively charged polymer [29, 38, 43].

4.2.1.2.3 Electroconductive Polymers for Cardiac Tissue Engineering

Electroconductive polymers studied for cardiac tissue engineering can be constructed in various forms: polymer blends or composites, polymer nanomaterials, electroconductive hydrogels, micro/nanopatterned polymeric substrates, and nanoparticle incorporated polymers (Figure 4.3). This section focuses on different forms of electroconductive polymers without nanoparticles. The following section, "nanomaterials," describes nanoparticles incorporated polymers.

Polypyrrole (PPy), polyaniline (PANI), and derivatives of polythiophene (PT) are among the extensively studied conductive polymers in the cardiac tissue engineering field due to their electrical properties compatible with the native myocardium [44–46].

PPy is a well-known electroconductive polymer with potential applications in cardiac tissue engineering. Previous studies conducted using different cell types such as endothelial cells [47, 48] and human keratinocytes [49] show that PPy has excellent biocompatibility, tunable surface properties [50], and stimuli-responsive properties [48]. Also, potential neural engineering applications of PPy have been widely explored [51–53]. Evidence from these studies inspires investigations on using PPy in cardiac tissue engineering. A paper published by Nishizawa et al. reports the formation of PPy-coated polyimide (PI) microelectrodes. The study further demonstrates the stimulation of chick embryonic cardiac myocytes without significant damage [33]. PPy was also used to develop interpenetrating networks in the polycaprolactone (PCL) matrix, which supported the formation of functional cardiac cell sheets from HL-1 atrial myocytes (mouse) [54]. Since the synthesis conditions, including current density, reactant concentrations, and dopant, significantly affect the properties of the resultant polymer, Puckert et al. conducted a study to optimize conditions for producing a PPy substrate suitable for mouse cardiac progenitor cells (CPCs) [34].

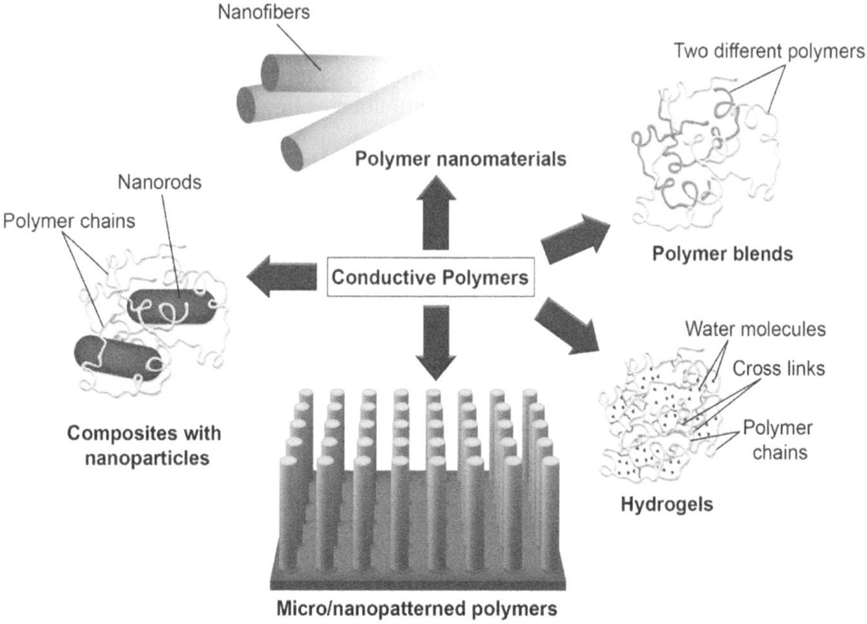

FIGURE 4.3 Common types of electroconductive polymer constructs studied for cardiac tissue engineering applications.

The study reveals that PPy films produced using dodecylbenzenesulfonate (DBS) dopant exhibited high biocompatibility and cell viability for CPCs. Adjary et al. prepared 3D-printed cardiac patches from nanocellulose, PPy, and PGS-based ink [55]. The electroconductivity of patches was 34 (±2.7) mS/cm when the PPy volume percentage was 5%. The data shows that the patch is compatible with H2c9 cardiac myoblasts and increases the proliferation.

PANI is another extensively studied electroconductive polymer due to its tunable electrical conductivity, low cost, convenient synthesis, and environmental stability [56]. Nevertheless, PANI has limited use in tissue engineering applications due to its drawbacks: low processability, low biodegradability, inflexibility, causing chronic inflammation, and releasing byproducts toxic to cells [57–59]. A few studies report potential applications of PANI in cardiac tissue applications. For example, a study reveals that substrates made from different forms of PANI support the adhesion and proliferation of H9c2 cardiac myoblasts [60]. Also, researchers pay significant attention to improving the properties of PANI by blending it with other polymers and developing nanomaterials of PANI.

Electroconductive polymer blends have been prepared by mixing PANI with other polymers. For instance, Borriello et al. published a study on incorporating electroconductive camphorsulfonic acid (CSA) and PANI with PCL to produce a conductive biodegradable polymer [61]. Here, the polymer contains CSA doped-PANI nanoneedles integrated into PCL substrates. The study showed the differentiation of human mesenchymal stem cells cultured on the fabricated substrates into cardiomyocyte-like cells [61]. Qazi et al. blended PANI with CSA and PGS to produce composite cardiac patches. Although they studied the cytocompatibility of the composite using skeletal muscle cells, they haven't shown the use of the fabricated material in cardiac tissue engineering-related applications [62].

PT and its derivatives are another group of electroconductive polymers. The derivatives of PT includes polyterthiophene (P3T), poly(3-methythiophene) (P3MT), poly(3,4-ethylenedioxythiophene) (PEDOT), and poly(3,4-proplenedioxy thiophene) (ProDOT). PEDOT is the most studied polymer in the PT family. The properties, such as solubility, of PEDOT can be improved by doping with PSS. Although poly(3,4-ethylene dioxythiophene:polystyrene sulfonate (PEDOT:PSS) has applications in bioelectronic devices [63, 64], investigations including PEDOT:PSS as a polymer in cardiac tissue engineering are limited. A few studies report the incorporation of PEDOT:PSS with other polymers as micro or nanostructures in cardiac tissue engineering applications [65, 66].

An essential aspect of tissue engineering is to mimic the macro- and micro-architecture of natural tissue. Thus, some studies report fabricating materials with architectural features similar to the natural heart. Patterning the substrate surface with nano topographical features such as grooves and pillars is an excellent strategy to mimic the myocardium extracellular matrix [67]. Tsui et al. conducted a study to fabricate a conductive acid-modified silk-PPy composite scaffold containing nanoscale grooves and ridges [68]. The anisotropic nanopattern and electroconductive cues present on silk-PPy scaffolds synergistically increased the cellular organization of human pluripotent stem cells-derived cardiomyocytes (hPSC-CMs), sarcomere development, an expression of CX43. Another study reports a conductive elastomer based on poly(glycerol sebacate) (PGS) and aniline trimer (AT) [69]. Here, the elastomer is a network polymer crosslinked with hexamethylene diisocyanate (HDI) and contains microscale grooves and ridges. The data shows improved proliferation of H2c9 rat cardiac myoblasts and micropattern-guided alignment of sarcomeric α-actinin of cardio myoblasts.

4.2.1.2.4 Electroconductive Hydrogels for Cardiac Tissue Engineering

As mentioned before, hydrogels are crosslinked polymers that retain a large quantity of water. Hydrogels can mimic natural tissue environments; thus, they are considered a good fit for tissue engineering applications. Hydrogels are widely studied in tissue engineering applications such as promoting differentiation of chondrocytes from hMSCs [70], neural tissue engineering [71], scaffolds in bone regeneration [72], adipose tissue engineering [73], and therapeutic repair of muscle injuries [74, 75]. A detailed review of the synthesis, trends, and applications of hydrogels is mentioned elsewhere [76]. Electroconductive hydrogels can be prepared using electroconductive polymers or by incorporating nanomaterials into non-conductive hydrogels. Electroconductive hydrogels have become promising in cardiac tissue engineering regardless of the preparation method.

A hydrogel made of collagen and alginate is usually not electroconductive but compatible with biological systems due to the presence of natural polymers. Roshanbinfar et al. modified a collagen/alginate hydrogel with PEDOT:PSS to introduce electroconductivity [66]. The biohybrid, electroconductive hydrogel they prepared facilitated the proliferation, survival, and unidirectional alignment of rat cardiomyocytes.

Evaluation of the behavior of human induced pluripotent stem cell-derived cardiomyocytes (hiPSC-CMs) indicates maturation of these cells, increased contraction speed and amplitude, and synchronous rhythmic beating [66]. Cui et al. produced injectable hydrogels from copolymers of carboxy tetraaniline (CTA), poly(D- or L-lactide) (PDLA or PLLA), and poly(ethylene glycol) (PEG), and they demonstrated that the hydrogel accelerated the proliferation of encapsulated rat cardiomyocytes [77]. Another study reported the synthesis of self-healing conductive hydrogels based on chitosan grafted with aniline tetramer (CS-AT) and dibenzaldehyde-terminated poly(ethylene glycol) (PEG-DA) [78]. The study demonstrates the use of the hydrogel as a delivery vehicle to deliver H9c2 cardiac myoblasts as evidence for potential applications in cardiac tissue engineering. Also, the subcutaneous injection of the hydrogel to rats shows its injectability and biodegradability. Wu et al. published a combined therapy for MI to improve cardiac functions using two conductive hydrogels: an injectable hydrogel and a self-adhesive conductive hydrogel [79]. The injectable hydrogel was made from oxidized sodium hyaluronic acid (HA-CHO) and hydrazided hyaluronic acid (HHA). The self-adhesive hydrogel contains a mixture of gelatin-dopamine (GelDa) and dopamine-modified polypyrrole (DA-PPy). The combined therapy starts with injecting the HA-CHO/HHA hydrogel into the MI site and then painting Gel-Da/DA-PPy hydrogel on the surface of the heart.

Electroconductive hydrogels can also be prepared by incorporating conductive nanoparticles such as gold nanoparticles [80, 81] and carbon nanotubes [82, 83] into non-conductive hydrogels [84]. Most studies investigate the application of these materials as platforms to evaluate cardiac functions of seeded cells in vitro, whereas some studies assess the performance of these hydrogels in vivo [85–87].

4.2.1.3 Nanomaterials

Substances with a size range from 1 to 100 nm (nanoscale) are generally considered nanomaterials. Nanomaterials may have a thickness in the nanoscale, but the length can range into more than 1 μm. Nanomaterials have become attractive because reducing a material's size to the nanoscale dramatically alters its properties, such as solubility, reactivity, spectroscopic, electrical, magnetic properties, and membrane diffusion [88]. Nanomaterials are fabricated using two techniques: by reducing a large material to nanosized particles – *top-down approach*, or by integrating individual atoms or molecules to assemble nanoscale particles – *bottom-up approach*) (Figure 4.4) [89]. The top-down methods use lithography, laser ablation, mechanical milling, and electro-explosion techniques. The bottom-up methods use supercritical fluid synthesis, spinning, sol-gel, chemical reduction, molecular condensation, chemical vapor deposition, and laser pyrolysis [90]. Other than the chemical and physical methods, biological synthesis methods such as plant extract-based reduction, bacterial synthesis, and fungal or algae-mediated processes are used for nanomaterial synthesis [91]. Those materials are considered nanoparticles if all external dimensions are in the nanoscale [92]. Nanomaterials are synthesized in different aspect ratios, the ratio of length (longest axis) to width (shortest axis) (Figure 4.5). Nanomaterials with an aspect ratio of one are called nanospheres. Nanorods have an aspect ratio greater than one, usually between 3 and 5. When the aspect ratio is much higher, they are usually called nanowires. Nanofibers are fiber-like structures with a

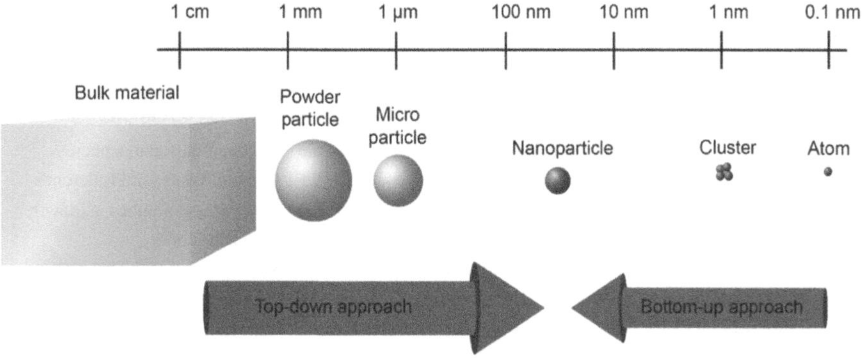

FIGURE 4.4 Top-down and bottom-up approaches in nanomaterial synthesis.

nanoscale diameter. These have a large surface area, high porosity, small pore size, and low density [93].

Nanomaterials can be classified based on the scale of their dimensions: Zero-dimensional (0-D) – have all three dimensions in the nanoscale; one-dimensional (1-D) – has two dimensions in the nanoscale and one extends beyond the nanoscale; two-dimensional (2-D) – have two dimensions outside nanoscale; three-dimensional (3-D) – all dimensions are not confined to the nanoscale, also called as bulk nanomaterials (see Table 4.1 for more details) [92]. Nanomaterials are generally categorized into inorganic-based, carbon-based, organic-based, and composite-based nanomaterials based on their composition [94]. The inorganic-based nanomaterials are based on metals or metal oxides, for example, metals such as gold, silver, aluminum, copper, zinc, iron, and cadmium; and metal oxides such as copper oxide, zinc oxide, titanium dioxide (TiO_2), iron oxide (Fe_2O_3 and Fe_3O_4). Also, metalloids and their oxides, such as silicon and silica (SiO_2) nanoparticles, are categorized into inorganic-based nanomaterials (Figure 4.6). Carbon-based nanomaterials comprise graphene,

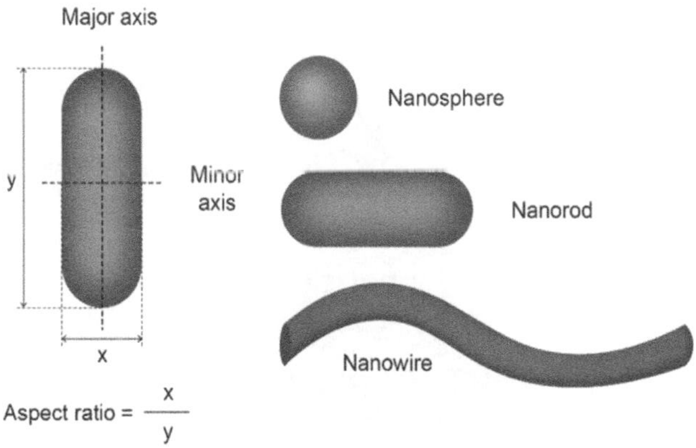

FIGURE 4.5 Major and minor axis of a nanorod (left) and different shapes of nanomaterials (right).

TABLE 4.1
Classification of Nanomaterials Based on Their Dimensions

Classification	Description	Examples
Zero-dimensional (0-D)	All dimensions are confined to nanoscale (1–100 nm)	Nanoparticles, nanospheres, quantum dots, and fullerenes
One-dimensional (1-D)	Two dimensions are in the nanoscale, and one extends beyond the nanoscale.	Nanorods, nanotubes, nanowires, and nanofibers
Two-dimensional (2-D)	One dimension is in the nanoscale, and the others extend beyond the nanoscale.	Nanofilms, nanosheets, and nanolayers
Three-dimensional (3-D)	All dimensions are not confined to the nanoscale.	Nanoparticle dispersions, nanowire arrays, and nanotube arrays

fullerene, single and multi-walled carbon nanotubes, carbon fiber, activated carbon, and carbon black [94]. Organic-based nanomaterials are made of organic materials, such as carbohydrates, proteins, lipids, and polymers [95]. Composite-based nanomaterials are a combination of any of the other three kinds [94].

4.2.1.4 Nanomaterials in Tissue Engineering

The nanoscale features of biological systems can interact with nanoscale materials, which opens many avenues to explore nanotechnology in regenerative medicine. Nanotechnology has developed desirable materials with controlled chemical,

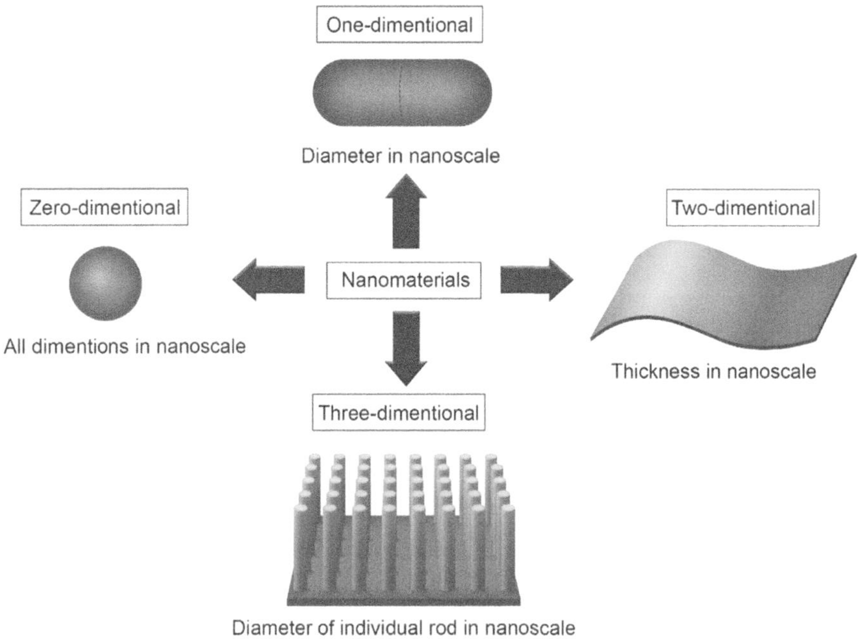

FIGURE 4.6 Classification of nanomaterials based on their dimensions.

biological, structural, and mechanical microenvironments to deliver cells successfully and more robust tissue regeneration. Fabrication of biomaterials with nanostructured surfaces may help to mimic the native micro and nano environment of the native tissue of the targeted site, which may lead to better cell adhesion, growth, proliferation, and differentiation [96]. Nanoparticles are also used in tissue engineering to improve the mechanical and biological performances of the scaffold. It has been shown that the cell proliferation rate increases with the introduction of specific nanoparticles. For example, introducing gold nanoparticles and TiO_2 nanoparticles has enhanced the cell proliferation rates of bone and cardiac tissues [97]. The mechanical properties of scaffolds can be tweaked by introducing nanoparticles. For example, a biodegradable patch (refer to Section 4.2.1.2.2 for more details of cardiac patches) made of nanocomposite polymers embedded with TiO_2 showed a higher tensile strength in reinforcing the infraction site. Compared to micro-sized particles, nanomaterials show enhanced dielectric and electrical properties [98]. Therefore, the electrical properties of scaffolds can be enhanced by introducing nanomaterials [99].

4.2.1.5 Applications of Electroconductive Bionanomaterials for Cardiac Tissue Engineering

As discussed in the early sections, after MI, reduced function of the myocardium due to loss of cardiomyocytes has to be managed using therapeutic approaches to maintain the proper function of the heart. The electrical pulse signaling, interrupted by the infraction, has to be restored, at least to some extent. This can be achieved by introducing electrical conductivity into biomaterials used in MI treatments, and it is a more practical approach. The bionanomaterials have become suitable candidates for this approach and have successfully incorporated into scaffolds that are used to seed with cardiomyocytes, such as cardiac patches, hydrogels, polymers, fibrous networks, polymer networks, Films, and 3D printed constructs. These nanomaterials can support the heart's biochemical, electrical, and mechanical needs and promote cardiomyocyte regeneration.

In MI treatment, it is crucial to establish quick and efficient electrical coupling between adjacent cells. This can be achieved using cardiac patches. Cardiac patches are a combination of seed cells and scaffold materials. Usually, cell communication and interactions improve by applying electrical stimulation. These patches provide temporary support to the infarcted site, and in the long term, they help restore the damaged tissue by delivering cells or bioactive factors [100]. Decellularized matrices, made by removing cellular tissue components with a combination of physical stress and chemical/enzymatic agents, are used as electrical patches in treatments of MI-damaged hearts [101, 102].

Gold nanorods can be synthesized in different shapes, for example, nanospheres, nanorods, nanocages, and nanocubes. Low cytotoxicity, biocompatibility, ideal electrical conductivity, nanotopography, innate optical properties, and easy modification of surfaces make them excellent candidates for tissue engineering [59]. Cardiac patches made by depositing gold nanoparticles on decellularized omental matrices showed improved morphology, greater striation, and organized electrical coupling proteins in cardiomyocytes [102]. In another study, cardiac patches were made by incorporating gold nanotubes/nanowires into biodegradable castor oil-based polyurethane and later seeded with cardiomyocytes. These nanocomposite scaffolds showed a significant increase in cell confluency. Moreover, after the electrical stimulation, the incorporation of the gold nanotubes/nanowires up-regulated the gene expression for some genes in cardiomyocytes [103]. Also, in a study, a scaffold made with gelatin methacrylate hydrogels incorporated with gold nanorods showed enhanced electrical and mechanical properties. The cardiomyocytes seeded onto this scaffold showed excellent cell retention, viability, and metabolic activity [104].

Carbon nanotubes have good mechanical and electrical properties, making them candidates for cardiac tissue engineering. By integrating carbon nanotubes into scaffolding materials, the tensile strength and Young's modulus can be increased. Carbon nanotubes can be synthesized using physical or chemical methods such as electric-arc techniques, laser ablation, and chemical vapor deposition [59]. When highly aligned poly(ethylene glycol)-poly(D, L-lactide) polymer fibers were loaded with carbon nanotubes, with enhanced conductivity, they showed higher cell viability, cell elongation, secretion of extracellular matrix, and beating rates for in vitro grown cardiomyocytes [105]. Also, several studies have shown the promoted differentiation of stem cells in the presence of carbon nanotubes [59].

Carbon nanofibers are also good candidates for tissue engineering applications of MI treatment. Carbon nanofibers are hollow cylinders with lengths in the range of microns and have suitable physical, mechanical, and electric conductive properties. The methods used to fabricate carbon nanofibers are catalytic thermal vapor deposition or electrospinning [59]. Studies have shown that carbon nanofibers can increase the conductivity and cytocompatibility of polymer scaffolds. For example, a study that incorporated carbon nanofibers into poly(lactic-co-glycolic acid) (PLGA) showed higher adhesion and proliferation of cardiomyocytes [106]. Another study showed that incorporating carbon nanofibers into PLGA can produce conductivities similar to the natural heart tissue [107].

Another carbon-based candidate for cardiac tissue engineering is graphene, an allotrope of carbon. Other than unique physical and electrical properties, graphene has a higher surface area, which can facilitate a high load of bioactive compounds [59]. Some studies show graphene can improve cardiogenic differentiation. For example, a hybrid scaffold of graphene and polyethylene glycol showed enhanced myofibrils, sarcomeric structure, and electrical coupling of cardiac cells [108].

Silicon nanomaterials show electroconductive properties in the presence of dopants in their lattice. It has been shown that a hybrid made of silicon nanowires with cardiac myofibroblasts can synchronize the cardiomyocytes' electrical activity with applied light pulses [109]. In an attempt to fabricate scaffold-free cardiac tissue engineering, Tan et al. showed that adding silicon nanowires created an electroconductive microenvironment that promotes enhanced cellular structures. This has been confirmed by the enhanced expression of sarcomeric α-actinin, Cx-43, and β-myosin heavy chains. Also, they have noticed a higher synchronization of spontaneous contraction and increased sarcomere alignment [110]. Silicon nanoparticles can be incorporated into polymers to enhance properties. For instance, Ezazi et al. blended silicon nanoparticles with PPy and poly(glycerol sebacate) (PGS) to produce biodegradable cardiac patches for MI treatments [111].

Polymer-based nanomaterials are another extensively studied group of materials for potential cardiac tissue engineering applications. A scaffold made of electrospun nanofibers of PPy/poly(ε-caprolactone)/gelatin composites promoted attachment and proliferation of primary rabbit cardiomyocytes and expression of cardiac-specific markers [45]. From the different concentrations of PPy used in the study, nanofibers made with 15% PPy exhibited conductivity, mechanical properties, biocompatibility, and biodegradability compatible with cardiac tissue. Also, electrospun PLGA nanofibers modified with chlorine-doped PPy were biocompatible with CPCs [112]. The properties of nanofibers made out of PANI, a synthetic polymer, can be improved by adding natural components. For example, a study done by Li et al. demonstrates the fabrication of scaffolds from PANI-gelatin electrospun nanofibers. The nanofibrous scaffolds supported the attachment, migration, and proliferation of H9c2 rat cardiac cells regardless of the composition of PANI and gelatin in the blend [113]. In another study, Fernandes et al. modified PANI nanofibers with hyperbranched poly-L-lysine dendrimers (HPLys), an adhesive peptide. The scaffold had biocompatible properties and supported the proliferation of neonatal rat heart cells. Also, they observed the differentiation of these cardiac cells when stimulated by an electric current [114]. Also, PANI nanotubes modified with polyglycerol dendrimers (PGLDs) exhibited differentiation of cardiac cells under the application of microcurrents [115]. Another study reported the use of composite PANI and PLGA nanofibrous meshes in rat neonatal cardiomyocyte cultures. The cells grown on the scaffold exhibited synchronous beating with an electric stimulation [116].

A cryogel formed by incorporating PPy nanoparticles with gelatin methacrylate and poly(ethylene glycol) diacrylate using a dopamine crosslinker was found to enhance the functionalization of cardiomyocytes as evident by the increase in expression of CX-43 [117].

4.3 CHALLENGES OF USING ELECTROCONDUCTIVE BIOMATERIALS FOR CARDIAC TISSUE ENGINEERING

Cytocompatibility and optimal biodegradation are two main factors that need to be evaluated to determine the use of a conductive biomaterial in the cardiac tissue engineering process [30]. Myocardium is a contractile active tissue undergoing polarization and depolarization cycles. It has been shown that pore geometry has a vital role in cardiac cell maturation and assembly. Moreover, substrate stiffness and flexibility are also crucial in designing a suitable scaffold. After all, the conductivity of the biomaterial should match with the conductivity of the natural tissue [118].

Carbon nanomaterials can provide an environment like the biological extracellular matrix due to their chemical composition and physical structure. Therefore, these materials are potential candidates for building scaffolds. Enhanced conductivity makes them better candidates for cardiac tissue engineering. However, the cytotoxicity of carbon nanotubes is a major drawback. Inflammation, T lymphocyte apoptosis, and rupture of cell membranes are some side effects of multi-walled carbon nanotubes. Most cytotoxic effects of carbon nanotubes are due to the aggregation of the nanotubes [119]. Surface modification is a strategy that can be used to overcome this hurdle [59, 120]. Biocompatibility of graphene can be improved by using methods such as oxidation, reduction, size control, and functionalization [59]. Graphene oxide is a highly oxidized species of graphene. Reducing graphene oxide can be used to enhance biocompatibility while maintaining good conductivity. Reduced graphene oxide can increase the hydrophobicity of scaffolds as well [59].

Silicon nanoparticles may induce endothelial dysfunction and facilitate the release of proinflammatory procoagulant factors. Silver and gold nanoparticles can migrate into the cell and reduce the cell viability. Therefore, the biocompatibility of nanoparticles needs to be thoroughly investigated to use them in tissue engineering applications [119]. However, it is shown that gold nanoparticles have better biocompatibility compared to most nanomaterials used in biological applications [30].

Although electroconductive polymers seem promising for cardiac tissue engineering, developing materials with properties that mimic the native heart is challenging. Therefore, applications of electroconductive polymers in real-life applications are limited. As mentioned previously, common issues with electroconductive polymers include mismatch of mechanical properties, degradability, and difficulty of handling. The scaffolding material should stay intact with the newly introduced tissue until it integrates with the native tissue. However, when the integration is completed, the scaffolding material should degrade successfully without producing toxic byproducts. Most proposed polymer materials do not confirm the successful degradation in vivo. Degradability may be achieved by combining degradable polymers/materials with conducting polymers. However, cleaning the degraded electroconductive byproducts through standard metabolic pathways would be difficult. Although synthesizing polymer blends improves the properties to a certain extent, their clinical applications are limited due to toxicity, incompatibility with the host tissue, and solubility [44, 121]. Also, fabricating electroconductive polymers to resemble the 3D microenvironment of the native cardiac tissue is necessary to achieve a better transition toward clinical applications.

ABBREVIATIONS

BS	benzene sulphonate
CSA	camphorsulphonic acid
CVD	cardiovascular disease
DBS	dodecylbenzenesulfonate
HA	hyaluronic acid
MI	myocardial infarction
PANI	polyaniline
PCL	polycaprolactone
PGLA	poly(lactic-co-glycolic acid)
PGS	poly(glycerol sebacate)
PPy	polypyrrole
PSS	polystyrene sulfonate
pTS	para-toluenesulphonate

REFERENCES

1. Chaudhry, R., J.H. Miao, and A. Rehman, Physiology, Cardiovascular. 2023, StatPearls Publishing: Treasure Island (FL).
2. Olvera Lopez, E., B. Ballard, and A. Jan, Cardiovascular Disease. 2023, StatPearls Publishing: Treasure Island (FL).
3. Ripa, R. et al., Physiology, Cardiac Muscle. 2023, StatPearls Publishing: Treasure Island (FL).
4. Huyer, L.D. et al., Biomaterial based cardiac tissue engineering and its applications. Biomedical Materials, 2015. 10(3): p. 034004.
5. Tran, D.B., C. Weber, and R.A. Lopez, Anatomy, Thorax, Heart Muscles. 2023, StatPearls Publishing: Treasure Island (FL).
6. Ojha, N., and A.S. Dhamoon, Myocardial Infarction. 2023, StatPearls Publishing: Treasure Island (FL).
7. Jenča, D. et al., Heart failure after myocardial infarction: Incidence and predictors. ESC Heart Failure, 2021. 8(1): p. 222–237.
8. Murry, C.E., H. Reinecke, and L.M. Pabon, Regeneration gaps: Observations on stem cells and cardiac repair. Journal of the American College of Cardiology, 2006. 47(9): p. 1777–1785.
9. Kosaraju, A. et al., Left Ventricular Ejection Fraction. 2023. StatPearls Publishing: Treasure Island (FL).
10. Chalise, U., M. Becirovic-Agic, and M.L. Lindsey, The cardiac wound healing response to myocardial infarction. WIREs mechanisms of disease, 2023. 15(1): p. e1584.
11. Patino-Guerrero, A. et al., Three-dimensional scaffold-free microtissues engineered for cardiac repair. Journal of Materials Chemistry B, 2020. 8(34): p. 7571–7590.
12. Segers, V.F., and R.T. Lee, Stem-cell therapy for cardiac disease. Nature, 2008. 451(7181): p. 937–942.
13. Pagano, F. et al., On the road to regeneration: "Tools" and "routes" towards efficient cardiac cell therapy for ischemic cardiomyopathy. Current Cardiology Reports, 2019. 21: p. 1–11.
14. Volarevic, V. et al., Ethical and safety issues of stem cell-based therapy. International Journal of Medical Sciences, 2018. 15(1): p. 36–45.
15. Zhang, J. et al., Can we engineer a human cardiac patch for therapy? Circulation Research, 2018. 123(2): p. 244–265.
16. Monteiro, L.M. et al., Restoring heart function and electrical integrity: Closing the circuit. NPJ Regenerative Medicine, 2017. 2(1): p. 9.
17. Li, Y. et al., Conductive biomaterials for cardiac repair: A review. Acta Biomaterialia, 2022. 139: p. 157–178.
18. Saberi, A. et al., Electrically conductive materials: Opportunities and challenges in tissue engineering. Biomolecules, 2019. 9(9):p. 448.
19. Gamboa, J. et al., Recent progress in biomedical sensors based on conducting polymer hydrogels. ACS Applied Bio Materials, 2023. 6(5): p. 1720–1741.
20. Chan, B.P., and K.W. Leong, Scaffolding in tissue engineering: General approaches and tissue-specific considerations. European Spine Journal, 2008. 17(Suppl 4): p. 467–479.
21. Bassett, C.A.L., R.J. Pawluk, and R.O. Becker, Effects of electric currents on bone in vivo. Nature, 1964. 204(4959): p. 652–654.
22. Tai, G., M. Tai, and M. Zhao, Electrically stimulated cell migration and its contribution to wound healing. Burns Trauma, 2018. 6: p. 20.
23. Hardy, J.G. et al., Electrical stimulation of human mesenchymal stem cells on biomineralized conducting polymers enhances their differentiation towards osteogenic outcomes. Journal of Materials Chemistry B, 2015. 3(41): p. 8059–8064.
24. Kohane, D.S., and R. Langer, Polymeric biomaterials in tissue engineering. Pediatric Research, 2008. 63(5): p. 487–491.

25. Dhandayuthapani, B., et al., Polymeric scaffolds in tissue engineering application: A review. International Journal of Polymer Science, 2011(1): p. 290602.
26. Tormos, C.J., and S.V. Madihally, Chapter 5 - Chitosan for cardiac tissue engineering and regeneration, in Chitosan Based Biomaterials Volume 2, J.A. Jennings and J.D. Bumgardner, Editors. 2017, Woodhead Publishing. p. 115–143.
27. K. N., and C.S. Rout, Conducting polymers: A comprehensive review on recent advances in synthesis, properties and applications. RSC Advances, 2021. 11(10): p. 5659–5697.
28. Guimard, N.K., N. Gomez, and C.E. Schmidt, Conducting polymers in biomedical engineering. Progress in Polymer Science, 2007. 32(8): p. 876–921.
29. Ghasemi-Mobarakeh, L. et al., Application of conductive polymers, scaffolds and electrical stimulation for nerve tissue engineering. Journal of Tissue Engineering and Regenerative Medicine, 2011. 5(4): p. e17–e35.
30. Esmaeili, H. et al., Electroconductive biomaterials for cardiac tissue engineering. Acta Biomaterialia, 2022. 139: p. 118–140.
31. Balint, R., N.J. Cassidy, and S.H. Cartmell, Conductive polymers: Towards a smart biomaterial for tissue engineering. Acta Biomaterialia, 2014. 10(6): p. 2341–2353.
32. Calvo, P.A. et al., Chemical oxidative polymerization of pyrrole in the presence of m-hydroxybenzoic acid- and m-hydroxycinnamic acid-related compounds. Synthetic Metals, 2002. 126(1): p. 111–116.
33. Nishizawa, M. et al., Electrodeposition of anchored polypyrrole film on microelectrodes and stimulation of cultured cardiac myocytes. Biomaterials, 2007. 28(8): p. 1480–1485.
34. Puckert, C. et al., Optimisation of conductive polymer biomaterials for cardiac progenitor cells. RSC Advances, 2016. 6(67): p. 62270–62277.
35. Tan, Y., and K. Ghandi, Kinetics and mechanism of pyrrole chemical polymerization. Synthetic Metals, 2013. 175: p. 183–191.
36. Armes, S.P., Optimum reaction conditions for the polymerization of pyrrole by iron(III) chloride in aqueous solution. Synthetic Metals, 1987. 20(3): p. 365–371.
37. Martins, N.C.T. et al., Electrodeposition and characterization of polypyrrole films on aluminium alloy 6061-T6. Electrochimica Acta, 2008. 53(14): p. 4754–4763.
38. Kaner, R.B., and A.G. MacDiarmid, Plastics that conduct electricity. Scientific American, 1988. 258(2): p. 106–111.
39. Le, T.-H., Y. Kim, and H. Yoon, Electrical and electrochemical properties of conducting polymers. Polymers, 2017. 9(4): p. 150.
40. Cui, X. et al., Surface modification of neural recording electrodes with conducting polymer/biomolecule blends. Journal of Biomedical Materials Research, 2001. 56(2): p. 261–72.
41. Wang, X. et al., Evaluation of biocompatibility of polypyrrole in vitro and in vivo. Journal of Biomedical Materials Research Part A, 2004. 68A(3): p. 411–422.
42. Finkenstadt, V.L., Natural polysaccharides as electroactive polymers. Applied Microbiology and Biotechnology, 2005. 67(6): p. 735–745.
43. Ravichandran, R. et al., Applications of conducting polymers and their issues in biomedical engineering. Journal of the Royal Society Interface, 2010. 7(suppl_5): p. S559–S579.
44. Wang, L. et al., Electrospun conductive nanofibrous scaffolds for engineering cardiac tissue and 3D bioactuators. Acta Biomaterialia, 2017. 59: p. 68–81.
45. Kai, D. et al., Polypyrrole-contained electrospun conductive nanofibrous membranes for cardiac tissue engineering. Journal of Biomedical Materials Research Part A, 2011. 99A(3): p. 376–385.
46. Ashtari, K. et al., Electrically conductive nanomaterials for cardiac tissue engineering. Advanced Drug Delivery Reviews, 2019. 144: p. 162–179.
47. Garner, B. et al., Human endothelial cell a. Journal of Materials Science: Materials in Medicine, 1999. 10(1): p. 19–27.

48. Garner, B. et al., Polypyrrole–heparin composites as stimulus-responsive substrates for endothelial cell growth. Journal of Biomedical Materials Research, 1999. 44(2): p. 121–129.
49. Culture of human keratinocytes on polypyrrole-based conducting polymers. Tissue Engineering, 2006. 12(4): p. 645–655.
50. Li, Y., K.G. Neoh, and E.-T. Kang, Plasma protein adsorption and thrombus formation on surface functionalized polypyrrole with and without electrical stimulation. Journal of Colloid and Interface Science, 2004. 275(2): p. 488–495.
51. Lee, J.Y., J.-W. Lee, and C.E. Schmidt, Neuroactive conducting scaffolds: Nerve growth factor conjugation on active ester-functionalized polypyrrole. Journal of the Royal Society Interface, 2009. 6(38): p. 801–810.
52. Gomez, N. et al., Micropatterned polypyrrole: A combination of electrical and topographical characteristics for the stimulation of cells. Advanced Functional Materials, 2007. 17(10): p. 1645–1653.
53. George, P.M. et al., Fabrication and biocompatibility of polypyrrole implants suitable for neural prosthetics. Biomaterials, 2005. 26(17): p. 3511–3519.
54. Spearman, B.S. et al., Conductive interpenetrating networks of polypyrrole and polycaprolactone encourage electrophysiological development of cardiac cells. Acta Biomaterialia, 2015. 28: p. 109–120.
55. Ajdary, R. et al., Multifunctional 3D-printed patches for long-term drug release therapies after myocardial infarction. Advanced Functional Materials, 2020. 30(34): p. 2003440.
56. Borah, R. et al., Surface functionalization-induced enhancement in surface properties and biocompatibility of polyaniline nanofibers. RSC Advances, 2015. 5(60): p. 48971–48982.
57. Huang, L. et al., Synthesis of biodegradable and electroactive multiblock polylactide and aniline pentamer copolymer for tissue engineering applications. Biomacromolecules, 2008. 9(3): p. 850–858.
58. Zhang, Q.-S. et al., Synthesis of a novel biodegradable and electroactive polyphosphazene for biomedical application. Biomedical Materials, 2009. 4(3): p. 035008.
59. Ashtari, K. et al., Electrically conductive nanomaterials for cardiac tissue engineering. Advanced Drug Delivery Reviews, 2019. 144: p. 162–179.
60. Bidez, P.R. 3rd et al., Polyaniline, an electroactive polymer, supports adhesion and proliferation of cardiac myoblasts. Journal of Biomaterials Science, Polymer Edition, 2006. 17(1–2): p. 199–212.
61. Borriello, A. et al., Optimizing PANi doped electroactive substrates as patches for the regeneration of cardiac muscle. Journal of Materials Science: Materials in Medicine, 2011. 22(4): p. 1053–1062.
62. Qazi, T.H. et al., Development and characterization of novel electrically conductive PANI–PGS composites for cardiac tissue engineering applications. Acta Biomaterialia, 2014. 10(6): p. 2434–2445.
63. Stříteský, S. et al., Printing inks of electroactive polymer PEDOT:PSS: The study of biocompatibility, stability, and electrical properties. Journal of Biomedical Materials Research Part A, 2018. 106(4): p. 1121–1128.
64. Hempel, F. et al., PEDOT:PSS organic electrochemical transistor arrays for extracellular electrophysiological sensing of cardiac cells. Biosensors and Bioelectronics, 2017. 93: p. 132–138.
65. Lei, Q., J. He, and D. Li, Electrohydrodynamic 3D printing of layer-specifically oriented, multiscale conductive scaffolds for cardiac tissue engineering. Nanoscale, 2019. 11(32): p. 15195–15205.
66. Roshanbinfar, K. et al., Electroconductive biohybrid hydrogel for enhanced maturation and beating properties of engineered cardiac tissues. Advanced Functional Materials, 2018. 28(42): p. 1803951.

67. Kim, D.H. et al., Nanoscale cues regulate the structure and function of macroscopic cardiac tissue constructs. Proceedings of the National Academy of Sciences of the United States of America, 2010. 107(2): p. 565–570.
68. Tsui, J.H. et al., Conductive silk-polypyrrole composite scaffolds with bioinspired nanotopographic cues for cardiac tissue engineering. Journal of Materials Chemistry B, 2018. 6(44): p. 7185–7196.
69. Hu, T. et al., Micropatterned, electroactive, and biodegradable poly(glycerol sebacate)-aniline trimer elastomer for cardiac tissue engineering. Chemical Engineering Journal, 2019. 366: p. 208–222.
70. Jayasinghe, H.G., and S.V. Madihally, Recent advances in promoting chondrogenesis of human mesenchymal stem cells using physically and chemically modified hydrogels. Nano LIFE, 2021. 11(02): p. 2130001.
71. Madhusudanan, P., G. Raju, and S. Shankarappa, Hydrogel systems and their role in neural tissue engineering. Journal of the Royal Society Interface, 2020. 17(162): p. 20190505.
72. Liu, J., et al., Hydrogel scaffolds in bone regeneration: Their promising roles in angiogenesis. Frontiers in Pharmacology, 2023. 14: p.1050954.
73. O'Halloran, N.A. et al., Hydrogels in adipose tissue engineering-potential application in post-mastectomy breast regeneration. Tissue Engineering and Regenerative Medicine, 2018. 12(12): p. 2234–2247.
74. Lev, R., and D. Seliktar, Hydrogel biomaterials and their therapeutic potential for muscle injuries and muscular dystrophies. Journal of the Royal Society Interface, 2018. 15(138): p. 20170380.
75. Volpi, M. et al., Hydrogel-based fiber biofabrication techniques for skeletal muscle tissue engineering. ACS Biomaterials Science & Engineering, 2022. 8(2): p. 379–405.
76. Madduma-Bandarage, U., and S.V. Madihally, Synthetic hydrogels: Synthesis, novel trends, and applications. Journal of Applied Polymer Science, 2021. 138(19): p. 50376.
77. Cui, H. et al., PLA-PEG-PLA and its electroactive tetraaniline copolymer as multi-interactive injectable hydrogels for tissue engineering. Biomacromolecules, 2013. 14(6): p. 1904–1912.
78. Dong, R. et al., Self-healing conductive injectable hydrogels with antibacterial activity as cell delivery carrier for cardiac cell therapy. ACS Applied Materials & Interfaces, 2016. 8(27): p. 17138–17150.
79. Wu, T. et al., Coadministration of an adhesive conductive hydrogel patch and an injectable hydrogel to treat myocardial infarction. ACS Applied Materials & Interfaces, 2020. 12(2): p. 2039–2048.
80. Baei, P. et al., Electrically conductive gold nanoparticle-chitosan thermosensitive hydrogels for cardiac tissue engineering. Materials Science and Engineering: C, 2016. 63: p. 131–141.
81. You, J.-O. et al., Nanoengineering the heart: Conductive scaffolds enhance connexin 43 expression. Nano Letters, 2011. 11(9): p. 3643–3648.
82. Shin, S.R. et al., Carbon-nanotube-embedded hydrogel sheets for engineering cardiac constructs and bioactuators. ACS Nano, 2013. 7(3): p. 2369–2380.
83. Yu, H. et al., Mechanically and electrically enhanced CNT-collagen hydrogels as potential scaffolds for engineered cardiac constructs. ACS Biomaterials Science & Engineering, 2017. 3(11): p. 3017–3021.
84. Lee, M., M.C. Kim, and J.Y. Lee, Nanomaterial-based electrically conductive hydrogels for cardiac tissue repair. International Journal of Nanomedicine, 2022. 17: p. 6181–6200.
85. Li, X. et al., A PNIPAAm-based thermosensitive hydrogel containing SWCNTs for stem cell transplantation in myocardial repair. Biomaterials, 2014. 35(22): p. 5679–5688.
86. Paul, A. et al., Injectable graphene oxide/hydrogel-based angiogenic gene delivery system for vasculogenesis and cardiac repair. ACS Nano, 2014. 8(8): p. 8050–8062.

87. Zhu, S. et al., Injectable conductive gelatin methacrylate/oxidized dextran hydrogel encapsulating umbilical cord mesenchymal stem cells for myocardial infarction treatment. Bioactive Materials, 2022. 13: p. 119–134.
88. Armarego, W.L.F., Chapter 5 - Nanomaterials, in Purification of Laboratory Chemicals (9th Edition), W.L.F. Armarego, Editor. 2022, Butterworth-Heinemann. p. 586–630.
89. Klinkova, A., and H. Thérien-Aubin, Chapter 3 - Inorganic nanoparticles, in Nanochemistry: Chemistry of Nanoparticle Formation and Interactions, A. Klinkova and H. Thérien-Aubin, Editors. 2024, Elsevier. p. 49–110.
90. Baig, N., I. Kammakakam, and W. Falath, Nanomaterials: A review of synthesis methods, properties, recent progress, and challenges. Materials Advances, 2021. 2(6): p. 1821–1871.
91. Dhumal, K., R. Dateer, and A. Mali, Recent catalytic advancements in organic transformations using biogenically synthesized palladium nanoparticles. Catalysis Letters, 2023. 154(2): pp. 329–351.
92. Joudeh, N., and D. Linke, Nanoparticle classification, physicochemical properties, characterization, and applications: A comprehensive review for biologists. Journal of Nanobiotechnology, 2022. 20(1): p. 262.
93. Nunes, C.S., and P. Philipps-Wiemann, Chapter 22 - Formulation of enzymes, in Enzymes in Human and Animal Nutrition, C.S. Nunes and V. Kumar, Editors. 2018, Academic Press. p. 429–440.
94. Majhi, K.C., and M. Yadav, Chapter 5 - Synthesis of inorganic nanomaterials using carbohydrates, in Green Sustainable Process for Chemical and Environmental Engineering and Science, Inamuddin, et al., Editors. 2021, Elsevier. p. 109–135.
95. Pan, K., and Q. Zhong, Organic nanoparticles in foods: Fabrication, characterization, and utilization. Annual Review of Food Science and Technology, 2016. 7: p. 245–266.
96. Mostafavi, E. et al., Electroconductive nanobiomaterials for tissue engineering and regenerative medicine. Bioelectricity, 2020. 2(2): p. 120–149.
97. Hasan, A. et al., Nanoparticles in tissue engineering: Applications, challenges and prospects. International Journal of Nanomedicine, 2018. 13: p. 5637–5655.
98. Gunasekaran, V., et al., Electrical and dielectric properties: Nanomaterials, in Handbook of Magnetic Hybrid Nanoalloys and Their Nanocomposites, S. Thomas and A. Rezazadeh Nochehdehi, Editors. 2022, Springer International Publishing: Cham. p. 783–800.
99. Jawad, H. et al., Assessment of cellular toxicity of TiO2 nanoparticles for cardiac tissue engineering applications. Nanotoxicology, 2011. 5(3): p. 372–380.
100. Zhang, Y. et al., Recent advances in cardiac patches: Materials, preparations, and properties. ACS Biomaterials Science & Engineering, 2022. 8(9): p. 3659–3675.
101. Kim, Y.S. et al., Applications of decellularized extracellular matrix in bone and cartilage tissue engineering. Bioengineering & Translational Medicine, 2019. 4(1): p. 83–95.
102. Shevach, M. et al., Gold nanoparticle-decellularized matrix hybrids for cardiac tissue engineering. Nano Letters, 2014. 14(10): p. 5792–5796.
103. Ganji, Y. et al., Cardiomyocyte behavior on biodegradable polyurethane/gold nanocomposite scaffolds under electrical stimulation. Materials Science and Engineering: C, 2016. 59: p. 10–18.
104. Navaei, A. et al., Gold nanorod-incorporated gelatin-based conductive hydrogels for engineering cardiac tissue constructs. Acta Biomaterialia, 2016. 41: p. 133–146.
105. Liu, Y. et al., Tuning the conductivity and inner structure of electrospun fibers to promote cardiomyocyte elongation and synchronous beating. Materials Science and Engineering: C, 2016. 69: p. 865–874.
106. Stout, D.A., B. Basu, and T.J. Webster, Poly (lactic-co-glycolic acid): Carbon nanofiber composites for myocardial tissue engineering applications. Acta Biomaterialia, 2011. 7(8): p. 3101–3112.

107. Asiri, A.M. et al., Greater cardiomyocyte density on aligned compared with random carbon nanofibers in polymer composites. International Journal of Nanomedicine, 2014. p. 5533–5539.
108. Smith, A.S. et al., Micro-and nano-patterned conductive graphene–PEG hybrid scaffolds for cardiac tissue engineering. Chemical Communications, 2017. 53(53): p. 7412–7415.
109. Rotenberg, M.Y. et al., Living myofibroblast–silicon composites for probing electrical coupling in cardiac systems. Proceedings of the National Academy of Sciences, 2019. 116(45): p. 22531–22539.
110. Tan, Y. et al., Silicon nanowire-induced maturation of cardiomyocytes derived from human induced pluripotent stem cells. Nano Letters, 2015. 15(5): p. 2765–2772.
111. Zanjanizadeh Ezazi, N. et al., Fabrication and characterization of drug-loaded conductive poly(glycerol sebacate)/nanoparticle-based composite patch for myocardial infarction applications. ACS Applied Materials & Interfaces, 2020. 12(6): p. 6899–6909.
112. Gelmi, A., et al., Electroactive 3D materials for cardiac tissue engineering. SPIE Smart Structures and Materials + Nondestructive Evaluation and Health Monitoring. Vol. 9430. 2015: SPIE.
113. Li, M. et al., Electrospinning polyaniline-contained gelatin nanofibers for tissue engineering applications. Biomaterials, 2006. 27(13): p. 2705–2715.
114. Fernandes, E.G.R., V. Zucolotto, and A. De Queiroz, Electrospinning of hyperbranched poly-l-lysine/polyaniline nanofibers for application in cardiac tissue engineering. Journal of Macromolecular Science, Part A, 2010. 47(12): p. 1203–1207.
115. Moura, R.M., and A.A. de Queiroz, Dendronized polyaniline nanotubes for cardiac tissue engineering. Artificial Organs, 2011. 35(5): p. 471–477.
116. Hsiao, C.-W. et al., Electrical coupling of isolated cardiomyocyte clusters grown on aligned conductive nanofibrous meshes for their synchronized beating. Biomaterials, 2013. 34(4): p. 1063–1072.
117. Wang, L. et al., Mussel-inspired conductive cryogel as cardiac tissue patch to repair myocardial infarction by migration of conductive nanoparticles. Advanced Functional Materials, 2016. 26(24): p. 4293–4305.
118. Solazzo, M. et al., The rationale and emergence of electroconductive biomaterial scaffolds in cardiac tissue engineering. APL Bioengineering, 2019. 3(4): 041501.
119. Pan, Q. et al., Nanoparticles: Promising tools for the treatment and prevention of myocardial infarction. International Journal of Nanomedicine, 2021. 16: p. 6719–6747.
120. Ku, S.H., M. Lee, and C.B. Park, Carbon-based nanomaterials for tissue engineering. Advanced Healthcare Materials, 2013. 2(2): p. 244–260.
121. Guo, B., and P.X. Ma, Conducting polymers for tissue engineering. Biomacromolecules, 2018. 19(6): p. 1764–1782.

5 Piezoelectric Fundamentals and Properties

Sujata Swain and P. Kumar

5.1 INTRODUCTION

The phenomenon of piezoelectricity of a material is defined as when a material is subjected to mechanical stress, an electrical field is produced. Also, the material experienced mechanical deformation when subjected to an electrical field [1]. This bidirectional behavior of piezoelectric material is used in different applications such as sensors, actuators, and energy harvesting technology. The term "piezoelectric" comes from the Greek word "piezin" which means the action of pressing or squeezing [2]. The piezoelectric effect was discovered by Pierre and Jacques Curie in 1880 [3]. It was observed that quartz and Rochelle salt could produce an electric charge when subjected to mechanical deformation.

During the Second World War, the first oxide polycrystalline ceramic (barium titanate) BaTiO3 was discovered. At first, it was used as a dielectric material for solid condensers. Roberts, in 1947 found that, when BT ceramic poled under a high voltage, it showed a piezoelectric value 100 times higher than quartz [4, 5]. Shirane et al. in 1952 studied the solid solution of $PbTiO_2$-$PbZrO_3$, and they reported that the piezoelectric constant was doubled as compared to BT, and the T_C (Curie temperature) was over 300°C [6]. Now the piezoelectric ceramic, i.e., the solid solution of $PbTiO_2$-$PbZrO_3$, abbreviated as PZT, although discovered after BT, dominated over market [7]. However, as BT is a lead-free piezoceramic, it is used as an environmentally friendly material.

5.2 ROLE OF FERROELECTRIC PROPERTIES IN PIEZOELECTRICITY

It is essential to study the contribution of ferroelectric properties in piezoelectricity as most of the piezoelectric materials are ferroelectric in nature. The ferroelectricity of a material can be defined as it possessing spontaneous polarization, which can be reversed back by the application of an external electric field.

As shown in Figure 5.1, ferroelectrics are the core subset of dielectrics. Dielectrics are characterized by electrical insulators that are polarized by an external electrical field when placed in between the parallel plate capacitor. Piezoelectrics are the subset of the big dielectric family, and the polarization is generated in a non-centro symmetry crystal as a result of the separation of positive and negative charges by the application of stress. Pyroelectrics are characterized by the ability to produce a voltage upon heating and cooling, as the magnitude of polarization changes thermally by the change in temperature. All ferroelectric materials exhibit pyroelectric properties,

DOI: 10.1201/9781003670995-5

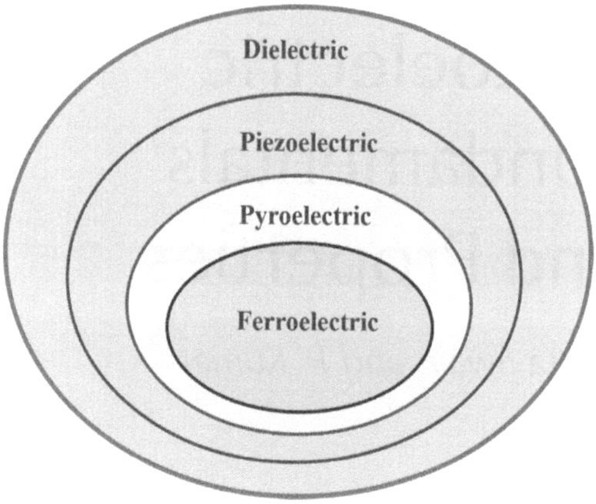

FIGURE 5.1 Venn diagram showing the relationship between dielectric, piezoelectric, pyroelectric, and ferroelectric materials.

and all pyroelectric materials exhibit piezoelectric properties. Nevertheless, not all piezoelectrics are pyroelectrics, and not all pyroelectrics are ferroelectrics.

5.2.1 Key Principles of Ferroelectricity

The spontaneous polarization exhibited by ferroelectric materials is characterized by the presence of asymmetrical configuration of electrical dipoles. These states represent various alignments of the dipoles within the crystal lattice. The capacity to transition between these states in response to an external electric field is the key characteristic that renders ferroelectric materials highly advantageous in diverse applications, including non-volatile memory systems. Ferroelectricity is commonly encountered in materials that possess a perovskite structure, characterized by the generic chemical formula ABX_3. Typically, in this arrangement, the A-site is filled by a bigger cation, the B-site by a smaller cation, and the X-site by an anion, usually oxygen. The spontaneous polarization found in ferroelectric materials is a result of the displacement of the B-site cation within the octahedral structure formed by the X-site anions.

Ferroelectric materials display a domain structure characterized by sections within the material that possess uniform polarization. The domains are divided by domain walls, which are the specific areas where the direction of polarization changes. Domain creation reduces depolarizing fields that would occur from a uniform polarization, therefore minimizing the overall energy of the material. Understanding the ferroelectric characteristics of the material relies heavily on understanding how these domains behave when subjected to an external electric field. Applying an electric field causes the domains that are aligned with the field to expand, while the misaligned domains decrease, resulting in a net increase in polarization. The process is reversible, indicating that the material can revert to its original condition or build a new domain structure with a distinct polarization pattern when the field is eliminated.

Ferroelectric materials exhibit hysteresis as a distinctive characteristic as shown in Figure 5.2. Upon the application and subsequent removal of an external electric field, the polarization does not instantaneously revert to zero. Instead, it traces a

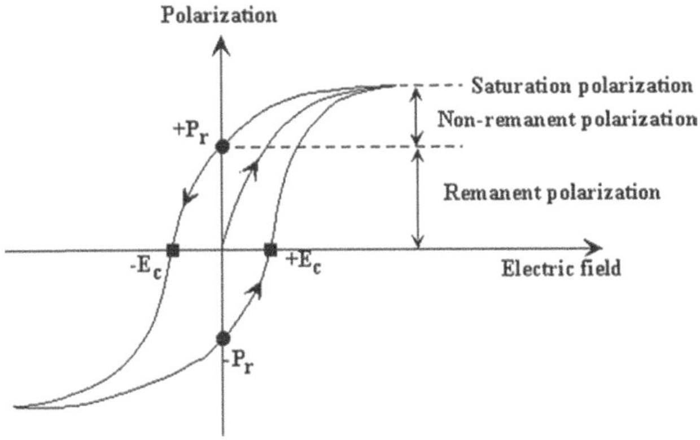

FIGURE 5.2 P~E hysteresis loop [8].

loop, referred to as the hysteresis loop. The presence of this loop is a characteristic feature of ferroelectric materials, and it gives information regarding their coercive field, E_c (the minimum field strength needed to change the direction of polarization) and remnant polarization, P_r (the polarization that remains even after the external field is eliminated).

The piezoelectric effect in ferroelectric materials improves as a result of their capacity to change polarization states when subjected to an external electric field. The switching process enables a more pronounced change in polarization when subjected to mechanical stress, resulting in a more robust piezoelectric response compared to non-ferroelectric piezoelectric materials.

Applying mechanical stress to a ferroelectric material can result in a reorientation of the dipoles, which in turn alters the polarization. The alteration in polarization leads to the production of an electric charge, which is the fundamental nature of the piezoelectric effect. The amplitude of this phenomenon in ferroelectric materials is generally greater than in non-ferroelectric piezoelectric materials because of the added contribution from domain switching.

5.3 FUNDAMENTAL PRINCIPLES OF PIEZOELECTRICITY

5.3.1 The Direct and Converse Piezoelectric Effect

Piezoelectric materials display distinctive relationships between mechanical stress and electrical charge. These relationships can be classified into two separate phenomena: direct piezoelectric and converse piezoelectric effects [9].

5.3.1.1 Direct Piezoelectric Effect

The generation of an electrical charge when the piezoelectric material is subjected to a mechanical force is called the direct piezoelectric effect. As shown in Figure 5.3, the arrangement of electrical charge present in the material gets separated upon the application of mechanical force. Therefore, a voltage is found across the material. The direct piezoelectric effect is applicable in various applications such as detecting sound, sensing acceleration, and measuring pressure by piezoelectric sensors.

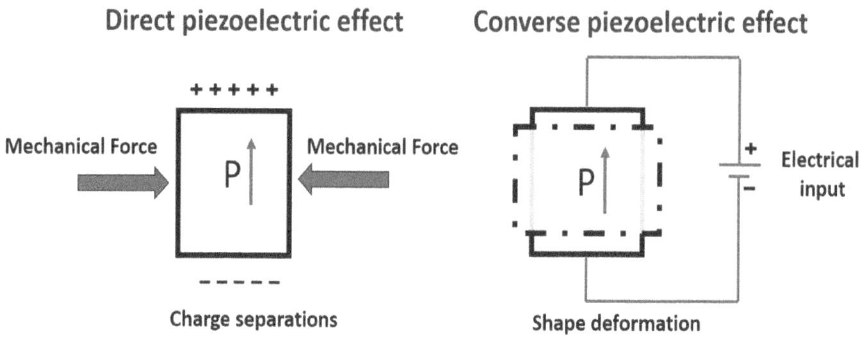

FIGURE 5.3 Mechanism of direct and converse piezoelectric effect.

5.3.1.2 Converse Piezoelectric Effect

Likewise, under the application of an electrical field, piezoelectric material experienced a mechanical strain or stress, which is termed the converse piezoelectric effect. Figure 5.3 shows a shape deformation experienced by the piezoelectric material when subjected to an electric field. The phenomenon of the converse piezoelectric effect is useful in various applications like optical devices, actuators, microelectromechanical systems (MEMs), precision positioning systems, etc.

Mathematically, direct and converse piezoelectric effects can be written as:

$$D = dT(\text{Direct})$$

$$S = dE(\text{Converse})$$

where d, D, T, E, and S represent piezoelectric charge coefficient, dielectric displacement, mechanical stress, electric field, mechanical strain, etc. [10].

5.3.2 Crystal Structure and Symmetry

The phenomenon of piezoelectricity possessed by the material is closely associated with their crystal lattice configuration and the non-centro symmetry structure. This asymmetry allows the material to polarize under mechanical stress.

5.3.2.1 Crystal Structure

The crystal structure is related to the orderly and repetitive arrangement of atoms and molecules within the piezoelectric material.

Unit cell: The smallest repeating unit of a crystal lattice is called the unit cell. In piezoelectric materials, the unit cell often has atoms positioned in such a way that they do not exhibit inversion symmetry.

Common crystal structures:

- Tetragonal: Exhibits piezoelectric properties when elongated along one axis.
- Hexagonal: Often found in materials like quartz.
- Orthorhombic: Exhibits different piezoelectric properties along different axes.

5.3.2.2 Symmetry

Symmetry in crystals refers to the invariance of the crystal structure under certain operations, such as rotations, reflections, or translations. For a material to exhibit piezoelectricity, it must lack certain symmetrical elements that would otherwise cancel out the polarization effects [11].

Crystal structures are classified into 32-point groups based on their symmetry elements. Out of these, 21 point groups lack a center of symmetry and 20 of these exhibit piezoelectricity. The absence of a center of symmetry is critical because it allows for the generation of a net dipole moment under stress.

Non-centro symmetry structures: These structures do not have a center of symmetry. When stress is applied, the asymmetry causes a redistribution of electric charges, resulting in a net polarization.

5.3.3 Piezoelectric Coefficients

Piezoelectric materials exhibit the unique property of generating electric charge in response to mechanical stress and, conversely, undergoing mechanical deformation when an electric field is applied. This behavior is quantified by piezoelectric coefficients, which are fundamental parameters in describing the efficiency and effectiveness of piezoelectric materials [12, 13].

Types of piezoelectric coefficient:

i. d-Coefficient (Direct piezoelectric effect): The d-coefficient (d_{ij}) quantifies the electric polarization generated per unit of mechanical stress applied where i stands for the direction of polarization generated in the material and j stands for the direction of applied stress. It is expressed in coulombs per newton (C/N) or meters per volt (m/V). For instance, d_{33} represents the polarization in the direction of the applied stress, which is called as longitudinal piezoelectric coefficient. d_{31} denotes the polarization in a perpendicular direction of the applied stress and is called a transverse piezoelectric coefficient [14]. d_{15} denotes shear piezoelectric co-efficient, describes that stress is applied along shear, and the response is observed in the plane of the material. Materials with high d-coefficients exhibit a high level of efficiency in transferring mechanical energy into electrical energy, which makes them well-suited for applications such as sensors and energy harvesting.

ii. g-Coefficient (Piezoelectric voltage coefficient): The g-coefficient (gij) is defined as the ratio between the electric field generated in response to mechanical stress. The unit of g is V.m/N (voltage. meter/Newton).

$$\mathrm{G} = \frac{\textit{Electrical field developed}}{\textit{Applied mechanical stress}}$$

Also, the g-constant can be derived from the piezoelectric charge coefficient (d) and the relative permittivity which can be stated as: $g = \frac{d}{\varepsilon}$ g-coefficient can be written as g_{33}, g_{31}, or g_{15} corresponding to d_{33}, d_{31}, or d_{15}, respectively depending on the directions.

iii. e-Coefficient (Strain coefficient): The e-coefficient (eij) is defined as the ratio between the mechanical strain generated to the applied electric field in a piezoelectric material, and the unit is meters per volt (m/V). Different applications like actuators and precision positioning systems signify the use of e-coefficients.
iv. h-Coefficient (Piezoelectric stress coefficient): The h-coefficient (hij) is defined as the ratio between the stress produced in a piezoelectric material to an electric field and the unit Pa.m^2/C. This coefficient is necessary to understand the ability of a piezoelectric material to generate mechanical stress when subjected to an electric field.
v. Tensor nature of piezoelectric coefficient: Piezoelectric materials possess anisotropic properties due to which these are expressed as tensors [15]. Therefore, the magnitude of this piezoelectric coefficient depends on the orientation of the applied stress and electric field in the crystallographic axes of the material.
vi. Material-specific coefficient: Also, piezoelectric coefficients can be determined by the structure, composition, and production of the material. For example, quartz possesses a low piezoelectric coefficient. However, due to its great thermal stability, it is used for applications requiring constant frequency control. PZT (Lead zirconate titanium) is used for transducers and actuators due to its high d-coefficient. PVDF (Polyvinylidene Fluoride) is a polymer having a lower d-coefficient than ceramics. However, it is used to manufacture thin films due to its flexible nature.

5.4 TYPES OF PIEZOELECTRIC MATERIAL

Piezoelectric materials are widely used in various applications like actuators, sensors, aerospace materials, medical devices, energy harvesting devices, etc. There are multiple no. of piezoelectric materials exist having distinct characteristics and uses each.

5.4.1 Natural Piezoelectric Material

Piezoelectric materials have the unique ability to generate an electric charge in response to applied mechanical stress. This phenomenon is known as the piezoelectric effect. Among the various types of piezoelectric materials, natural piezoelectric materials inherently possess this property without any need for artificial processing or manufacturing [16].

Key natural piezoelectric materials:

i. Quartz (SiO_2): Quartz is one of the most well-known natural piezoelectric materials. It is highly stable, has a high melting point, and exhibits excellent mechanical properties. Quartz is commonly used in applications such as oscillators, frequency control devices, and timekeeping instruments like watches.
ii. Rochelle salt (sodium potassium tartrate): Rochelle salt has a high piezoelectric coefficient, producing a significant electrical response to mechanical

stress. It was historically used in early microphones and phonograph pick-ups. However, it is sensitive to humidity and temperature changes, which limits its modern applications.

iii. Tourmaline: Tourmaline is a mineral that exhibits piezoelectric properties. It is used in pressure sensors and can withstand high temperatures. Tourmaline is also valued in geological and material science studies due to its complex crystal structure and varied compositions.

Natural piezoelectric materials, with their intrinsic properties, play a vital role in various scientific and industrial applications. Their stability, especially in the case of quartz, makes them invaluable for precise and reliable devices in electronics and instrumentation.

5.4.2 Ceramic Piezoelectric Materials

Ceramic piezoelectric materials are engineered substances that exhibit the piezoelectric effect, generating an electric charge in response to mechanical stress. These materials like PZT, BT, BZT-BCT, BNT, KNN, etc. are particularly valued for their high piezoelectric coefficients, mechanical strength, and versatility, making them suitable for various applications, including sensors, actuators, and medical devices [17].

Key characteristics:

- High piezoelectric coefficients: These materials have the ability to produce a substantial electric charge when subjected to mechanical stress.
- Thermal stability: Ceramic piezoelectrics exhibit excellent thermal stability, allowing them to function efficiently across a broad temperature spectrum [18].
- Mechanical strength: These materials are robust and can endure significant mechanical stress without deteriorating.
- Ease of fabrication: These materials may be easily produced in a wide range of forms and sizes to suit diverse applications.

Typical ceramic materials:

i. Lead zirconate titanate (PZT): PZT is considered the most widely used piezoelectric material. It has a high piezoelectric constant and possesses enhanced electrochemical coupling. PZT has a d_{33} value of ~360 pC/N. It retains its high piezoelectric properties at a high Curie temperature ~350°C [19]. PZT is used in several applications such as actuators, sensor devices, and ultra transducers [20]. However, PZT has a major drawback that it contains lead oxide, which is hazardous and toxic to the natural environment. Thus, recent research has been made to develop lead-free piezoelectric to substitute materials containing lead.

ii. Barium titanate ($BaTiO_3$): Lead-free piezoelectric BT is mainly used as a dielectric material due to its high capacitance. It possesses a high piezoelectric constant and dielectric constant [21, 22]. A piezoelectric constant of value ~190 pC/N was found for pure BT, synthesized by a conventional solid-state reaction route [22]. However, by controlling the grain size of sintered BT ceramics, an enhanced piezoelectric coefficient was found. d_{33} of value ~460 pC/N was found for BT ceramic with a grain size of 1–2 micrometer order [19]. Also, the piezoelectric coefficient of BT can be enhanced by substituting A and B sites with perovskite crystals. By substituting Zr and Ca, a binary compound was formed of $Ba(Zr_{0.2}Ti_{0.8}O_3)$-$(Ba_{0.7}Ca_{0.3})TiO_3$ (BZT-BCT) that exhibits a high d_{33} value of ~620 pC/N [22]. BT has a low Curie temperature of ~130°C [19]. Different applications like MLCC, actuators, and piezoelectric microphones use BT as the piezoelectric material [23].

iii. Lead-free ceramics: These ceramics are used to substitute lead-based material and are environment-friendly. Bismuth sodium titanate (BNT), potassium sodium niobate (KNN), lithium sodium potassium niobate (LKNN), zinc oxide (ZnO), etc. are examples of lead-free ceramics. BNT ($Bi_{0.5}Na_{0.5}TiO_3$) based lead-free ceramics have favorable piezoelectric properties and remanent polarization. However, the high coercive field and conductivity make BNT ceramics difficult to pole, and results allow a d_{33} value of ~ 73–95 pC/N [22]. KNN and LKNN are the two promising piezoelectric ceramics having d_{33} values of ~63 pC/N and ~98 pC/N, respectively [24]. The incorporation of lithium into KNN has significantly increased the piezoelectric properties. Both KNN and LKNN possess high Curie temperature and very good thermal stability, which makes them used for high-temperature applications.

5.4.3 Polymeric Piezoelectric Material

Piezoelectric polymer possesses piezoelectric properties along with the advantages of being lightweight, flexible, and easy to fabricate [25]. Due to its lightweight, it is applicable in portable and mobile applications. Polymers have the ability to bend and flex without undergoing breakage, which can be used for flexible sensors and wearable devices. Piezoelectric polymers have some structural requirements like:

i. permanent molecular dipoles are present.
ii. the ability to align the orientation of the molecular dipoles.
iii. the ability to sustain the alignment after it is achieved.
iv. when mechanically stressed, the ability to undergo large strains.

Common polymeric piezoelectric materials

- PVDF: Polyvinylidene fluoride (PVDF) and its co-polymer are widely used in the field of polymeric piezoelectric material [26]. Among all the piezoelectric polymers, PVDF exhibits a relatively high piezoelectric coefficient around ~ 20 pC/N [24]. Also, PVDF possesses high dielectric constant and breakdown strength. PVDF exhibits several phases, among which α and β phases are the two prominent phases. The α phase of PVDF polymer is the most stable phase and non-polar in structure, resulting in a zero net polarization. However, the β phase possesses a non-zero dipole moment and is polar in structure [25]. PVDF is used in tissue engineering applications due to its non-cytotoxic, biocompatible, and flexible nature. Due to the robust piezoelectric and pyroelectric properties of PVDF polymer, it is used in several applications like actuators, pressure sensors, and energy harvesting devices [27].

- PVDF-TrFE: Polyvinylidene fluoride-trifluoroethylene (PVDF-TrFE) is a co-polymer of PVDF. It exhibits enhanced piezoelectric properties as compared to PVDF. It has a d_{33} value of ~30 pC/N [24]. The incorporation of trifluoroethylene (TrFE) into PVDF polymer improves the stabilization of the β phase, which is essential for piezoelectric performances. This co-polymer possesses enhanced piezoelectric properties and crystallinity. It is extensively used in actuators, flexible electronic devices, and precision sensor applications.
- Polylactic acid (PLA): It has gained attention due to its biodegradable and biocompatible nature. It has lower piezoelectric properties as compared to PVDF. It is used in medical implants, eco-friendly sensors, tissue engineering applications, etc.
- Polyimides and co-polymers: These materials have enhanced thermal stability and mechanical properties. They are well-suited for applications that include high temperatures and flexible electronics.

5.4.4 Composite Piezoelectric Materials

Piezocomposite materials include piezoceramic along with polymer in order to enhance different properties due to their tailored mechanism. The geometry of the piezocomposite can be categorized depending on the connectivity between the two phases, i.e., 1-, 2-, and 3-dimensionally [28]. The properties of composite materials depend on the proportion of both ceramic and polymer materials and their structural connectivity. Piezocomposite offers various applications in the field of material research by increasing flexibility, enhanced durability, and tailored properties to fit the requirements of the targeted applications [29, 30]. The combination of the high piezoelectric coefficient of brittle ceramic and the low piezoelectric coefficient of flexible polymer can make a suitable composite needed for various applications [31]. The advantages of piezocomposites are low acoustic impedance, well-matching with human tissue, high coupling factors, etc. Also, piezocomposites are widely used in underwater sonar, medical implantation, diagnostics, etc.

Types of composite materials:

i. 1–3 Composites: In this structure, the ceramic rods are inserted within the polymer matrix. The ceramic rod possesses piezoelectric properties, whereas flexibility and resilience come from the piezoelectric polymer matrix.

ii. 0–3 Composites: This structure consists of piezoceramic filler particles that are evenly dispersed within the polymer matrix. It can be said that the piezoceramic particles are three-dimensionally disconnected from each other.

iii. 2–2 Composites: This structure is a layered structure consisting of piezoelectric materials with non-piezoelectric materials by a lamination process.

5.5 PROPERTIES OF PIEZOELECTRIC MATERIAL

5.5.1 Electromechanical Coupling Factor

The electromechanical coupling factor (k^2) is defined as the ratio between electrical energy stored in response to the applied mechanical energy and vice versa [32]. k^2 can be written by the following equation:

$$k^2 = \frac{\text{mechanical energy stored}}{\text{electrical energy stored}}$$

$$k^2 = \frac{\text{electrical energy stored}}{\text{mechanical energy stored}}$$

A higher coupling coefficient signifies a more effective conversion of energy, which is important for high-performance transducers and actuators applications.

5.5.2 Dielectric Permittivity

The dielectric constant (ε_r) of a material is described as the ability to store electrical energy. When a material is placed in an electrical field, its relative permittivity defines its ability to polarise [33]. Piezoelectric materials benefit from high dielectric permittivity since they amplify their sensitivity and responsiveness to electrical inputs. This characteristic is advantageous for applications such as sensors and capacitors. Mathematically, the dielectric constant can be written as $\varepsilon_r = \frac{\varepsilon}{\varepsilon_0}$, where ε represents the permittivity of the material and ε_0 represents the permittivity of free space with value of 8.85×10^{-12} F/m.

5.5.3 Curie Temperature

The Curie temperature (T_C) is the threshold temperature at which a piezoelectric material undergoes a phase transition, resulting in the loss of its piezoelectric capabilities [34, 35]. Materials with higher Curie temperatures are more desirable for high-temperature applications because they retain their piezoelectric characteristics throughout a wider range of temperatures [36, 37].

5.5.4 Mechanical Quality Factor (Q_M)

It is necessary to study the Q_m of the piezoelectric materials, which describes the efficiency of a material to store mechanical energy without minimum losses for an oscillatory system. Mathematically, Q_m can be written as the ratio between energy stored in mechanical energy in the system (E_s) to energy lost per cycle due to mechanical vibration (E_d).

$$Q_m = 2\pi \frac{E_s}{E_d}$$

The mechanical loss factor represented as "η" is inversely proportional to Q_m, i.e

$$\eta = \frac{1}{Q_m}$$

A high value of Q_m represents a low loss factor, which signifies minimal energy dissipation per each vibration cycle. A low value of Q_m represents a high loss factor, indicating higher energy dissipation.

5.6 APPLICATION OF PIEZOELECTRIC MATERIALS

Piezoelectric materials play a crucial role in various technological applications because of their distinct features.

5.6.1 Key Applications

5.6.1.1 Sensors

Piezoelectric sensors are employed to detect different types of mechanical alterations, including pressure, acceleration, and sound. These sensors transform mechanical stress into an electrical signal, allowing for precise measurement and analysis. Different uses include pressure sensors, microphones, and accelerometers [38].

5.6.1.2 Actuators

Piezoelectric actuators convert an electrical signal into mechanical movement, which allows precisely controlled small displacements. These actuators are used in different applications that require precise motion control like precision robotics, engineering, and medical equipment [38, 39]. In optical equipment like microscopes, piezoelectric motors are used to precise the position of the system.

5.6.1.3 Energy Harvesting

The ability of the piezoelectrical material to convert mechanical energy to electrical energy at a small magnitude, i.e., from milli to micro energy level, is called piezoelectric energy harvesting [40]. Mechanical effects come from different ambient sources like changes in pressure and vibrations. The energy harvesting systems used this potential to produce power low-energy electronics by supporting sustainable and self-powered systems [41, 42]. It can be used as a source of power supply by reducing the chemical waste that comes from conventional batteries. Also, for wearable and wireless sensor applications, it can be used as a power source.

5.6.1.4 Medical Devices

Piezoelectric materials are utilized in medical equipment, such as ultrasound transducers, to produce sound waves for imaging using the converse piezoelectric effect [43]. In addition, piezoelectric injectors employ accurate mechanical activation to administer precise doses of medication.

5.7 CONCLUSIONS

Piezoelectric materials are essential in current technology as they possess distinctive capacities to convert mechanical energy into electrical energy and vice versa. Comprehending the basic principles of piezoelectricity, the distinct properties of various piezoelectric materials, and their wide-ranging uses is crucial for the progress of the discipline. Continuing research and development efforts hold the potential to improve performance and increase the range of applications for piezoelectric materials, stimulating innovation and extending their influence on technology and society.

ACKNOWLEDGMENT

Dr. Sujata Swain expresses gratitude to the Department of Science and Technology (DST), New Delhi, India (Sanction Code: DST/WISE-PDF/PM-13/2023 (G)) for providing the necessary funding for the current research project.

REFERENCES

1. R.C. Garimella, V.R. Sastry, M.S. Mohiuddin, Piezo-Gen - An approach to generate electricity from vibrations, Procedia Earth Planet. Sci. 11 (2015) 445–456. https://doi.org/10.1016/j.proeps.2015.06.044
2. N. More, G. Kapusetti, Piezoelectric material – A promising approach for bone and cartilage regeneration, Med. Hypotheses 108 (2017) 10–16. https://doi.org/10.1016/j.mehy.2017.07.021
3. J.J. Thomson, Piezo-electricity and its application, Sci. Am. 87 (1919) 412–413. https://doi.org/10.1038/scientificamerican06281919-412supp
4. K. Uchino, Fundamentals of piezoelectrics, Encycl. Smart Mater. (2021) 1–21. https://doi.org/10.1016/B978-0-12-803581-8.12129-0
5. S. Roberts, Dielectric and piezoelectric properties of barium titanate, Phys. Rev. 71 (1947) 890–895. https://doi.org/10.1103/PhysRev.71.890
6. G. Shirane, A. Takeda, Phase transitions in solid solutions of $PbZrO_3$ and $PbTiO_3$ (I) small concentrations of $PbTiO_3$, J. Phys. Soc. Japan 7 (1952) 5–11. https://doi.org/10.1143/JPSJ.7.5
7. P. Kumari, R. Rai, S. Sharma, M. Shandilya, A. Tiwari, State-of-the-art of lead free ferroelectrics: A critical review, Adv. Mater. Lett. 6 (2015) 453–484. https://doi.org/10.5185/amlett.2015.4086
8. N. Izyumskaya, Y.I. Alivov, S.J. Cho, H. Morkoç, H. Lee, Y.S. Kang, Processing, structure, properties, and applications of PZT thin films, Crit. Rev. Solid State Mater. Sci. 32 (2007) 111–202. https://doi.org/10.1080/10408430701707347
9. S. Das Mahapatra, P.C. Mohapatra, A.I. Aria, G. Christie, Y.K. Mishra, S. Hofmann, V.K. Thakur, Piezoelectric materials for energy harvesting and sensing applications: Roadmap for future smart materials, Adv. Sci. 8 (2021). https://doi.org/10.1002/advs.202100864
10. M.T. Todaro, F. Guido, V. Mastronardi, D. Desmaele, G. Epifani, L. Algieri, M. De Vittorio, Piezoelectric MEMS vibrational energy harvesters: Advances and outlook, Microelectron. Eng. 183–184 (2017) 23–36. https://doi.org/10.1016/j.mee.2017.10.005
11. A. Safari, Piezoelectric and Acoustic Materials for Transducer Applications 1 2 3, n.d. https://link.springer.com/content/pdf/10.1007%2F978-0-387-76540-2.pdf
12. B.I. Oladapo, Q. Zhao, Enhancing tissue regeneration with self-healing elastic piezoelectricity for sustainable implants, Nano Energy 120 (2024) 109092. https://doi.org/10.1016/j.nanoen.2023.109092

13. J. Nunes-Pereira, P. Costa, S. Lanceros-Mendez, Piezoelectric Energy Production, Elsevier Ltd., 2018. https://doi.org/10.1016/B978-0-12-809597-3.00324-2
14. X. Mo, H. Zhou, W. Li, Z. Xu, J. Duan, L. Huang, B. Hu, J. Zhou, Piezoelectrets for wearable energy harvesters and sensors, Nano Energy 65 (2019) 104033. https://doi.org/10.1016/j.nanoen.2019.104033
15. W.N. Zou, C.X. Tang, E. Pan, Symmetry types of the piezoelectric tensor and their identification, Proc. R. Soc. A Math. Phys. Eng. Sci. 469 (2013). https://doi.org/10.1098/rspa.2012.0755
16. R. Wang, J. Sui, X. Wang, Natural piezoelectric biomaterials: A biocompatible and sustainable building block for biomedical devices, ACS Nano 16 (2022) 17708–17728. https://doi.org/10.1021/acsnano.2c08164
17. M. Acosta, N. Novak, V. Rojas, S. Patel, R. Vaish, J. Koruza, G.A. Rossetti, J. Rödel, $BaTiO_3$-based piezoelectrics: Fundamentals, current status, and perspectives, Appl. Phys. Rev. 4 (2017). https://doi.org/10.1063/1.4990046
18. S. Swain, P.K. Sonia, Microstructural, mechanical and electrical properties of BT, BZT-BCT, and BNT-BT-BKT ferroelectrics synthesized by mechanochemical route, Ceram. Int. 47 (2021) 26511–26518. https://doi.org/10.1016/j.ceramint.2021.06.064
19. M. Habib, I. Lantgios, K. Hornbostel, A review of ceramic, polymer and composite piezoelectric materials, J. Phys. D. Appl. Phys. 55 (2022). https://doi.org/10.1088/1361-6463/ac8687
20. H. Allik, K. M. Webman, J. T. Hunt, Vibrational response of sonar transducers using piezoelectric finite elements. J. Acoust. Soc. Am. 56 (6) (1974) 1782–1791. https://doi.org/10.1121/1.1903513.
21. C. Micela, M. Cioangher, Microstructure and properties of barium titanate ceramics prepared by mechanochemical synthesis, Rom. J. Inf. Sci. Technol. 10 (2007) 335–345.
22. J. Wu, Perovskite lead-free piezoelectric ceramics, J. Appl. Phys. 127 (2020) 190901. https://doi.org/10.1063/5.0006261
23. H. Zhang, T. Wei, Q. Zhang, W. Ma, P. Fan, D. Salamon, S.T. Zhang, B. Nan, H. Tan, Z.G. Ye, A review on the development of lead-free ferroelectric energy-storage ceramics and multilayer capacitors, J. Mater. Chem. C 8 (2020) 16648–16667. https://doi.org/10.1039/d0tc04381h
24. J. Jacob, N. More, K. Kalia, G. Kapusetti, Piezoelectric smart biomaterials for bone and cartilage tissue engineering, Inflamm. Regen. 38 (2018) 1–11. https://doi.org/10.1186/s41232-018-0059-8
25. A.P.K. Parida, S. Swain, R. Sahu, R.R. Negi, B. Samanta, P. Kumar, Phase formation and electrical properties study of PVDF thick films synthesized by solution casting method, Int. J. Mater. Res. 114 (2023) 344–350. https://doi.org/10.1515/ijmr-2022-0229
26. O. Hamdi, F. Mighri, D. Rodrigue, Piezoelectric cellular polymer films: Fabrication, properties and applications, AIMS Mater. Sci. 5 (2018) 845–869. https://doi.org/10.3934/MATERSCI.2018.5.845
27. M. Smith, S. Kar-Narayan, Piezoelectric polymers: Theory, challenges and opportunities, Int. Mater. Rev. 67 (2022) 65–88. https://doi.org/10.1080/09506608.2021.1915935
28. K. Uchino, Piezoelectric composite materials, Adv. Piezoelectric Mater. Sci. Technol. (2010) 318–346. https://doi.org/10.1533/9781845699758.1.318
29. S. Swain, R. Bhaskar, B. Mishra, M.K. Gupta, S.P.S.P.S. Sonia, P. Dasgupta, Kumar, Microstructural, dielectric, mechanical, and biological properties of hydroxyapatite (HAp)/BZT-BCT (0.5Ba(Zr0.2Ti0.8)O3-0.5(Ba0.7Ca0.3)TiO3) bio-composites with improved mechano-electrical properties for bone repair, Ceram. Int. 48 (2022) 24505–24516. https://doi.org/10.1016/j.ceramint.2022.05.084
30. S. Swain, R. Bhaskar, K.B. Narayanan, M.K. Gupta, S. Sharma, Biological properties of sintered hydroxyapatite/barium titanate nanocomposites for bone regeneration

of sintered hydroxyapatite/barium titanate nanocomposites for bone regeneration, Biomed. 18(2) (2023) 025016. https://doi.org/10.1088/1748-605X/acb8f1
31. L. Zhang, Z.-Y. Cheng, Development of polymer-based 0–3 composites with high dielectric constant, J. Adv. Dielectr. 01 (2011) 389–406. https://doi.org/10.1142/s2010135x11000574
32. Y. Yan, L.D. Geng, H. Liu, H. Leng, X. Li, Y.U. Wang, S. Priya, Near-ideal electromechanical coupling in textured piezoelectric ceramics, Nat. Commun. 13 (2022) 1–10. https://doi.org/10.1038/s41467-022-31165-y
33. M. Rahman, J. Haider, T. Akter, M.S.J. Hashmi, Techniques for Assessing the Properties of Advanced Ceramic Materials, Elsevier, 2014. https://doi.org/10.1016/B978-0-08-096532-1.00124-2
34. Y. Meng, G. Chen, M. Huang, Piezoelectric materials: Properties, advancements, and design strategies for high-temperature applications, Nanomaterials 12 (2022). https://doi.org/10.3390/nano12071171
35. H. Somaily, S. Kolesnik, J. Mais, D. Brown, K. Chapagain, B. Dabrowski, O. Chmaissem, Strain-induced tetragonal distortions and multiferroic properties in polycrystalline Sr1-x B axMn O3 (x=0.43-0.45) perovskites, Phys. Rev. Mater. 2 (2018). https://doi.org/10.1103/PhysRevMaterials.2.054408
36. P.Y. Foeller, J.S. Dean, I.M. Reaney, D.C. Sinclair, Design of a bilayer ceramic capacitor with low temperature coefficient of capacitance, Appl. Phys. Lett. 109 (2016). https://doi.org/10.1063/1.4961616
37. G. Kerridge, D.C. Sinclair, J.S. Dean, Resource efficient exploration of ternary phase space to develop multi-layer ceramic capacitors, Acta Mater. 207 (2021) 116690. https://doi.org/10.1016/j.actamat.2021.116690
38. A. Zaszczyńska, A. Gradys, P. Sajkiewicz, Progress in the applications of smart piezoelectric materials for medical devices, Polymers (Basel) 12 (2020) 1–19. https://doi.org/10.3390/polym12112754
39. D. Yang, W. Zhang, Y. Wang, L. Li, F. Yao, L. Miao, W. Zhao, X. Kong, Q. Feng, D. Hu, Formation mechanisms and electrical properties of perovskite mesocrystals, Ceram. Int. 47 (2021) 1479–1512. https://doi.org/10.1016/j.ceramint.2020.08.274
40. M. Sunar, Piezoelectric materials, Compr. Energy Syst. 1–5 (2018) V2-696–V2-719. https://doi.org/10.1016/B978-0-12-809597-3.00248-0
41. H. Shaukat, A. Ali, S. Bibi, W.A. Altabey, M. Noori, S.A. Kouritem, A review of the recent advances in piezoelectric materials, energy harvester structures, and their applications in analytical chemistry, Appl. Sci. 13 (2023). https://doi.org/10.3390/app13031300
42. M. Safaei, H.A. Sodano, S.R. Anton, A review of energy harvesting using piezoelectric materials: State-of-the-art a decade later (2008-2018), Smart Mater. Struct. 28 (2019). https://doi.org/10.1088/1361-665X/ab36e4
43. R. Lay, G.S. Deijs, J. Malmström, The intrinsic piezoelectric properties of materials-a review with a focus on biological materials, RSC Adv. 11 (2021) 30657–30673. https://doi.org/10.1039/d1ra03557f

6 Piezoelectric Materials in Cardiac Patches for Cardiovascular Disease

Rakesh Bhaskar, Soon Mo Choi, and Sung Soo Han

6.1 INTRODUCTION

Cardiovascular diseases (CVDs) encompass a range of illnesses affecting the heart and/or blood vessels. They are responsible for a significant proportion of deaths in industrialized countries, estimated to account for around 31% of all fatalities [1]. CVDs cause injury and/or illness to cardiac tissues including coronary artery diseases (ischemia), infarction, and cardiomyopathies (necrotic and dilated), which have a limited capacity for regeneration [2, 3]. The injured cardiac tissues usually become non-functional and affect the ability of the heart to contract later causing catastrophic failure of heart functioning. CVDs mainly affect the cardiac cells, blood arteries, and heart valves resulting in structural or functional alterations in the cardiovascular system [4–7]. With few approaches, CVDs can be treated using a variety of therapeutic modalities, such as drugs/medicines, angioplasty, bypass graft surgery, and heart transplantation [8, 9].

Chemical therapeutics such as pathway inhibitors, nitrogen oxides, cardiac-specific blockers, membrane stabilizers, antiplatelet drugs, and blood thinners are among the contemporary and mainstream CVD treatment agents [10–14]. However, the existing drugs have a series of adverse effects including unintended bleeding, hypersensitivity, dizziness, and liver damage [11, 15]. Interventional techniques such as coronary bypass grafting, valve repair or replacement surgery, coronary angioplasty, valvuloplasty, and stenting are regularly used in acute and complex CVDs [16–18]. To restore heart functions in these situations, transplantation is necessary, but donor availability severely restricts its use. The heart is a complex organ system with very little capacity for adult cardiac cells or cardiomyocytes (CMs) to self-renew or regenerate, and CVDs bring additional challenges to replacing the damaged CMs [3]. Moreover, the loss of CMs disrupts the transmission of electrical signals between cardiac, fibroblasts, and other cells, leading to the creation of scar tissue as well as uneven electrical signal propagation [19]. Hence, the significant improvement in the therapeutic management of CVDs remains a highly risky and high rate of mortality. Another procedure used in earlier attempts to restore normal cardiovascular functions was cardiomyoplasty [20–22]. In this method, various types of cardiac cells collected from individual patients were injected into the injured heart. However, this methodology carried several limitations, including high cell mortality, low retention, induced inflammatory responses, myocardial damage, as well as artery blockage after cellular injections [21].

DOI: 10.1201/9781003670995-6

CTE has arisen as a viable option for the replacement of impaired CMs, presenting a potential alternative to address the damage caused by heart functions [23]. The design and fabrication of CMs-compatible scaffolds have revealed significant advantages in CTE application. However, the production of fully mature CMs in vitro is still challenging. The creation of cardiac complex structures is one of the most difficult tasks in tissue engineering applications. Cardiac patches based on conductive polymers can be implanted into the heart as part of tissue-engineered therapy, facilitating electrical signaling and integration with host cells. Considerable effort has been devoted to exploring new piezoelectric nanomaterials (PNMs) and piezopolymers that exhibit excellent cytocompatibility and therapeutic potential for novel strategies in CTE. PNMs possess the advantage of generating electricity when subjected to deformations such as stress and strain, eliminating the need for an external source of energy. It has recently been explored to facilitate interactions between cardiac cells and piezo materials [24, 25]. Therefore, these piezoelectric materials can also imitate the mechanoelectrical transduction channels of CMs [26–28]. The overview begins with a brief understanding of the physiological challenges associated with the regeneration of cardiac cells, followed by a discussion of the intrinsic piezoelectric properties of biological tissues. This book chapter provides a comprehensive review of novel piezoelectric strategies in the treatment and management of CVDs.

6.2 MECHANISM OF PIEZOELECTRICITY

Piezoelectric biomaterials belong to a class of advanced materials that demonstrate electromechanical behavior by converting energy into electrical polarization with the help of external stimulus [29]. In this context, the term "pressure control energy" can be utilized to describe the phenomenon of piezoelectricity [30, 31]. Jacques and Pierre Currie discovered piezoelectricity in 1880 while conducting tests on Rochelle salt and quartz crystals. The piezoelectric behaviors can be explained by the generation of electric charges or voltages in response to applied mechanical stress or deformation, as well as the mechanical deformation that occurs in response to applied electric fields. These behaviors are essential for various applications such as sensors, actuators, transducers, and energy harvesting devices [32]. The piezoelectric substances undergo polarization and crystallite reorientation when subjected to a strong electric field aligning themselves with the direction of the electric field's vectors [33]. Piezoelectricity is quantified by the piezoelectric coefficient d, which is the ratio between applied stress and charge (Formula 1), or between strain and applied electric field (Formula 2).

$$\text{Formula 1}\ P = Q/A = dX$$

$$\text{Formula 2}\ X = dE$$

where P is the polarization (Cm^{-2}), Q is the charge (C), A is the area (m^2), d is the piezoelectric coefficient (CN^{-1} for the direct effect and $m\ V^{-1}$ for the converse effect), X is the stress (Nm^{-2}), x is the mechanical strain (unitless), and E is the electric field ($V\ m^{-1}$) [34].

The piezoelectric coefficient (d_{33}) is the most frequently used variable to measure the charge produced by a piezoelectric material in stress-related applications. The transverse coefficient (d_{31}) and longitudinal coefficient (d_{33}) are the coefficients that are most frequently applied to quantify the piezoelectric characteristics. The d_{31} quantifies the electric polarization when it is created in a perpendicular direction against the given stress. Whereas the d_{33} quantifies the electric polarization when given stress is in an equal direction. The degree of transduction (mechanical-electrical) efficiency is also measured by the electromechanical coupling coefficient [35, 36].

The electromechanical connectivity in the CMs is extremely sensitive to ion concentration fluctuations in their transmembrane [37]. The electrical activities regulate excitation-contraction coupling mechanics in CMs by an intracellular calcium-dependent mechanism and extracellular matrix (ECM)-based mechanotransduction pathways (Figure 6.1) [38]. The contraction-relaxation activities of CMs

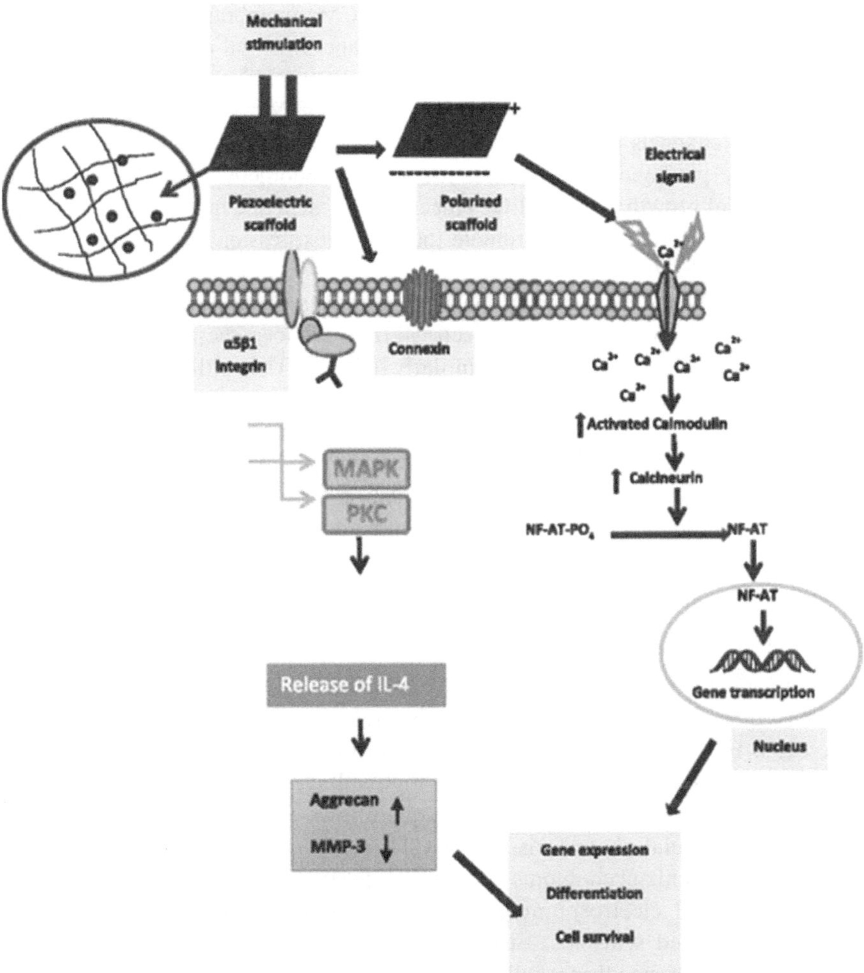

FIGURE 6.1 Illustrated diagrams showing the Ca^{2+} signaling pathways and other pathways that respond to electrical and mechanical stimuli: When mechanical stimulation is applied to piezoelectric scaffolds, it generates electrical signals that stimulate voltage-gated Ca^{2+} channels. This leads to an increase in intracellular Ca^{2+} concentration, which subsequently activates calmodulin, a protein regulated by calcium. Reproduced with open access permission [47].

for synchronous contraction are due to the membrane potential differences and action potential transfer through gap junctions [39]. The cytoplasmic calcium (Ca^{2+}) concentration encourages the sliding of actin-myosin filaments and CM-contraction and is required for the depolarization of the cell membrane [38, 40]. This behavior depends on the translation of environmental mechanical stresses into electrochemical signals that activate different signaling pathways [41]. The electrical transmembrane potential induces the opening and closure of voltage-gated ion channels that facilitate the entry of ions leading to depolarization [42]. This encourages transmembrane receptor integrins to link to various ECM domains [38, 41]. These ECM domains then translate external stimuli into various cellular functions like adhesion, differentiation, and maturation (Figure 6.1). The production of action potentials by ion influx/efflux across CMs membranes serves to explain their electrical characteristics [43]. The membrane potential crosses the threshold of action potential (70 mV) and voltage-gated sodium (Na^+) channels open to depolarize the membrane [44]. Following the closure of Na^+ channels, voltage-gated L-type Ca^{2+} channels open and allow Ca^{2+} to diffuse into the cell [42]. EMS also enhances the proangiogenic response of vascular endothelial cells through vascular endothelial growth factor (VEGF) receptors. In ischemic myocardium, the EMS of 25 and 50 Hz voltage may promote the VEGF expression and induce capillary angiogenesis [45, 46].

On the other hand, piezoelectric materials may overcome this limitation by inducing EMS in cells through mechanoelectrical transduction. These materials respond to environmental cues and function similarly to ECM. The cardiac ECM undergoes constant remodeling and adaptation in response to the environment, influencing the cellular organization and myofibril extension, which makes it a highly dynamic structure [48]. Piezoelectric materials have been employed extensively in energy generation and harvesting, sensing, and actuation applications [49]. This approach has recently shifted its focus toward the design and fabrication of nanofibers-based patches that incorporate piezoelectric properties.

6.3 PIEZOELECTRIC ELECTROSPUN FIBERS

Recent studies have focused on the development of nanodevices and fibrous patches that can induce piezoelectric behavior in electromechanically sensitive cells. Electrospinning is a straightforward process used to produce nanofibers, wherein a strong electric field and high voltage are employed to charge the polymeric solution [50–54]. This technique allows for the creation of scaffolds that possess crucial characteristics for CTE including piezoelectricity, biocompatibility, and enhanced biomechanical properties (Figure 6.2). These inherent properties of electrospinning make it a promising tool for the production of nanofiber-based scaffolds. Electrospinning parameters primarily encompass voltage, flow rate, needle-to-collector distance, needle/nozzle shape and dimensions, and collector type. Additionally, parameters related to the polymer solution such as molecular weight, concentration, surface tension, viscosity, conductivity, and boiling point of the solvent play a significant role in the fabrication process [55]. These parameters influence the diameter, morphology, and even topography

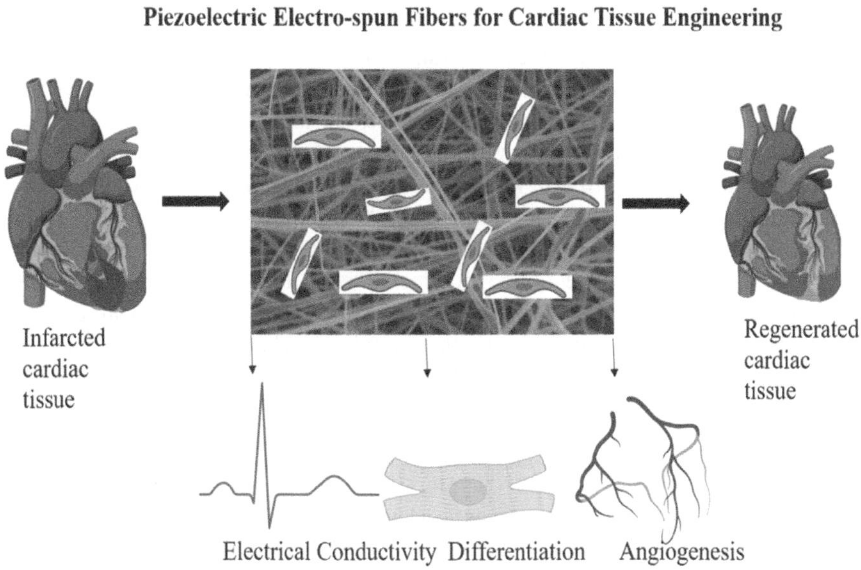

FIGURE 6.2 The strategy of electromechanical stimulation can facilitate the regeneration of damaged cardiac tissue.

of the fibers (temperature, humidity, airflow) during the process of electrospinning [24]. High electric fields encourage the transition of individual crystallites' dipole moments from a dispersed to an aligned distribution [56]. To achieve the optimal fiber diameter, it is essential to effectively control and optimize several key parameters related to environmental factors, electrospinning, and polymer solutions [47, 56, 57].

Coaxial electrospinning allows for the incorporation of additional functionalities to enhance fiber and cell responses. It is crucial to prioritize improved multifunctionality and mechanical properties during the fabrication of fibers [58]. The coaxial fibers also can incorporate remaining un-spinnable polymers, high control over core-shell thickness and dimension ratios as well as encapsulation of useful molecules and nanomaterials [59]. These fibers have been employed to transport medicine, molecules that encourage differentiation into the cardiac lineage in CTE [60]. In addition, in situ polymerization is a further process before electrospinning enabling the creation of coaxial electrospun scaffolds used in CTE [61]. In electrospinning, in situ polymerization enables controlled and homogenous modification of the surface chemical and physical properties to mimic the cardiac ECM without affecting its mechanical qualities [61, 62]. Although piezoelectricity is a naturally occurring phenomenon, certain materials from the ceramic and polymer families have demonstrated significant piezoelectric effects. The choice of materials used for electrospinning the fibers has a crucial influence on the level of piezoelectric performance exhibited by the scaffold [29]. These materials could primarily be split into piezopolymers and piezoceramics.

6.4 NATURAL PIEZOPOLYMERS

Piezoelectricity has been detected in a range of natural materials such as collagen, poly(lactic acid), poly(3-hydroxybutyrate-co-3-hydroxyvalerate) (PHBV), cellulose, chitosan, and silk, etc. These materials possess advantageous mechanical properties and biocompatibility. However, their piezoelectric response typically falls within the range of 0.1–10 pm V^{-1}, which is relatively low for numerous potential applications [63]. When considering the comparable piezoelectric coefficients, one of the commonly observed contributions is the d_{14} coefficient, which is influenced by the crystalline structure of the polymer. Piezopolymers are known for their mechanical flexibility, lightweight nature, and low electromechanical coupling factor. Furthermore, they exhibit excellent durability, chemical stability, and cost-effectiveness, making them promising materials for a wide range of applications.

6.4.1 Collagen

Collagen, as a fibrous structure, serves as a key component in bone and cartilage and plays a crucial role in their piezoelectric properties. Due to its piezoelectric characteristics, electrical signals generated by collagen in response to internal stresses are subsequently transmitted to voltage-gated channels located in the cell membrane, and this transmission occurs through the ECM [64]. Its piezoelectric coefficient, which ranges from 0.2 to 2.0 pC N^{-1}, is which causes the piezoelectric behavior of ligaments, bone cartilage, etc. The longitudinal reorientation of dipole moments of amino acids in the polypeptide chain due to mechanical stimulation causes a modification of polarization [47]. Previous research has indicated that the orientation of the peptide chain has the potential to enhance electrical conductivity. These interactions contribute to the conductivity properties of the peptide-based materials making them suitable for applications requiring electrical conductivity [65]. However, it is still challenging to create ultrashort peptides with specific supramolecular structures that have high piezoelectric responses.

Strong impacts of piezoelectricity have been observed in biological pathways, particularly when collagen is involved in the action. Voltage-gated calcium channels are activated in response to the electrical charge generated by the stimulation of the cell. This electrical charge triggers the opening of the voltage-gated calcium channels, allowing calcium ions to enter the cell. A recent study has documented that electrical stimulation may stimulate TGF-β through the calcium/calmodulin pathway. It is considered a significant factor in promoting various biological processes, including cell proliferation and differentiation, ECM formation, inflammation, and tissue repair. It plays a crucial role in regulating these processes and is involved in the complex signaling pathways that govern cellular behavior and tissue remodeling. The piezoelectric collagen fibers have high biocompatibility and provide support for expression of the important CM-biomarkers, such as cardiac troponin I, GATA binding protein, and myosin heavy chain. Additionally, Ravichandran and colleagues investigated coaxial electrospinning to create fibers with a PGS (core) and collagen (shell) composition for the differentiation of CMs from MSCs [66]. The collagen electrospun scaffold that was created exhibited an elastic modulus within the range of 10–15 kPa, which is comparable to that of the host cardiac muscles. This similarity in elastic modulus makes the scaffold suitable for promoting cardiac regeneration, as it can provide a supportive environment that mimics the mechanical properties of native cardiac tissue [67].

6.4.2 Poly-3-hydroxybutyrate-3-hydroxy Valerate (PHBV)

The PHBV is a member of the poly-hydroxyalkanoate (PHA) class polyesters, which is formed by bacteria (*Cupriavidus Necator*) and *archaea* via fermentation of a carbon substrate inside a microorganism. They are less expensive, biodegradable, non-toxic, thermo-plasticity, and biodegradability. These properties make them well-suited for use in implants, as they can interact harmoniously with biological systems, can be easily molded or shaped, and eventually degrade or be absorbed by the body as new tissue forms [68]. Indeed, PHBV has certain drawbacks, such as poor mechanical performance, high crystallinity, inherent rigidity, brittleness, and hydrophobicity. However, these flaws can be mitigated by blending PHBV with hydrophilic polymers such as gelatin, chitosan, PLA, and polyethylene oxide (PEO). By incorporating these hydrophilic polymers, the overall properties of the composite material can be improved, including enhanced mechanical properties, reduced crystallinity, increased flexibility, and improved hydrophilicity. This approach allows for the elimination or reduction of the limitations associated with pure PHBV [64]. Due to changes in the surface charge, the PHBV exhibits the piezoelectric coefficient and functions similarly to the human bone (1.2 pCN^{-1}) [65]. Recently, reports on the processing of novel highly porous PHBV and PHBV/PEO blend fibers by electrospinning examined the effectiveness for tissue regeneration [69]. In contrast, when comparing the adhesion and expansion of MSCs, CMs, and cardiac fibroblasts, it was observed that these cell types exhibited better attachment and growth on PCL and PHB fibers. Moreover, PHB fibers demonstrated a significant promoting angiogenesis and function of the damaged heart.

6.4.3 Poly(Lactic Acid) and Its Co-Polymer

Poly(lactic acid) (PLA) is a highly innovative material that is currently being developed for a wide range of biological and medicinal applications [70, 71]. PLA and its copolymers might be utilized in vascular grafts, biodegradable stents, drug delivery, and cardiac patches for the treatment of CVD, specifically in myocardial infarction [72]. Furthermore, cardiac patches composed of PLA-based scaffolds have been developed to promote revascularization and aid in cardiac regeneration [70]. PLA exists in various stereoisomeric forms, including poly(L-lactic acid) (PLLA), poly(D,L-lactic acid) (PDLLA), and poly(D-lactic acid) (PDLA). The specific isomeric configuration of the monomer typically determines the form of PLA [70, 73]. PLLA may comprise one of three distinct crystalline phases (α, β, γ) depending on the manufacturing conditions [69, 74]. The crystalline phases that are present in PLLA have a significant impact on its mechanical, thermal, and electrical properties [70]. Recently, the PLA-based nanofiber facilitated the growth of contractile cells and seamlessly integrated with the surrounding host tissue. Specifically, tubular

PLA nanofiber scaffolds were utilized to create tissue-engineered vascular grafts (TEVGs), which were implanted as aortic intervening tubes in mice with positive outcomes. Additionally, the inclusion of gelatin in the composite scaffolds resulted in enhanced proliferation and functionality of smooth muscle cells [72, 75, 76]. The electrospun fiber PLGA, PLGA/collagen poly(1,8-octanediol-cocitrate) (POC), and PLLA-PCL were employed to construct scaffolds appropriate for cardiac TE which resembles natural cardiac tissue in terms of its mechanical features [60, 77, 78].

In another study, novel drug delivery by emulsion electrospinning was developed to promote angiogenesis and heart regeneration in cases of myocardial infarction patients [79]. Flaig and his colleagues conducted a study examining the effects of incorporating poly(glycerol sebacate) (PGS) into electrospun PLA fibers. Their findings revealed that the addition of PGS led to an increase in both the crystallinity and stiffness of the PLA fibers [80]. These fibers also served as excellent scaffolds for cardiac regeneration since they did not trigger unfavorable inflammatory reactions. The scaffold exhibited exceptional properties including electroconductivity, interconnected pores, and a large surface area, which facilitated the adhesion and proliferation of rat CMs. The investigations further demonstrated that CMss cultured on PLLA scaffolds exhibited mature contractile machinery [81]. A PLGA-based scaffold expressing the cardiovascular growth factor neuregulin-1 was also inserted into a rat model of myocardial ischemia [82]. The main drawbacks of PLA fibers have a lower piezoelectric coefficient than PVDF-TrFE (10 pCN^{1}). Myocardial cells synchronized contractile response to ongoing electrical inputs that cause the heartbeat. One of the key challenges is getting the correct patches to contract synchronously, whether biological or synthetic material. Researchers have employed a variety of strategies, including the incorporation of inorganic components like carbon nanotubes (CNT), $BaTO_3$, gold, and electroactive polymers (such as polypyrrole; PPy) to address these problems [83, 84]. Ghai et al. investigate the functional survivability of CMs on conductive scaffolds fabricated by PLGA embedded with CNTs [85]. Incorporating conducting polymers like PPy and polyaniline (PANi) is another approach frequently utilized to increase conductivity [86]. It was discovered that these scaffolds offer cardiac-imitating cues that guide differentiate MSCs into CMs. Furthermore, the hydrophobic nature of PLA may hinder cell attachment, and its brittleness can limit its application in soft tissues. However, PLA-based polymers offer a promising scaffold that has the potential to enhance cardiomyocyte development and activity, mimicking the contraction of normal cardiac muscle. Despite these promising aspects, further studies are required to investigate and optimize for CVD treatments.

6.4.4 Chitosan

Chitin, a naturally occurring polysaccharide, can be easily converted into chitosan through a process called N-deacetylation. Chitin consists of repeating units of 2-amino-2-deoxy-D-glucopyranose, which has numerous biological applications, including controlled drug delivery and tissue engineering [87, 88]. This biomaterial can potentially be used for cardiovascular prostheses, promote cell growth, and deliver drugs in a controlled manner [89, 90]. A recent study has explored the piezoelectric, dielectric, and physicochemical properties of this biomaterial [91]. The electrospun fibers were fabricated using a different concentration of PLA/chitosan, enhancing hydrophilicity, promoting CM adhesion, and increasing the elongation, Young's modulus, and tensile strength of the scaffold. This combination of materials and fabrication technique shows promise for developing scaffolds that support CM regeneration [92, 93]. Chitosan thin film processing is crucial for piezoelectric applications [94, 95].

6.5 SYNTHESIS PIEZOPOLYMERS

6.5.1 Poly(Vinylidene Fluoride) and Its Copolymers

PVDF and its copolymers like poly(vinylidene fluoride-co-trifluoroethylene), poly(vinylidene fluoride-co-trifluoroethylene), poly(vinylidene fluoride-co-hexafluoropropylene), poly(vinylidene fluoride-cochlorotrifluoroethylene) (PVDF-CTFE)), and poly(vinylidene fluoride-co-hexafluoropropylene) (PVDF-HFP) are extensively researched due to their notably high piezoelectric constants [96, 97]. The PVDF is a semi-crystalline dielectric polymer with sufficient electrical stability and biocompatibility for use in different TE applications. Due to their high dielectric constant and electroactive response, which encompasses piezo-, pyro-, and ferroelectric effects, PVDF and its copolymers find a broad range of applications in energy generation and storage, sensors, and biomedical fields [97–99]. Several types of PVDF-based scaffolds have been fabricated including films, membranes, and electrospun fibers. PVDF has been studied for uses in bone, neural, CTE, etc. [27, 100].

PVDF has five distinct crystalline appearances (α, β, γ, δ, and ε) similar with multiple dielectric properties due to the coexistence of fluorine and hydrocarbon segments. Among them, α, β, and γ phases exhibit better dielectric properties. The β-phase in particular is in charge of PVDF's electroactive (piezoelectric, ferroelectric, and pyroelectric) reactions. The α-phase of PVDF is the thermodynamically most stable phase. Therefore, certain methods such as annealing, poling, and mechanical stretching have been investigated to enhance the piezoelectric activity of this polymer to change the non-polar α-phase into its polar β-phase [97]. During electrospinning, the creation of the β-phase is encouraged by inducing the in situ poling and stretching of polymer chains. Trifluoroethylene (TrFE) and PVDF copolymerize with more crystallinity than PVDF. The PVDF-further added TrFE's fluorine atoms encourage steric hindrance to urge the polymer towards the development of an aligned crystalline structure having trans-conformations [101].

Moreover, electrospinning provides a convenient method for fabricating piezoelectric PVDF nanofibers with a high content of electroactive phase through in situ poling and stretching. With the significant improvement in the presence of the electroactive β-phase, various additives have been utilized for electrospinning in the production of piezoelectric PVDF films. The PVDF-TrFE scaffolds were successfully utilized as a platform for the differentiation of induced pluripotent stem cells (iPSCs) into CMs [102]. In the study, Arumugam et al. developed an electrospun nanocomposite using PVDF and polymethyl methacrylate (PMMA) as the matrix materials, with the addition of nanofillers such as hydroxyapatite (Hap) and titanium dioxide (TiO_2) [103]. These cardiac patches provided the necessary tensile strength (77–88 MPa) and maximal elongation (80%) to withstand CM's relaxation–contraction, which was implanted in MI patients. The piezoelectric P(VDF-TrFE) scaffolds helped to develop well-organized sarcomeres, exhibited fast contractility, and expressed traditional cardiac-specific markers of CMs. Furthermore, contractility could be maintained for more than a week in CMs cultivated on poly(caprolactone) nanofilm coated with P(VDF-TrFE) microfibres [104]. The combination of stem cells and piezoelectric scaffolds holds great promise for various applications in the field of CTE. These innovative platforms have the potential to facilitate stem cell proliferation, enhance differentiation, promote cardiomyocyte adhesion, and enable synchronized contractile activity, thus offering a potential therapeutic approach for repairing myocardial infarction patients.

6.6 PIEZOCERAMICS

In recent years, the potential of piezoceramics for biomedical applications has rapidly grown in the interdisciplinary research fields [34]. They have better electromechanical, piezoelectric, and dielectric coefficients than piezopolymers, which are crucial for CTE applications. Thus, they can be used to mimic the cardiac ability to generate electrical potentials under mechanical stress, eliminating the requirement for an external power source [105]. Piezoceramics prevent electrospinning from working properly on its own; hence, electrospinning is typically used in conjunction to create nanofibers. Their piezoelectric response is temperature-dependent, and thermal movements can change the material's polarization, impairing piezoelectricity [106, 107].

The various piezoceramics nanomaterials such as $Pb(Zr,Ti)O_3$ (PZT), Boron nitride nanotubes (BNNTs), $(BaCa)(ZrTi)O_3$ (BCZT), and Barium titanate ($BaTiO_3$, BT), ZnO ceramics have shown piezoelectric properties with [108, 109]. Therefore, efforts are now focused on creating cardiac patches that combine the greatest qualities of piezoceramics. These materials are ferroelectric character with a high piezoelectric coefficient, which is also suitable for biomedical applications. The production of dipole moments and polarization are caused by the mechanical stimulation's promotion of the Ti^{4+} and O_2 movements to Ba^{2+} at the active site. The piezoelectricity of BT could also be improved through various modifications such as doping, calcification, poling, and crystal grain size. The crystalline structure of BT-based ceramics is rapidly altered by the modulation of the morphotropic phase, which enhances their chemical composition along with mechanical pressure. These materials achieved a longitudinal piezoelectric value of about 700 30 pCN^1. In a recent study, BT was applied as a coating to porous Ti alloy scaffolds to stimulate osteogenesis. As another example, ZnO nanoparticles placed on titanium modified with TiO_2 are utilized effectively for biomedical applications especially TE. In addition, BNNTs are also ceramic piezoelectric materials with high piezoelectricity [110]. Furthermore, BNNTs have ideal mechanical qualities while being low in weight. A recent study suggested that adding 1% of BNNTs into a piezopolymer (PVDF-TrFE) composites may help to increase the piezoelectric coefficient (d_{31}) [111, 112]. This improves cell differentiation and cartilage tissue regeneration.

The wurtzite family of piezoceramic nanomaterials, another nanomaterial ZnO, exhibits an asymmetric hexagonal structure and polar crystal surface. Combining piezopolymers with ZnO nanoparticles can enhance their piezoelectric response. Through electrostatic interactions, ZnO altered the PVDF chain orientation and increased the scaffold's piezoelectric activity [113, 114]. There have been some developments in cardiac monitoring and a revolutionary battery-free pacemaker made from ZnO/reduced graphene oxide (rGO) [115, 116]. Researchers revealed that the local electric field during electrospinning was improved by the addition of BNNTs into piezopolymer (PVDF-TrFE) electrospun fibers by bringing the synergistic effects with PVDF fibers [117]. The most promising use for this type of adaptable energy harvester is to power pacemakers, which aims to reduce surgical risks and eliminate the need for battery replacement. This material has received a great deal of use in CTE and biomedical applications because of its remarkable electromechanical performance and biocompatibility.

6.7 CONCLUSIONS AND PERSPECTIVE

Current treatment and management modalities for cardiovascular disease, such as optimal pharmacotherapy, cardiac resynchronization therapy, and implantable cardioverter-defibrillators, effectively slow down disease progression, improve systolic function, and prevent life-threatening arrhythmias. However, these methods are unable to enhance cell regeneration for the repair of impaired functional cardiac muscle. To overcome these limitations, stem cell transplantation has emerged as a promising strategy in CVD management. However, stem cell-based therapies raise concerns regarding histocompatibility, immune tolerance of regenerated CM, and the risk of proarrhythmic stimulations. Electrical stimulation presents a potential solution to address certain challenges in tissue engineering, regenerative medicine, and other biomedical fields. It can promote aligned and oriented tissue growth, opening new possibilities for the creation of three-dimensional tissue-specific cardiac tissue.

Piezoelectric materials have recently shown innovative applications in sensing, actuation, and energy generation within the biomedical field. A deeper understanding of the relationship between piezoelectric electrical stimulation and cellular activity holds great potential for advancements in regeneration therapy for electrically excitable tissues, which play a significant role in CTE applications. Piezoelectric materials can simulate cardiac potentials without the need for an external power source when subjected to mechanical stress. The EMS treatment of cardiac cells has been found to encourage cellular alignment, differentiation, and sarcomere formation. However, improper exposure to EMS can lead to apoptosis and cell death. To address these challenges, further research is needed to gain a comprehensive understanding of piezoelectric testing and the underlying mechanisms of cellular behavior influenced by piezoelectric activity. Electrospinning technology has garnered scientific interest in fabricating fibrous scaffolds with piezoelectric properties. These fibrous piezoelectric tissues facilitate bioelectrical signaling, and cell-to-cell communication, and support ECM. Studies have demonstrated that piezoelectric stimulation induces calcium influx, which controls gene transcription, cell polarization, proliferation, and differentiation of CMs. The utilization of piezoelectric materials, such as collagen, chitosan, PLA, PHBV, PVDF, $BaTiO_3$, and ZnO, in electrospun fiber scaffolds for cardiac tissue engineering (CTE) applications has been extensively discussed which is highlighting their benefits and drawbacks. Ceramics exhibit strong piezoelectric activity but face limitations due to their stiffness and temperature sensitivity, limiting their widespread use in CTE. On the other hand, piezoelectric polymers like PVDF and PVDF-TrFE offer greater flexibility, biocompatibility, and a wider application window in CTE due to their strong piezoelectric activity. However, nanofiber piezoelectric materials have limitations such as low electrical output, poor surface conditions, and the risk of infection after implantation, necessitating the development of optimized strategies. Overall, the utilization of piezoelectric materials in the field of CTE opens up new avenues for electrical stimulation-based applications to address CVDs. Therefore, it is expected that piezoelectric electrospun nanofibers will receive increased attention in the future for the treatment and management of CVDs.

FUNDING STATEMENT

This research was supported by the National Research Foundation of Korea (NRF) (Grant No. RS-2023-00278268).

CONFLICT OF INTEREST

Authors declare no conflict of interest.

REFERENCES

1. H. C. Kim, "Epidemiology of cardiovascular disease and its risk factors in Korea," *Glob. Heal. Med.*, vol. 3, no. 3, pp. 134–141, 2021. doi: 10.35772/ghm.2021.01008.
2. O. Bergmann *et al.*, "Evidence for cardiomyocyte renewal in humans," *Science*, Vol. 324, no. 5923, pp.98–102, 2009. doi:10.1126/science.1164680.
3. R. Gong, Z. Jiang, N. Zagidullin, T. Liu, and B. Cai, "Regulation of cardiomyocyte fate plasticity: A key strategy for cardiac regeneration," *Signal Transduct. Target. Ther.*, vol. 6, no. 1, 2021. doi: 10.1038/s41392-020-00413-2.
4. J. N. Cohn, "Prevention of cardiovascular disease," *Trends Cardiovasc. Med.*, vol. 25, no. 5, pp. 436–442, 2015. doi: 10.1016/j.tcm.2014.12.005.
5. P. W. Siri-Tarino, and R. M. Krauss, "Diet, lipids, and cardiovascular disease," *Curr. Opin. Lipidol.*, vol. 27, no. 4, pp. 323–328, 2016. doi: 10.1097/MOL.0000000000000310.
6. S. Costantino, F. Paneni, and F. Cosentino, "Ageing, metabolism and cardiovascular disease," *J. Physiol.*, vol. 594, no. 8, pp. 2061–2073, 2016. doi: 10.1113/JP270538.
7. D. P. Leong *et al.*, "Reducing the global burden of cardiovascular disease, part 2: Prevention and treatment of cardiovascular disease," *Circ. Res.*, vol. 121, no. 6, pp. 695–710, 2017. doi: 10.1161/CIRCRESAHA.117.311849.
8. M. F. Tenreiro, A. F. Louro, P. M. Alves, and M. Serra, "Next generation of heart regenerative therapies: Progress and promise of cardiac tissue engineering," *Npj Regen. Med.*, vol. 6, no. 1, 2021. doi: 10.1038/s41536-021-00140-4.
9. S. Francula-Zaninovic, and I. A. Nola, "Management of measurable variable cardiovascular disease' risk factors," *Curr. Cardiol. Rev.*, vol. 14, no. 3, pp. 153–163, 2018. doi: 10.2174/1573403x14666180222102312.
10. R. V. Patel, B. M. Mistry, S. K. Shinde, R. Syed, V. Singh, and H. S. Shin, "Therapeutic potential of quercetin as a cardiovascular agent," *Eur. J. Med. Chem.*, vol. 155, pp. 889–904, 2018. doi: 10.1016/j.ejmech.2018.06.053.

11. A. K. Malakar, D. Choudhury, B. Halder, P. Paul, A. Uddin, and S. Chakraborty, "A review on coronary artery disease, its risk factors, and therapeutics," *J. Cell. Physiol.*, vol. 234, no. 10, pp. 16812–16823, 2019. doi: 10.1002/jcp.28350.
12. A. Alfaddagh *et al.*, "Inflammation and cardiovascular disease: From mechanisms to therapeutics," *Am. J. Prev. Cardiol.*, vol. 4, no. November, p. 100130, 2020. doi: 10.1016/j.ajpc.2020.100130.
13. C. Recio, F. Maione, A. J. Iqbal, N. Mascolo, and V. De Feo, "The potential therapeutic application of peptides and peptidomimetics in cardiovascular disease," *Front. Pharmacol.*, vol. 7, no. JAN, pp. 1–11, 2017. doi: 10.3389/fphar.2016.00526.
14. M. Simons, and J. A. Ware, "Therapeutic angiogenesis in cardiovascular disease," *Nat. Rev. Drug Discov.*, vol. 2, no. 11, pp. 863–871, 2003. doi: 10.1038/nrd1226.
15. M. Abdelsayed, E. J. Kort, S. Jovinge, and M. Mercola, "Repurposing drugs to treat cardiovascular disease in the era of precision medicine," *Nat. Rev. Cardiol.*, vol. 19, no. 11, pp. 751–764, 2022. doi: 10.1038/s41569-022-00717-6.
16. G. Cai, H. Huang, F. Li, G. Shi, X. Yu, and L. Yu, "Distal transradial access: A review of the feasibility and safety in cardiovascular angiography and intervention," *BMC Cardiovasc. Disord.*, vol. 20, no. 1, pp. 1–12, 2020. doi: 10.1186/s12872-020-01625-8.
17. S. Waxman, F. Ishibashi, and J. E. Muller, "Detection and treatment of vulnerable plaques and vulnerable patients: Novel approaches to prevention of coronary events," *Circulation*, vol. 114, no. 22, pp. 2390–2411, 2006. doi: 10.1161/CIRCULATIONAHA.105.540013.
18. R. C. Neely, M. Leacche, C. R. Byrne, A. V. Norman, and J. G. Byrne, "New approaches to cardiovascular surgery," *Curr. Probl. Cardiol.*, vol. 39, no. 12, pp. 427–466, 2014. doi: 10.1016/j.cpcardiol.2014.07.006.
19. Y. Kim, Z. Zharkinbekov, M. Sarsenova, G. Yeltay, and A. Saparov, "Recent advances in gene therapy for cardiac tissue regeneration," *Int. J. Mol. Sci.*, vol. 22, no. 17, 2021. doi: 10.3390/ijms22179206.
20. T. Reffelmann, and R. A. Kloner, "Cellular cardiomyoplasty - cardiomyocytes, skeletal myoblasts, or stem cells for regenerating myocardium and treatment of heart failure?" *Cardiovasc. Res.*, vol. 58, no. 2, pp. 358–368, 2003. doi: 10.1016/S0008-6363(02)00739-3.
21. E. A. Bocchi, "Cardiomyoplasty for treatment of heart failure," *Eur. J. Heart Fail.*, vol. 3, no. 4, pp. 403–406, 2001. doi: 10.1016/S1388-9842(01)00162-3.
22. T. Akita, and K. Bando, "Cardiomyoplasty for treatment of heart failure," *Nippon Rinsho. Japanese J. Clin. Med.*, vol. 65, no. Suppl 5, pp. 231–235, 2007.
23. Y. Zhao, G. Eng, B. W. Lee, M. Radisic, and G. Vunjak-Novakovic, *Cardiac tissue engineering*, INC, 2020. doi: 10.1016/B978-0-12-818422-6.00033-2.
24. M. R. Gomes, F. Castelo Ferreira, and P. Sanjuan-Alberte, "Electrospun piezoelectric scaffolds for cardiac tissue engineering," *Biomater. Adv.*, vol. 137, no. March, p. 212808, 2022. doi: 10.1016/j.bioadv.2022.212808.
25. N. A. Kamel, "Bio-piezoelectricity: Fundamentals and applications in tissue engineering and regenerative medicine," *Biophys. Rev.*, vol. 14, no. 3, pp. 717–733, 2022. doi: 10.1007/s12551-022-00969-z.
26. R. Balint, N. J. Cassidy, and S. H. Cartmell, "Electrical stimulation: A novel tool for tissue engineering," *Tissue Eng. - Part B Rev.*, vol. 19, no. 1, pp. 48–57, 2013. doi: 10.1089/ten.teb.2012.0183.
27. C. Ribeiro, V. Sencadas, D. M. Correia, and S. Lanceros-Méndez, "Piezoelectric polymers as biomaterials for tissue engineering applications," *Colloids Surf. B Biointerfaces*, vol. 136, pp. 46–55, 2015. doi: 10.1016/j.colsurfb.2015.08.043.
28. N. Tandon *et al.*, "Electrical stimulation systems for cardiac tissue engineering," *Nat. Protoc.*, vol. 4, no. 2, pp. 155–173, 2009. doi: 10.1038/nprot.2008.183.
29. R. M. Lec, "Piezoelectric biosensors: recent advances and applications," *2001 IEEE Int. Freq. Control Symp. PDA Exhib. PIEZOELECTRIC*, no. 215, 2001.

30. H. Jaffe, "Piezoelectric ceramics," *J. Am. Ceram. Soc.*, vol. 41, no. 11, pp. 494–498, 1958. doi: 10.1111/j.1151-2916.1958.tb12903.x.
31. M. T. Chorsi *et al.*, "Piezoelectric biomaterials for sensors and actuators," *Adv. Mater.*, vol. 31, no. 1, pp. 1–15, 2019. doi: 10.1002/adma.201802084.
32. W. Qian, W. Yang, Y. Zhang, C. R. Bowen, and Y. Yang, *Piezoelectric materials for controlling electro-chemical processes*, vol. 12, no. 1. Springer Singapore, 2020. doi: 10.1007/s40820-020-00489-z.
33. M. Pohanka, "The piezoelectric biosensors: Principles and applications, a review," *Int. J. Electrochem. Sci.*, vol. 12, no. 1, pp. 496–506, 2017. doi: 10.20964/2017.01.44.
34. R. Lay, G. S. Deijs, and J. Malmström, "The intrinsic piezoelectric properties of materials-a review with a focus on biological materials," *RSC Adv.*, vol. 11, no. 49, pp. 30657–30673, 2021. doi: 10.1039/d1ra03557f.
35. A. Zaszczyńska, A. Gradys, and P. Sajkiewicz, "Progress in the applications of smart piezoelectric materials for medical devices," *Polymers (Basel)*, vol. 12, no. 11, pp. 1–19, 2020. doi: 10.3390/polym12112754.
36. S. Panda *et al.*, "Piezoelectric energy harvesting systems for biomedical applications," *Nano Energy*, vol. 100, no. June, p. 107514, 2022. doi: 10.1016/j.nanoen.2022.107514.
37. J. L. Ruan *et al.*, "Mechanical stress conditioning and electrical stimulation promote contractility and force maturation of induced pluripotent stem cell-derived human cardiac tissue," *Circulation*, vol. 134, no. 20, pp. 1557–1567, 2016. doi: 10.1161/CIRCULATIONAHA.114.014998.
38. H. Liao, Y. Qi, Y. Ye, P. Yue, D. Zhang, and Y. Li, "Mechanotranduction pathways in the regulation of mitochondrial homeostasis in cardiomyocytes," *Front. Cell Dev. Biol.*, vol. 8, no. January, pp. 1–17, 2021. doi: 10.3389/fcell.2020.625089.
39. L. T. Izu *et al.*, "mechano-electric and mechano-chemo-transduction in cardiomyocytes," *J. Physiol.*, vol. 598, no. 7, pp. 1285–1305, 2021. https://doi.org/10.1113/JP276494.
40. A. Amar, S. Zlochiver, and O. Barnea, "Mechano-electric feedback effects in a three-dimensional (3D) model of the contracting cardiac ventricle," *PLoS One*, vol. 13, no. 1, pp. 1–13, 2018. doi: 10.1371/journal.pone.0191238.
41. R. Peyronnet, O. Solovyova, G. Iribe, and L. B. Katsnelson, "Editorial: mechano-calcium, mechano-electric, and mechano-metabolic feedback loops: Contribution to the myocardial contraction in health and diseases," *Front. Physiol.*, vol. 12, no. April, pp. 10–13, 2021. doi: 10.3389/fphys.2021.676826.
42. A. O. Grant, "Cardiac ion channels," *Circ. Arrhythmia Electrophysiol.*, vol. 2, no. 2, pp. 185–194, 2009. doi: 10.1161/CIRCEP.108.789081.
43. D. Miller, L. Wang, and J. Zhong, *Sodium channels, cardiac arrhythmia, and therapeutic strategy*, 1st ed., vol. 70. Elsevier Inc, 2014. doi: 10.1016/B978-0-12-417197-8.00012-2.
44. D. A. Eisner, J. L. Caldwell, K. Kistamás, and A. W. Trafford, "Calcium and excitation-contraction coupling in the heart," *Circ. Res.*, vol. 121, no. 2, pp. 181–195, 2017. doi: 10.1161/CIRCRESAHA.117.310230.
45. A. F. Kanaan, and A. P. Piedade, "Electro-responsive polymer-based platforms for electrostimulation of cells," *Mater. Adv.*, vol. 3, no. 5, pp. 2337–2353, 2022. doi: 10.1039/d1ma01012c.
46. A. Hidmark *et al.*, "Electrical muscle stimulation induces an increase of VEGFR2 on circulating hematopoietic stem cells in patients with diabetes," *Clin. Ther.*, vol. 39, no. 6, pp. 1132–1144.e2, 2017. doi: 10.1016/j.clinthera.2017.05.340.
47. J. Jacob, N. More, K. Kalia, and G. Kapusetti, "Piezoelectric smart biomaterials for bone and cartilage tissue engineering," *Inflamm. Regen.*, vol. 38, no. 1, pp. 1–11, 2018. doi: 10.1186/s41232-018-0059-8.
48. Q. Xu *et al.*, "Construction of bio-piezoelectric platforms: From structures and synthesis to applications," *Adv. Mater.*, vol. 33, no. 27, 2021. doi: 10.1002/adma.202008452.

49. S. Das Mahapatra *et al.*, "Piezoelectric materials for energy harvesting and sensing applications: Roadmap for future smart materials," *Adv. Sci.*, vol. 8, no. 17, 2021. doi: 10.1002/advs.202100864.
50. Y. P. Singh, S. Dasgupta, and R. Bhaskar, "Preparation, characterization and bioactivities of nano anhydrous calcium phosphate added gelatin–chitosan scaffolds for bone tissue engineering," *J. Biomater. Sci. Polym. Ed.*, vol. 30, no. 18, pp. 1756–1778, 2019. doi: 10.1080/09205063.2019.1663474.
51. Y. P. Singh, S. Dasgupta, R. Bhaskar, and A. K. Agrawal, "Monetite addition into gelatin based freeze-dried scaffolds for improved mechanical and osteogenic properties," *Biomed. Mater.*, vol. 16, no. 6, 2021. doi: 10.1088/1748-605X/ac2e17.
52. Y. P. Singh, S. Dasgupta, S. Nayar, and R. Bhaskar, "Optimization of electrospinning process & parameters for producing defect-free chitosan/polyethylene oxide nanofibers for bone tissue engineering," *J. Biomater. Sci. Polym. Ed.*, vol. 31, no. 6, pp. 781–803, 2020. doi: 10.1080/09205063.2020.1718824.
53. Y. P. Singh *et al.*, "Gelatin/monetite electrospun scaffolds to regenerate bone tissue: Fabrication, characterization, and in-vitro evaluation," *J. Mech. Behav. Biomed. Mater.*, vol. 137, no. October 2022, p. 105524, 2023. doi: 10.1016/j.jmbbm.2022.105524.
54. Y. P. Singh, S. D. Purohit, M. K. Gupta, R. Bhaskar, S. S. Han, and S. Dasgupta, "Preparation, characterization, and bioactivity of reinforced monetite with chitosan-gelatin electrospun composite scaffold for bone tissue engineering," *Biomed. Mater.*, vol. 18, no. 5, 2023. doi: 10.1088/1748-605X/ace7a3.
55. M. R. Gomes, F. F. F. Garrudo, P. Sanjuan-Alberte, and F. C. Ferreira, "Novel Coaxial Fibers Combining Piezoelectrical and Electrical Conductive Polymers towards Cardiac Tissue Engineering," p. 74, 2022, doi: 10.3390/materproc2022008074.
56. J. S. Park, "Electrospinning and its applications," *Adv. Nat. Sci. Nanosci. Nanotechnol.*, vol. 1, no. 4, 2010. doi: 10.1088/2043-6262/1/4/043002.
57. B. Oh, and C. H. Lee, "Nanofiber for cardiovascular tissue engineering," *Expert Opin. Drug Deliv.*, vol. 10, no. 11, pp. 1565–1582, 2013. doi: 10.1517/17425247.2013.830608.
58. J. Yoon, H. S. Yang, B. S. Lee, and W. R. Yu, "Recent progress in coaxial electrospinning: New parameters, various structures, and wide applications," *Adv. Mater.*, vol. 30, no. 42, pp. 1–23, 2018. doi: 10.1002/adma.201704765.
59. Y. Lu *et al.*, "Coaxial electrospun fibers: Applications in drug delivery and tissue engineering," *Wiley Interdiscip. Rev. Nanomed. Nanobiotechnol.*, vol. 8, no. 5, pp. 654–677, 2016. doi: 10.1002/wnan.1391.
60. G. Zhao, X. Zhang, T. J. Lu, and F. Xu, "Recent advances in electrospun nanofibrous scaffolds for cardiac tissue engineering," *Adv. Funct. Mater.*, vol. 25, no. 36, pp. 5726–5738, 2015. doi: 10.1002/adfm.201502142.
61. P. H. Kim, and J. Y. Cho, "Myocardial tissue engineering using electrospun nanofiber composites," *BMB Rep.*, vol. 49, no. 1, pp. 26–36, 2016. doi: 10.5483/BMBRep.2016.49.1.165.
62. P. T. Bertuoli *et al.*, "Electrospun conducting and biocompatible uniaxial and core-shell fibers having poly(lactic acid), poly(ethylene glycol), and polyaniline for cardiac tissue engineering," *ACS Omega*, vol. 4, no. 2, pp. 3660–3672, 2019. doi: 10.1021/acsomega.8b03411.
63. N. D. Sharma, R. Maranganti, and P. Sharma, "On the possibility of piezoelectric nanocomposites without using piezoelectric materials," *J. Mech. Phys. Solids*, vol. 55, no. 11, pp. 2328–2350, 2007. doi: 10.1016/j.jmps.2007.03.016.
64. E. Fukada, "History and recent progress in piezoelectric polymers," *IEEE Trans. Ultrason. Ferroelectr. Freq. Control*, vol. 47, no. 6, pp. 1277–1290, 2000. doi: 10.1109/58.883516.
65. S. Bera *et al.*, "Molecular engineering of piezoelectricity in collagen-mimicking peptide assemblies," *Nat. Commun.*, vol. 12, no. 1, 2021. doi: 10.1038/s41467-021-22895-6.
66. R. Ravichandran, "Cardiogenic differentiation of mesenchymal stem cells on elastomeric poly (glycerol sebacate)/collagen core/shell fibers," *World J. Cardiol.*, vol. 5, p. 3, p. 28, 2013. doi: 10.4330/wjc.v5.i3.28.

67. P. M. Maria Kitsara, O. Agbulut, D. Kontziampasis, and Y. Chen, "Fibers for hearts: A critical review on electrospinning for cardiac tissue engineering," Acta biomaterialia., Vol. 48, pp. 20–40, 2017. doi.org/10.1016/j.actbio.2016.11.014.
68. A. L. Rivera-Briso, and Á. Serrano-Aroca, "Poly(3-hydroxybutyrate-co-3-hydroxyvalerate): Enhancement strategies for advanced applications," *Polymers (Basel)*, vol. 10, no. 7, pp. 1–28, 2018. doi: 10.3390/polym10070732.
69. S. N. Hanumantharao, and S. Rao, "Multi-functional electrospun nanofibers from polymer blends for scaffold tissue engineering," *Fibers*, vol. 7, no. 7, 2019. doi: 10.3390/fib7070066.
70. V. DeStefano, S. Khan, and A. Tabada, "Applications of PLA in modern medicine," *Eng. Regen*, vol. 1, no. April, pp. 76–87, 2020. doi: 10.1016/j.engreg.2020.08.002.
71. M. S. Singhvi, S. S. Zinjarde, and D. V. Gokhale, "Polylactic acid: Synthesis and biomedical applications," *J. Appl. Microbiol.*, vol. 127, no. 6, pp. 1612–1626, 2019. doi: 10.1111/jam.14290.
72. A. J. Guerra, P. Cano, M. Rabionet, T. Puig, and J. Ciurana, "3D-printed PCL/PLA composite stents: Towards a new solution to cardiovascular problems," *Materials (Basel)*, vol. 11, no. 9, pp. 1–13, 2018. doi: 10.3390/ma11091679.
73. S. Pisani, R. Dorati, B. Conti, T. Modena, G. Bruni, and I. Genta, "Design of copolymer PLA-PCL electrospun matrix for biomedical applications," *React. Funct. Polym.*, vol. 124, no. October 2017, pp. 77–89, 2018. doi: 10.1016/j.reactfunctpolym.2018.01.011.
74. X. Zhang *et al.*, "Electroactive electrospun nanofibers for tissue engineering," *Nano Today*, vol. 39, p. 101196, 2021. doi: 10.1016/j.nantod.2021.101196.
75. R. Ahuja *et al.*, "Biocompatibility analysis of PLA based candidate materials for cardiovascular stents in a rat subcutaneous implant model," *Acta Histochem.*, vol. 122, no. 7, p. 151615, 2020. doi: 10.1016/j.acthis.2020.151615.
76. M. Santoro, S. R. Shah, J. L. Walker, and A. G. Mikos, "Poly(lactic acid) nanofibrous scaffolds for tissue engineering," *Adv. Drug Deliv. Rev.*, vol. 107, pp. 206–212, 2016. doi: 10.1016/j.addr.2016.04.019.
77. J. H. Wee *et al.*, "Stem cell laden nano and micro collagen/PLGA bimodal fibrous patches for myocardial regeneration," *Biomater. Res.*, vol. 26, no. 1, pp. 1–17, 2022. doi: 10.1186/s40824-022-00319-w.
78. Z. Jing, X. Shi, G. Zhang, and J. Gu, "Synthesis and properties of poly(lactide)/poly(ε-caprolactone) multiblock supramolecular polymers bonded by the self-complementary quadruple hydrogen bonding," *Polymer (Guildf)*, vol. 121, pp. 124–136, 2017. doi: 10.1016/j.polymer.2017.06.019.
79. H. J. Chung *et al.*, *Epicardial delivery of VEGF and cardiac stem cells guided by 3-dimensional PLLA mat enhancing cardiac regeneration and angiogenesis in acute myocardial infarction*, vol. 205. Elsevier B.V., 2015. doi: 10.1016/j.jconrel.2015.02.013.
80. F. Flaig *et al.*, "Design of functional electrospun scaffolds based on poly(glycerol sebacate) elastomer and poly(lactic acid) for cardiac tissue engineering," *ACS Biomater. Sci. Eng.*, vol. 6, no. 4, pp. 2388–2400, 2020. doi: 10.1021/acsbiomaterials.0c00243.
81. S. Pascual-Gil, T. Simón-Yarza, E. Garbayo, F. Prósper, and M. J. Blanco-Prieto, "Cytokine-loaded PLGA and PEG-PLGA microparticles showed similar heart regeneration in a rat myocardial infarction model," *Int. J. Pharm.*, vol. 523, no. 2, pp. 531–533, 2017. doi: 10.1016/j.ijpharm.2016.11.022.
82. T. Simoń-Yarza *et al.*, "Functional benefits of PLGA particulates carrying VEGF and CoQ10 in an animal of myocardial ischemia," *Int. J. Pharm.*, vol. 454, no. 2, pp. 784–790, 2013. doi: 10.1016/j.ijpharm.2013.04.015.
83. W. Zhang, J. Yu, and H. Chang, "Two dimensional nanosheets as conductive, flexible elements in biomaterials," *J. Mater. Chem. B*, vol. 3, no. 25, pp. 4959–4964, 2015. doi: 10.1039/c5tb00087d.
84. Y. Liang, A. Mitriashkin, T. T. Lim, and J. C. H. Goh, "Conductive polypyrrole-encapsulated silk fibroin fibers for cardiac tissue engineering," *Biomaterials*, vol. 276, no. June, p. 121008, 2021. doi: 10.1016/j.biomaterials.2021.121008.

85. P. Ghai, T. Mayerhofer, and R. K. Jha, "Exploring the effectiveness of incorporating carbon nanotubes into bioengineered scaffolds to improve cardiomyocyte function," *Expert Rev. Clin. Pharmacol.*, vol. 13, no. 12, pp. 1347–1366, 2020. doi: 10.1080/17512433.2020.1841634.
86. H. Esmaeili *et al.*, "Electroconductive biomaterials for cardiac tissue engineering," *Acta Biomater.*, vol. 139, pp. 118–140, 2022. doi: 10.1016/j.actbio.2021.08.031.
87. E. Vunain, A. K. Mishra, and B. B. Mamba, *Fundamentals of chitosan for biomedical applications*, vol. 1. Elsevier, 2017. doi: 10.1016/B978-0-08-100230-8.00001-7.
88. E. Szymańska, and K. Winnicka, "Stability of chitosan - A challenge for pharmaceutical and biomedical applications," *Mar. Drugs*, vol. 13, no. 4, pp. 1819–1846, 2015. doi: 10.3390/md13041819.
89. M. Dash, F. Chiellini, R. M. Ottenbrite, and E. Chiellini, "Chitosan - A versatile semi-synthetic polymer in biomedical applications," *Prog. Polym. Sci.*, vol. 36, no. 8, pp. 981–1014, 2011. doi: 10.1016/j.progpolymsci.2011.02.001.
90. T. A. Ahmed, and B. M. Aljaeid, "Preparation, characterization, and potential application of chitosan, chitosan derivatives, and chitosan metal nanoparticles in pharmaceutical drug delivery," *Drug Des. Devel. Ther.*, vol. 10, pp. 483–507, 2016. doi: 10.2147/DDDT.S99651.
91. E. S. Hosseini, L. Manjakkal, D. Shakthivel, and R. Dahiya, "Glycine-chitosan-based flexible biodegradable piezoelectric pressure sensor," *ACS Appl. Mater. Interfaces*, vol. 12, no. 8, pp. 9008–9016, 2020. doi: 10.1021/acsami.9b21052.
92. Y. Liu, S. Wang, and R. Zhang, "Composite poly(lactic acid)/chitosan nanofibrous scaffolds for cardiac tissue engineering," *Int. J. Biol. Macromol.*, vol. 103, pp. 1130–1137, 2017. doi: 10.1016/j.ijbiomac.2017.05.101.
93. J. Feng, D. Zhang, M. Zhu, and C. Gao, "Poly(l-lactide) melt spun fiber-aligned scaffolds coated with collagen or chitosan for guiding the directional migration of osteoblasts in vitro," *J. Mater. Chem. B*, vol. 5, no. 26, pp. 5176–5188, 2017. doi: 10.1039/c7tb00601b.
94. F. B. Ahmad, M. H. Maziati Akmal, A. Amran, and M. H. Hasni, "Characterization of chitosan from extracted fungal biomass for piezoelectric application," *IOP Conf. Ser. Mater. Sci. Eng.*, vol. 778, no. 1, 2020. doi: 10.1088/1757-899X/778/1/012034.
95. A. Hänninen, E. Sarlin, I. Lyyra, T. Salpavaara, M. Kellomäki, and S. Tuukkanen, "Nanocellulose and chitosan based films as low cost, green piezoelectric materials," *Carbohydr. Polym.*, vol. 202, no. May, pp. 418–424, 2018. doi: 10.1016/j.carbpol.2018.09.001.
96. Y. Higashihata, J. Sako, and T. Yagi, "Piezoelectricity of vinylidene fluoride-trifluoroethylene copolymers," *Ferroelectrics*, vol. 32, no. 1, pp. 85–92, 1981. doi: 10.1080/00150198108238678.
97. P. Ueberschlag, "PVDF piezoelectric polymer," *Sens. Rev.*, vol. 21, no. 2, pp. 118–125, 2001. doi: 10.1108/02602280110388315.
98. W. Xia, and Z. Zhang, "PVDF-based dielectric polymers and their applications in electronic materials," *IET Nanodielectr.*, vol. 1, no. 1, pp. 17–31, 2018. doi: 10.1049/iet-nde.2018.0001.
99. B. Neese *et al.*, "Piezoelectric responses in poly(vinylidene fluoride/hexafluoropropylene) copolymers," *Appl. Phys. Lett.*, vol. 90, no. 24, pp. 2005–2008, 2007. doi: 10.1063/1.2748076.
100. Y. Li, C. Liao, and S. C. Tjong, "Electrospun polyvinylidene fluoride-based fibrous scaffolds with piezoelectric characteristics for bone and neural tissue engineering," *Nanomaterials*, vol. 9, no. 7, 2019. doi: 10.3390/nano9070952.
101. Z. Y. Wang, H. Q. Fan, K. H. Su, X. Wang, and Z. Y. Wen, "Structure, phase transition and electric properties of poly(vinylidene fluoride-trifluoroethylene) copolymer studied with density functional theory," *Polymer (Guildf)*, vol. 48, no. 11, pp. 3226–3236, 2007. doi: 10.1016/j.polymer.2007.04.015.
102. N. Adadi *et al.*, "Electrospun fibrous PVDF-TrFe scaffolds for cardiac tissue engineering, differentiation, and maturation," *Adv. Mater. Technol.*, vol. 5, no. 3, pp. 1–11, 2020. doi: 10.1002/admt.201900820.

103. R. Arumugam *et al.*, "Scalable novel PVDF based nanocomposite foam for direct blood contact and cardiac patch applications," *J. Mech. Behav. Biomed. Mater.*, vol. 88, pp. 270–280, 2018. doi: 10.1016/j.jmbbm.2018.08.020.
104. P. Hitscherich, S. Wu, R. Gordan, L. H. Xie, T. Arinzeh, and E. J. Lee, "The effect of PVDF-TrFE scaffolds on stem cell derived cardiovascular cells," *Biotechnol. Bioeng.*, vol. 113, no. 7, pp. 1577–1585, 2016. doi: 10.1002/bit.25918.
105. K. Kapat, Q. T. H. Shubhra, M. Zhou, and S. Leeuwenburgh, "Piezoelectric nano-biomaterials for biomedicine and tissue regeneration," *Adv. Funct. Mater.*, vol. 30, no. 44, 2020. doi: 10.1002/adfm.201909045.
106. Q. Zhou, S. Lau, D. Wu, and K. Kirk Shung, "Piezoelectric films for high frequency ultrasonic transducers in biomedical applications," *Prog. Mater. Sci.*, vol. 56, no. 2, pp. 139–174, 2011. doi: 10.1016/j.pmatsci.2010.09.001.
107. Y. Zeng *et al.*, "Recent progress in 3D printing piezoelectric materials for biomedical applications," *J. Phys. D. Appl. Phys.*, vol. 55, no. 1, 2021. doi: 10.1088/1361-6463/ac27d2.
108. K. K. Poon, M. C. Wurm, D. M. Evans, M. A. Einarsrud, R. Lutz, and J. Glaum, "Biocompatibility of (Ba,Ca)(Zr,Ti)O3 piezoelectric ceramics for bone replacement materials," *J. Biomed. Mater. Res. - Part B Appl. Biomater.*, vol. 108, no. 4, pp. 1295–1303, 2020. doi: 10.1002/jbm.b.34477.
109. J. L. Pons, E. Rocon, A. Forner-Cordero, and J. Moreno, "Biomedical instrumentation based on piezoelectric ceramics," *J. Eur. Ceram. Soc.*, vol. 27, no. 13–15, pp. 4191–4194, 2007. doi: 10.1016/j.jeurceramsoc.2007.02.126.
110. J. Zhang *et al.*, "3D printed piezoelectric BNNTs nanocomposites with tunable interface and microarchitectures for self-powered conformal sensors," *Nano Energy*, vol. 77, no. August, p. 105300, 2020. doi: 10.1016/j.nanoen.2020.105300.
111. J. H. Kang *et al.*, "Multifunctional electroactive nanocomposites based on piezoelectric boron nitride nanotubes," *ACS Nano*, vol. 9, no. 12, pp. 11942–11950, 2015. doi: 10.1021/acsnano.5b04526.
112. G. G. Genchi *et al.*, "P(VDF-TrFE)/BaTiO3 nanoparticle composite films mediate piezoelectric stimulation and promote differentiation of SH-SY5Y neuroblastoma cells," *Adv. Healthc. Mater.*, vol. 5, no. 14, pp. 1808–1820, 2016. doi: 10.1002/adhm.201600245.
113. R. Kumar, R. Singh, M. Singh, and P. Kumar, "On ZnO nano particle reinforced PVDF composite materials for 3D printing of biomedical sensors," *J. Manuf. Process.*, vol. 60, no. June, pp. 268–282, 2020. doi: 10.1016/j.jmapro.2020.10.027.
114. L. H. Gaabour, and K. A. Hamam, "The change of structural, optical and thermal properties of a PVDF/PVC blend containing ZnO nanoparticles," *Silicon*, vol. 10, no. 4, pp. 1403–1409, 2018. doi: 10.1007/s12633-017-9617-y.
115. M. Spasova, N. Manolova, N. Markova, and I. Rashkov, "Tuning the properties of PVDF or PVDF-HFP fibrous materials decorated with ZnO nanoparticles by applying electrospinning alone or in conjunction with electrospraying," *Fibers Polym.*, vol. 18, no. 4, pp. 649–657, 2017. doi: 10.1007/s12221-017-1189-3.
116. R. S. Sabry, and A. D. Hussein, "PVDF: ZnO/BaTiO3 as high out-put piezoelectric nanogenerator," *Polym. Test.*, vol. 79, no. July, 2019, doi: 10.1016/j.polymertesting.2019.106001.
117. W. Deng, Y. Zhou, A. Libanori, G. Chen, W. Yang, and J. Chen, "Piezoelectric nanogenerators for personalized healthcare," *Chem. Soc. Rev.*, vol. 51, no. 9, 2022. doi: 10.1039/d1cs00858g.

7 Biomaterial-driven Differentiation and Maturation of Cardiomyocytes

Advancements in Cardiac Tissue Engineering

Kannan Badri Narayanan, Surya Prakash Pandey, Sung Soo Han, and Mukesh Kumar Gupta

7.1 INTRODUCTION

Cardiovascular diseases (CVDs) encompass a wide range of illnesses affecting the heart and blood vessels, contributing to a significant proportion of global mortality. In industrialized countries, CVDs account for approximately 31% of all fatalities, making them a leading cause of death [1]. These conditions, including coronary artery diseases (ischemia), myocardial infarction, and various forms of cardiomyopathy, not only impose a heavy financial burden but also result in significant morbidity and mortality worldwide. CVDs cause injury to cardiac tissues, which have a limited capacity for regeneration, often leading to the development of non-functional scar tissue that impairs the heart's ability to contract, eventually leading to heart failure [2, 3]. Current therapeutic approaches for CVDs include pharmacological treatments, surgical interventions such as coronary artery bypass grafting and heart transplantation, and interventional techniques like angioplasty and stenting. While these methods can alleviate symptoms and improve survival, they often fail to fully restore cardiac function and are associated with significant risks and side effects. For example, chemical therapeutics, including pathway inhibitors, antiplatelet drugs, and blood thinners [4, 5]. Moreover, the limited availability of donor hearts severely restricts the use of transplantation as a viable treatment option [6–9]. Given the limited regenerative capacity of adult cardiomyocytes and the challenges posed by CVDs in replacing damaged heart tissue, there has been significant interest in developing alternative strategies, such as tissue engineering (TE). Cardiomyoplasty, an early approach that involved injecting various types of cardiac cells into the injured heart, faced several limitations, including high cell mortality, low retention rates, and adverse reactions such as inflammatory responses and myocardial damage. These challenges have driven the

DOI: 10.1201/9781003670995-7

exploration of more sophisticated TE techniques, where cardiomyocytes are seeded onto biodegradable scaffolds and implanted into the infarcted myocardium [10–12].

Cardiac tissue engineering (CTE) has emerged as a promising strategy for the replacement of impaired cardiomyocytes, offering a potential alternative to conventional therapies. However, the production of fully mature cardiomyocytes in vitro remains a significant challenge. One of the primary obstacles in CTE is the creation of complex cardiac structures that can replicate the functional properties of native heart tissue. An ideal biomaterial for CTE would be an injectable nanofiber scaffold with elasticity matching that of the native extracellular matrix (ECM), capable of supporting the rhythmic contraction and relaxation of the myocardium. Additionally, such a biomaterial should promote cell proliferation, immune compatibility, and differentiation into functional cardiomyocytes while possessing bioelectrical properties conducive to cardiac functions [13]. Recent advancements in biomaterials science have highlighted the potential of conducting-based polymers and piezoelectric nanomaterials (PNMs) in CTE applications. Conducting polymers can provide suitable ECM support and electrical stimulation for cardiac cells, facilitating the development of electrically active cardiac tissue. Cardiac patches based on these materials can be implanted into the heart, promoting electrical signaling and integration with host cells. PNMs, which generate electricity in response to mechanical stress, have shown promise in mimicking the mechanoelectrical transduction channels of cardiomyocytes, further enhancing the maturation and functionality of engineered cardiac tissues [14, 15].

This chapter explores the mechanistic role of biomaterials in the differentiation and maturation of cardiomyocytes, with a particular focus on the application of novel biomaterials such as conducting polymers and PNMs in CTE. It examines how these materials interact with cardiac cells at the molecular level, influencing signaling pathways, cellular organization, and the development of functional cardiac tissue. By understanding these mechanisms, researchers can design more effective biomaterials that closely replicate the native cardiac microenvironment, ultimately improving the outcomes of regenerative therapies for CVDs. The chapter also provides a comprehensive review of the latest advancements in stem cell therapy, CTE, and the novel piezoelectric strategies that hold promise for the treatment and management of CVDs [16–18]. The overview begins with a brief understanding of the physiological challenges associated with the regeneration of cardiac cells, followed by a discussion of the intrinsic piezoelectric properties of biological tissues. This article provides a comprehensive review on stem cell therapy, CTE, and novel piezoelectric strategy in the treatment and management of CVDs. Along with, we also discuss the most common ceramics and polymers used for electrospinning piezoelectric fibers for CTE.

7.2 CLASSICAL METHODS OF TREATMENT OF CARDIAC DISEASE

Current medications for CVDs incorporate conventional medical treatment and surgery [19]. Although Both strategies relieve symptoms and reduce mortality, the strategies have certain drawbacks [2, 6, 10, 15]. Routine drugs are less obtrusive but can impair the liver, kidneys, and other organs along with several side effects [20, 21]. Despite its incredible efficacy, the difficult procedure and potential post-operative problems have consistently limited the clinical applicability of heart surgery [21]. Subsequently, there is an urgent and neglected ought to create novel, helpful, and effective approaches to treat cardiovascular disease. Treatment of heart disease depends on its condition and severity. For instance, serious heart rhythm problems may require an implanted device like a pacemaker, whereas coronary illnesses may be treated with a change in lifestyle, medicine, and stent. The coronary stent has influenced on cardiovascular disease in recent years [20, 21]. It clearly emphasizes that improvements in both stent placement techniques and therapeutic medications, such as statins, beta-blockers, diuretics, and others, are crucial for the treatment of cardiovascular disease.

Drugs commonly utilized to treat heart diseases include anticoagulants, to diminish the blood's capacity to clot, and are utilized to treat certain vascular diseases and heartbeat disorders [22]. These medications help to prevent harmful blood clots from forming in blood arteries and can also prevent the clots from growing and leading to more serious issues with heart function. Drugs called pro-inhibitors have made blood vessels wider by lowering the amounts of hormones that control blood flow, lowering resistance, and enabling blood to circulate more efficiently throughout the body. Beta-blockers help to slow the heart rate and minimize the effects of adrenaline on the heart, lowering blood pressure and reducing the workload on the heart [23]. Other drugs based on Calcium (Ca) channel blockers unwind the vessels of the heart and cardiovascular system to moderate the heartbeat rate [24–26]. Our review highlights the difficulty of obtaining reflective drug molecules (ACE inhibitors, blockers, calcium channel blockers, thiazide/thiazide-like diuretics, and statins) from all of the key pharmacological classes used to treat CVD (Table 7.1). However, the effectiveness of the available early detection and improved treatment options for CVDs is limited and uncertain.

TABLE 7.1
Some Commonly Prescribed Medications for Cardiovascular Disease

S.No.	Medication Class	Medication Names	Purpose/Indication
1	Angiotensin-Converting Enzyme (ACE) Inhibitors	Ramipril, Enalapril, Lisinopril	Lower blood pressure, treat heart failure
2	Angiotensin II Receptor Blockers (ARBs)	Losartan, Valsartan, Olmesartan	Lower blood pressure, treat heart failure
3	Beta Blockers	Metoprolol, Atenolol, Carvedilol	Reduce heart rate and blood pressure
4	Calcium Channel Blockers	Amlodipine, Diltiazem, Verapamil	Relax blood vessels, lower blood pressure
5	Diuretics	Hydrochlorothiazide, Furosemide, Spironolactone	Reduce fluid buildup, lower blood pressure
6	Statins	Atorvastatin, Simvastatin, Rosuvastitin	Lower cholesterol levels
7	Antiplatelet Agents	Aspirin, Clopidogrel, Prasugrel	Prevent blood clots, reduce risk of heart attack
8	Anticoagulants	Warfarin, Apixaban, Rivaroxaban	Prevent blood clots, reduce stroke risk
9	Nitroglycerin	Nitroglycerin tablets, sprays	Relieve chest pain (angina)
10	Digoxin	Digoxin	Improve heart function, treat heart failure
11	Antiarrhythmics	Amiodarone, Flecainide, Propafenone	Control abnormal heart rhythms

7.3 STEM CELL THERAPY FOR CVDS

Current treatment and management strategies for CVDs, such as pharmacotherapy, cardiac resynchronization therapy, and implantable cardioverter-defibrillators, aim to slow down the progression of diseases, enhance systolic function, and prevent life-threatening arrhythmias. These approaches play a crucial role in improving patient outcomes and quality of life by effectively managing CVDs and reducing the associated risks. However, these methodologies fail to enhance the regeneration of cells to fulfill the damage of functional CMs [27, 28]. Recently, stem cell-based therapeutic strategies have created excitement by regenerating the cardiac tissues and replacing or rejuvenating the lost and damaged CMs [28–30]. These strategies for CMs regeneration have additional advantages and may improve the rate of recovery several folds [31]. The use of regenerative stem cell-based therapies becomes ideal for a number of issues affecting the heart, including complexity in its anatomical and functional structure, inability to recover from negative effects, and insufficient repair mechanisms (Figure 7.1).

However, effective cardiac repair strategies to treat cardiovascular disease remain very challenging. It is believed that mammalian CMs, very less proliferate however recent studies have revealed the capacity of differentiation in mature CMs [3, 4, 31, 33]. These findings have provided evidence of the existence of a self-renewing population of cardiac stem cells (CSCs) within the adult mammalian myocardium [4].

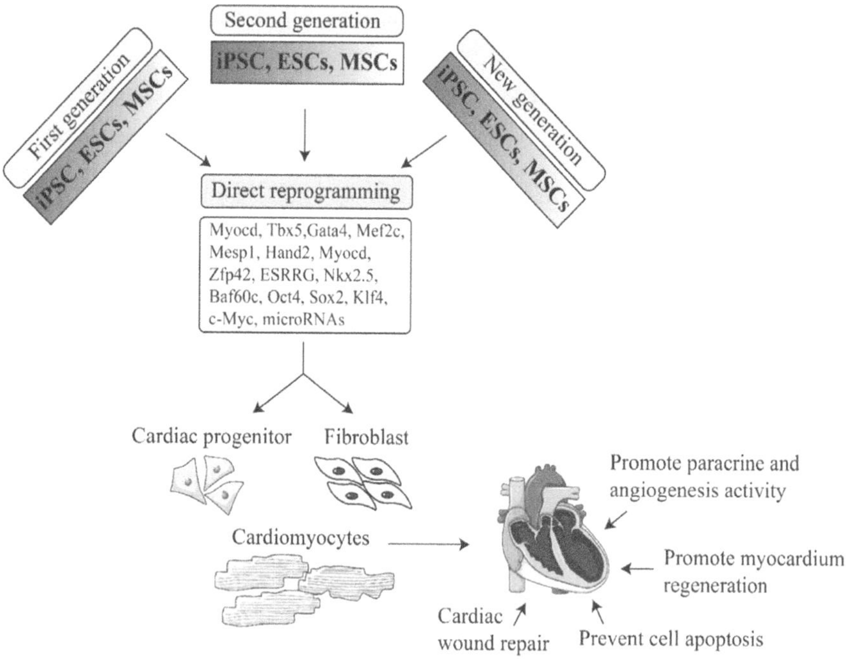

FIGURE 7.1 Reprogramming stem cells into cardiac muscle cells (CMs) and their role in heart repair. Reproduced with open access permission [32].

Various cell-based therapies are direct transplants into the myocardium, epicardial, and coronary arteries, which is suitable for chronic heart failure and acute myocardial infarction/MI patients [34, 35]. The bone mesenchymal stem cells (BMCs) moderately improved the left ventricle functions and decreased the diastolic volume, results suggest that the stem cells significantly improved the recovery in acute MI patients [36, 37]. The advantages of BMCs failed to identify the underlying stem cell mechanism of action, which would have allowed us to distinguish between the donor cells and the host myocardium. Although MSC therapy has the potential to cure cardiac disorders like MI in the future, its current use is severely constrained by biological and technological obstacles. Stem cell-based therapies do not promote myocardial regeneration largely because of more cell loss; lack of a sufficient ability of regeneration is one of the main issues [31, 36]. Many studies have shown that the majority of cells that are effectively transported to the heart die within the first few weeks. Another safety remains a principal concern with stem cell application in the repair of cardiac tissues.

In addition, after undergoing stem cell transplantation for cardiac healing, proarrhythmic consequences must be addressed from a safety perspective. Early therapeutic experiments performed with BM-derived stem cells have not yet shown proarrhythmic effects. However, it is unknown whether the proarrhythmic response is induced by an increase in the number of viable cells or an increase in the number of cells injected.

7.4 CARDIAC TISSUE ENGINEERING

The stem cell-based therapies remain concerned about the histocompatibility of regenerated CMs and stem cell-derived proarrhythmic substrates [38]. These concerns have limited the use of stem cell-based therapies in the treatment of CVDs. Stem cells on novel biomaterials and immune tolerance are emerging as promising strategies to overcome these limitations for CVDs management [13]. The CTE may provide more suitable therapeutic approaches for CVDs treatment. It aims to create contractile myocardial tissue to replace defects (due to congenital heart disease) or malfunctioning parts of the heart (due to MI) and guide heart repair. The primary targets of CTE are blood vessels, heart tissue, and heart valves. Although adult allogeneic and autologous stem cell transplants are found to be beneficial in select cardiac treatment cases, CTE has not yet been completely utilized for routine therapeutic practices. In order to produce grafts that can restore normal heart function, the best transplantation procedures for cardiac repair may need to use a variety of cell types and/or biomaterials. Additionally, they are also supported by the native myocardial ECM, and substitute materials used in TE must meet specific requirements in order to provide the right physical signals that activate gene regulatory networks and produce the desired structural and functional properties.

We firmly believe that TE will likely contribute significantly to the development of regenerative medicine. These procedures mostly involve the transplanting of stem cells that have been seeded on 3-D scaffolds and stimulated via mechanical, electrical, or chemical methods [39, 40]. These strategies are currently being employed to promote stem cell differentiation in tissue-engineered heart transplantation, which promotes the recovery of diseased CMs [41, 42]. An ideal scaffold in CTE is required to be a biodegradable, biocompatible, and biomimetic material that could create a live and functional construct for implantation into the host heart. Several bio-ingredients, polymers, and non-polymers have been used to fabricate the patches for CTE application [43].

7.5 IDEAL PROPERTY OF SCAFFOLDS

Developing standards for the successful replication of native tissue function is a key contest in the area of CTE, particularly given the rising demand for patient-relevant tissue models made from human stem cells. To generate certain in vivo responses and tissue development in designed tissues intended for transplantation, it is also necessary to tune biochemical characteristics, degradation kinetics, and bioactive components. We first need to precisely characterize the important morphology that constitutes normal physiological function in order to build biomimetic tissues that imitate cardiac function. It is a crucial characteristic of native tissue that artificial scaffolds must imitate to promote self-assembly, but the chemical and mechanical characteristics of native tissue also serve as design criteria for cardiac scaffolds.

This makes it clear that these materials must meet a number of criteria before fabricating CM scaffolds. This includes the capacity for the surface molecule to improve cell functions (grip, elongation, segregation, etc.). As shown in Figure 7.2, measurements of physical properties and functional outcomes are used to establish target values that serve as quality control measures to determine how closely scaffolds resemble their natural mimics.

Appropriate pore size (~10–100 μm) and pore connectivity are other requirements for scaffolds to allow proper growth of cells, developmental variables, supplements, and oxygen vascularization. They should also have an adequate biodegradation rate and high biocompatibility with a suitable rate within the CMs. The mechanical properties such as anisotropy, contractility (E ~ 0.2–0.5 MPa in systole and E ~ 0.01–0.02 MPa in diastole), and versatility are always considered to be important for scaffold in the application of CTE [45, 46].

Lastly, a balanced electrical conductivity (~10^5–10^3 S cm^{-1}) within the CMs is the most valuable parameter for fabricated scaffolds to empower and synchronize the bioelectrical properties in the host heart [47]. The unique intricacy of damaged heart tissue must be recreated, which is a significant challenge for the field of CTE [47]. A set of design criteria for the fabrication of cardiac tissue is based on three main features of native myocardium: (i) stem cell sources, (ii) electrical and mechanical stimulation (EMS), and (iii) design and fabrication of fiber scaffolds by using appropriate biomaterial. Here, we provide a general overview of some of the most pressing issues facing the area of CTE as well as some critical avenues for future research (Figure 7.3).

7.5.1 Stem Cell Sources for CTE

Therefore, an optimal stem cell source remains important for establishing a CTE application setup. Sources of stem cells are covered in this review for creating cardiac

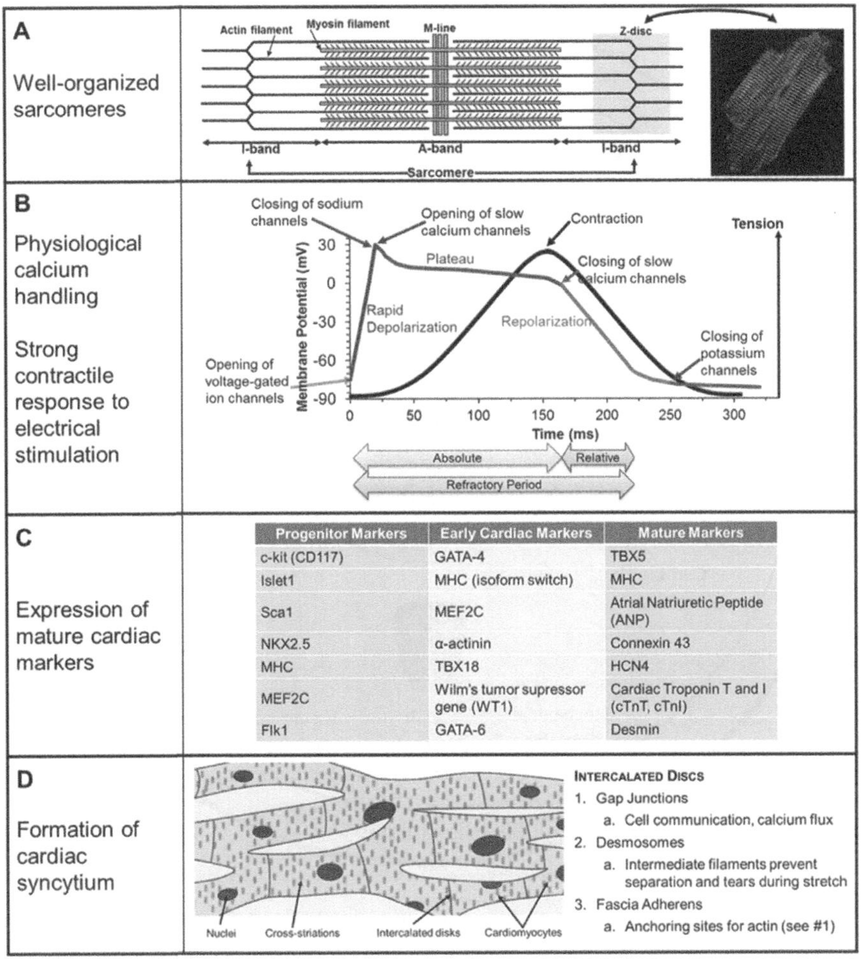

FIGURE 7.2 Valuable markers of CMs. (A) Well-structured sarcomeres are crucial for effective muscle contraction. (B) Physiological calcium regulation is essential for proper CMs function. The action potential activation aligns with the contractile apparatus, and the manipulation of cultured CMs can be achieved through electrical stimulation. (C) Assessing the expression of CM-specific markers (genes or proteins) provides a valuable method for determining whether a new biomaterial, culture conditions, or stimulation regimen promotes enhanced maturation compared to a control or static culture environment. (D) The coordination of contraction in the heart requires the formation of the cardiac syncytium. Reproduced with permission [44].

tissue constructions. Under ideal conditions, stem cells should be sufficient with their source and able to grow to beat CMs after transplantation. Various cell types such as embryonic stem cells (ESCs), iPSCs, mesenchymal stem cells (MSCs), and CSCs are important sources of stem cells which differentiated into CMs [49, 50]. In addition to muscles and non-muscle supporting cells, which include endothelial, fibroblasts are also required during CMs regeneration [51]. The biomaterials are used to create

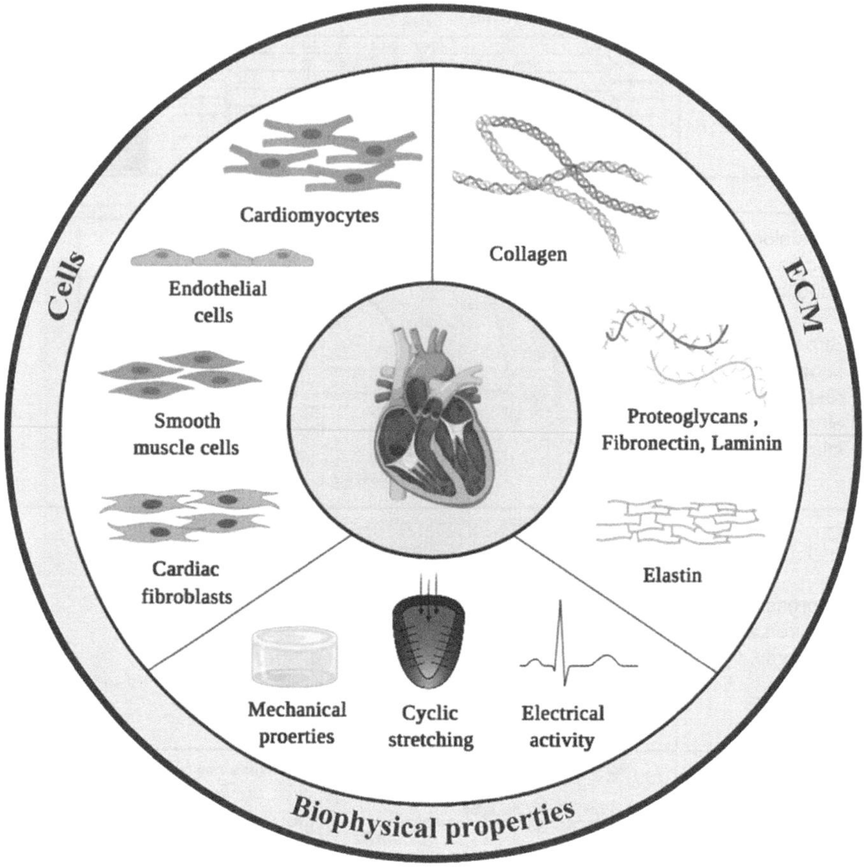

FIGURE 7.3 Schematic diagram of essential components is required for the fabrication of cardiac tissue in cardiac tissue engineering (CTE). Reproduced with permission from Ref. [48].

a scaffold that provides a 3-D physiological environment to optimize the support for accurate cellular attachment, growth, and proliferation to achieve functional cells. Additionally, cells on the scaffold can regenerate damaged cells with new ones and prevent anoikis and apoptosis, which improves cardiac function [52, 53]. Stem cells must coexist in harmony with the host's myocardium. This stem cell-myocardium could be grown on electrospun fibers, macro-porous scaffolds, or micro-templated scaffolds. These culture cells must be immune-compatible, non-allergic, and electrophysiologically suitable within the native heart tissue [53]. Utilizing adult stem cells from different sources has been encouraged by the benefits of alleviating concerns about immunological rejection or disease transmission. Although adult stem cells were first discovered in the bone marrow, more recent research has shown that they can also be found in adipose tissue, tooth pulp, circulating blood, amniotic fluid, and other extramedullary organs [54–61]. A subset of stem cell types, including ESCs, iPSCs, MSCs, and CSCs, may differentiate into beating CMs, replace the damaged

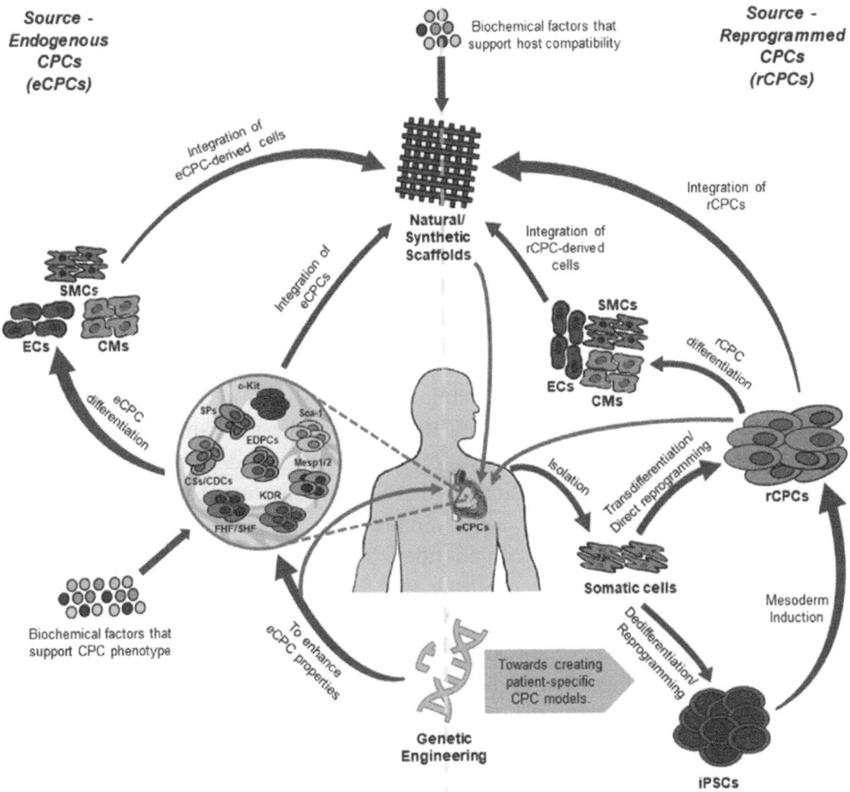

FIGURE 7.4 A subset of endogenous or reprogrammed cardiac progenitor cells (CPCs) can differentiate into beating CMs, replace the damaged myocardial tissue, and enhance cardiac function. Reproduced with permission [62].

myocardial tissue, and enhance cardiac function (Figure 7.4). The ability of stem cells to promote myogenesis but not necessarily vasculogenesis and the difficulty in electrical connection with cardiac myocytes are the main limitations. A potential approach to heart regeneration would be to mobilize native cardiac cells; however, obtaining enough of these cells remains challenging.

7.5.1.1 Embryonic Stem Cells (ESCs)

ESCs are proliferating pluripotent cells extracted from the inner cell mass of undifferentiated embryos. Recent studies have suggested that ESC-CMs distinguish mature CMs from other undifferentiated and undesirable cellular types, and reports have linked DNA methylation in ESCs to the discovery of novel regulators of cardiomyogenesis [63]. For CTE, the ESCs are the most valuable cell source due to their differentiation capacity into any other known cell types. The process of creating CMs from ESCs or iPSCs by adding differentiation stage-specific genes (Figure 7.5). Numerous research groups have succeeded in creating cardiac patches using ESCs, which could be placed directly into damaged regions of the host heart [64]. We still have concerns regarding moral issues as well as the possibility of immunogenicity rise on application of ESC-derived CMs, development of teratomas, and unregulated differentiation in CVDs therapeutic [65]. Due to the aforementioned problems, currently, the clinical application of CMs produced from ESC is essentially disallowed worldwide.

7.5.1.2 Induced Pluripotent Stem Cells (iPSCs)

Induced pluripotent stem cells (iPSCs) are used as a substitute of ESCs for CTE procedures because they are pluripotent stem cells that could be produced in vitro directly from somatic cells. A direct reprogramming of patient's autologous somatic cells could be used to produce iPSCs by employing different reprogramming factors. Human iPSCs have been differentiated into cardiac cells using histone deacetylase inhibitors, BMP4, trichostatin A (TSA), and activin A. Numerous investigations and research projects have begun using an alternative of iPSCs against ESCs in CVDs management and treatment on the basis of the published results [66]. As with the use of ESCs, fully reprogrammed iPSCs do not develop into a teratoma. In recent study that suggested cultivated iPSCs on an electrospun fiber, matrigel-coated, PCL-aligned nanofiber, which improved cellular proliferation, adhesion, and alignment over the matrix of nanofibers [67]. Shadrin et al. created 3-D iPSC cultures to differentiate CMs, resulting in enhanced electromechanical coupling and the expression of markers comparable to those found in adult myocardium [68]. Recently, using EMS methodologies, a laboratory-grown polypyrrole-coated PLGA fiber scaffold has been found to coordinate with electrical, mechanical, and topographical signals during the differentiation of human iPSCs into beating CMs. The sheet thickness remains a significant issue in cell sheet engineering, which is another important issue for CTE. However, utilizing temperature-responsive culture dishes, huge cardiac tissue sheets have been created. When these cardiac sheets were implanted in pig's infracted MCs, they were able to restore heart functions after the infarction. The iPSCs applications have the advantages of employing autologous cells, which reduces any possibility of immunological rejection and gets beyond the moral, legal, and social problems associated with ESCs [64, 69, 70]. However, the determination of the precise iPSCs reprogramming mechanisms, their functionalities after being reprogrammed and producing differentiated cells in *in vitro* settings is still challenging.

7.5.1.3 Mesenchymal Stem Cells (MSCs)

Several preclinical and clinical investigations have documented an effective role in the formation of CMs from MSCs [71]. The transplant of MSCs into cardiac patients has enhanced the left ventricle's volume and blood-pump efficiency. Recently, the researcher investigated the ability of menstrual- and bone marrow-derived MSCs to differentiate into CMs on Bombyx mori silk scaffolds to build cardiac patches with appropriate physical and mechanical properties during the CTE [72, 73]. Differentiation of MSCs into CMs has been achieved by using the pharmacological compounds (5-azacytidine and DMSO) as well as growth factors (BMP, angiotensin-II, platelet-derived growth factor, platelet-rich plasma (PRP), and TSA) [49, 50]. The nanofibers scaffolds made of hemoglobin, gelatin, and fibrinogen have been reported to differentiate MSCs into cardiac cells after being treated with

5-azacytidine. The MSCs-induced improved cardiac function is largely because of exosome generation, paracrine chemicals as well as immune response regulation.

7.5.1.4 Cardiac Stem Cells (CSCs)

A CSCs have multipotent and self-renewing properties, which allow the development of beating cardiac cells [74, 75]. CSCs are typically located in the atrium, where cell density remains relatively low (1 CSC/10,000 CMs). In the atrium, CSCs are mostly found in the neural crest and cardiac during fetal development [76, 77]. Unfortunately, due to their relatively low prevalence and the absence of genuine CSC-specific markers, isolation of pure CSC-population is still a challenge. The developing cardiac progenitor cells (CPCs) make CSCs have beneficial effects. Recently, cardiac cells have been grown on a nanofiber, and cardiac adipose tissue has inherent cardiac and angiogenic capacities [78, 79]. Recently, researcher was demonstrated to differentiate CSCs into beating CMs [80]. Combined administration of CSCs and pericytes restored heart muscle and vesicles by secreting various growth factors, angiopoietins, and microRNAs in infarcted mice [81, 82]. CSCs continue to be a highly argumentative issue in the field of CTE.

7.5.2 Electrical and Mechanical Phenomena

The bioelectricity is correlated to nearly all physical mechanisms in human, including muscular contraction, heartbeat, and neuronal activities, proving that bioelectrical phenomena are one of the most important fundamental life activities [83]. It was discovered in the early, many investigations have revealed that electric fields can modulate cell physiological behavioral mechanisms [84, 85]. EMS is an important bioelectrical phenomenon which is used as a physical therapy method to modulate the function and shape of muscle cells/tissues (Figure 7.5).

Recently, EMS has been widely used for therapeutic applications in wound healing, fracture repair, neuromuscular injury, and other clinical conditions [87–89]. The EMS promotes the release of angiogenic factors and reduces the inflammatory response in wound healing application [88], more recent advancements in the treatment of CVDs have been made through the EMS strategy. The EMS promotes angiogenesis, regulating autophagy, and apoptosis, inhibiting inflammatory responses and oxidative stress; it may therefore inhibit the development and progression of CVDs [44, 90]. The electromechanical connectivity in the CMs is extremely sensitive to ion concentration fluctuations in their transmembrane [90]. The electrical activities regulate excitation-contraction coupling mechanics in CMs by an intracellular calcium-dependent mechanism and ECM-based mechano-transduction pathways [91]. The contraction-relaxation activities of CMs for synchronous contraction are due to the membrane potential differences and action potential transfer through gap junctions [92]. The cytoplasmic calcium (Ca^{2+}) concentration encourages the sliding of actin-myosin filaments and CM-contraction and is required for the depolarization of the cell membrane [91, 93]. This behavior depends on the translation of environmental mechanical stresses into electrochemical signals that activate different signaling pathways [94]. The electrical transmembrane potential induces the opening and closure of voltage-gated ion channels that facilitates the entry of ions leading

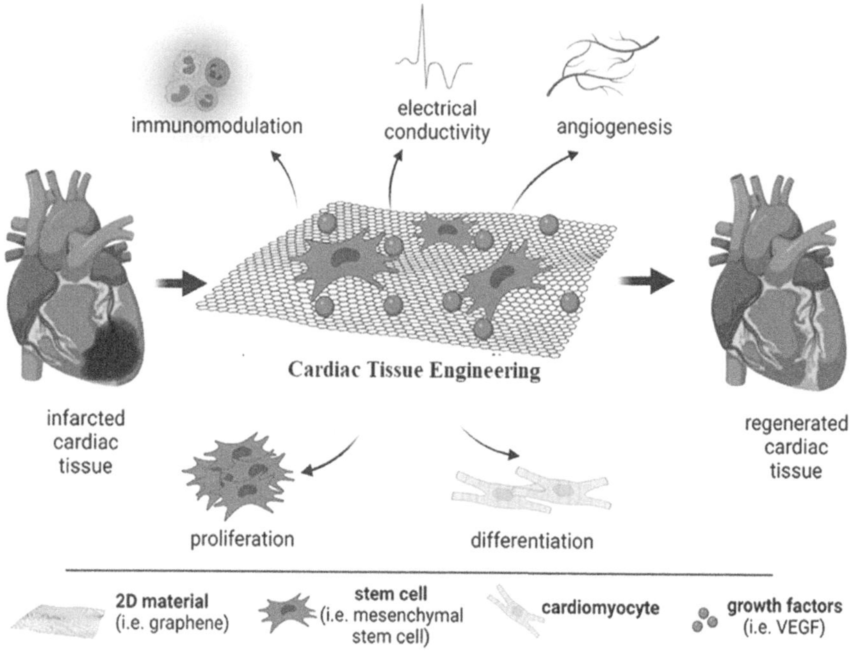

FIGURE 7.5 The strategy of electromechanical stimulation can facilitate the regeneration of damaged cardiac tissue. Reproduced with permission [86].

to depolarization [95]. This encourages transmembrane receptors integrins to link to various ECM-domains [91, 94]. These ECM-domains then translate external stimuli into various cellular functions like adhesion, differentiation, and maturation (Figure 7.6). The production of action potentials by ion influx/efflux across CMs' membranes serves to explain their electrical characteristics [96]. The membrane potential crosses the threshold of action potential (70 mV) and voltage-gated sodium (Na^+) channels open to depolarize the membrane [97]. Following the closure of Na^+ channels, voltage-gated L-type Ca^{2+} channels open and allow Ca^{2+} to diffuse into the cell [95]. EMS has been popularly applied in TE to improve muscle conduction and contractility [98]. Macrophages have been found to play roles in electrical conduction in the heart beyond the atrioventricular node, atrial fibrillation, and ischemic ventricular arrhythmias. CVD results in abnormal conduction of heart functions. Stimulation of the carotid artery affects blood flow to the site of myocardial ischemia to relieve angina. The atherosclerosis-induced narrowing of the coronary lumen causes up to 99% of CVDs cases, including myocardial ischemia and hypoxia pathophysiology. Currently, EMS is used to reduce myocardial ischemia-reperfusion injury [99]. EMS could also attenuate the macrophage inflammatory responses along with the reduction of lipid accumulation in adipose cells and atherosclerosis plaque areas. Though the specific mechanism of action EMS is still not much clear, it has provided a new frontier in the management for the treatment of CVDs. Electroactive polymers are fascinating smart biomaterials for CTE applications. A

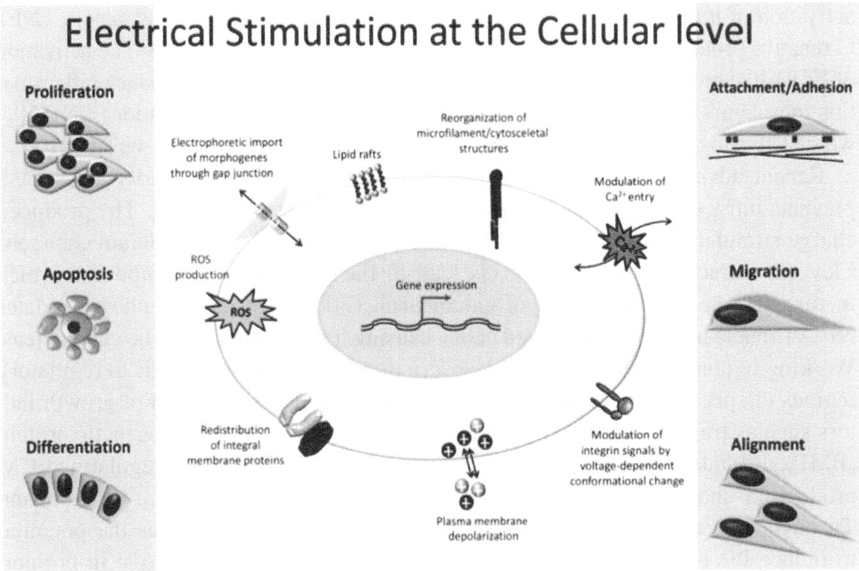

FIGURE 7.6 The strategy of electromechanical stimulation can facilitate cellular mechanisms such as proliferation, apoptosis, differentiation, and alignment of cardiac cells. Reproduced with permission [107].

direct application of EMS is feasible by using conductive polymers, such as poly (aniline), poly(pyrrole), poly(3,4-ethyl-enedioxythiophene), etc., for the fabrication of smart cardiac patches. However, when cells come into contact with them, they may disrupt the normal signaling process. Furthermore, conductive polymers have a drawback in that they are not compatible with high throughput platforms as they require external energy sources for the electrical activation of cells.

On the other hand, piezoelectric materials may overcome this limitation by inducing EMS in cells through mechanoelectrical transduction. These materials respond to environmental cues and function similarly to ECM. The cardiac ECM undergoes constant remodeling and adaptation in response to the environment, influencing the cellular organization and myofibril extension, which makes it a highly dynamic structure [100]. Piezoelectric materials have been employed extensively in energy generation and harvesting, sensing, and actuation applications [101]. This approach has recently shifted its focus toward the design and fabrication of scaffolds, including cardiac patches, nanofibers, and hydrogels, that incorporate piezoelectric properties. Additionally, there is limited information on how piezoelectric properties affect cardiac regeneration.

7.5.3 EMS Based Mechanism

This enhances the reparative effect on damaged CMs and myocardial functions. As a result, EMS regulates multiple signaling pathways in CMs and holds potential in the treatment of CVDs [102]. The prevention of myocardial hypertrophy in rats by EMS stimulation is correlated with the modulation of the ERK signaling pathway [103]. The activation of inflammatory pathways was effect to alter tumor necrosis factor (TNF), C-reactive protein, interleukin 1 beta (IL-1β), and interleukin 6 (IL-6). The activation of NOD-like receptor family protein 3 (NLRP3) is also reported to enhance inflammation in ischemic CM tissue [104]. EMS might be modulating the activation of NLRP3, which helps to maintain the inflammatory homeostasis in ischemic tissue [105, 106].

Recent advancements in CVDs management have provided evidence of EMS prevents intracellular Ca^+ and maintaining Ca^+ homeostasis [93, 94]. The produced charge stimulates the cell electrically, which opens voltage-gated calcium channels. Elevated intracellular calcium levels lead to the activation of calmodulin, which in turn triggers the activation of calcineurin. Calcineurin then dephosphorylates NF-AT (nuclear factor of activated cells), causing it to translocate to the cell nucleus. Working in conjunction with other transcription factors, NF-AT binds to regulatory regions of specific genes, including those involved in the production of growth factors such as transforming growth factor β (TGFβ) and bone morphogenetic protein (BMP), ultimately promoting their translation. They are involved in regulating ECM production and up/down-regulation of several proteins and cellular metabolism. Through the calcium/calmodulin pathway, electrical stimulation has the potential to induce the production of TGF-β, which in turn plays a crucial role in promoting various cellular activities including divisions, differentiation, ECM synthesis, etc. The diverse effects of TGF-β can be attributed to its involvement in modulating several common regulatory pathways responsible for regulating cellular events, either by inhibition or stimulation. Another mechanism involves the regulation of neuroendocrine pathways to anticipate myocardial hypertrophy. Though the exact neuroendocrine pathways of actions are unclear, it is believed that angiotensin II and endothelin regulate the ERK signaling pathway to induce anti-apoptotic effects in CMs [108, 109]. Therefore, further investigations will provide newer insights into EMS-induced regulation of apoptosis [110]. In addition to apoptosis, recent investigations have reported that EMS stimulates FGF2 secretion and facilitates the angiogenesis in endothelial cells of the umbilical vein through the MAPK/ERK signaling pathway [111]. In addition, the VEGF gene expression is also reported to upregulate in skeletal muscles of electrically stimulated rats. EMS also enhances the proangiogenic response of vascular endothelial cells through VEGF receptors. In ischemic myocardium, the EMS of 25 Hz and 50 Hz voltage may promote the VEGF expression and induce capillary angiogenesis [112, 113]. Further studies are required to provide more insights into specific actions of EMS on angiogenesis as well as VEGF and FGF2 downstream pathways [114]. This may provide a new, practically simple, and cost-effective method to enhance angiogenesis in ischemic myocardium. Restoration of cardiac contractile function requires electromechanical connection of cells to the host myocardium with synchronized contractile activity.

7.5.4 Advance Nanofibers Based on Piezoelectricity

Traditional TE approaches involve fabricating scaffolds to grow tissue-like structures. The process entails scaffold fabrication, in vitro cell seeding to generate the tissue, and subsequent implantation. Metrics are established at each stage to ensure success in TE applications.

These include evaluating the mechanical and chemical characteristics of the initial scaffold, assessing the effectiveness of the seeded cells, and considering the ultimate purpose of the implantation in vivo. Notably, we also discuss the crucial structural and functional properties of the myocardium and heart valves, providing evidence for the design and fabrication strategies in CTE.

The myocardium is surrounded by epiphyseal fibers, while myocardial cells are surrounded by perimysial fibers, and individual myocardial cells are encircled by endomysial fibers (Figure 7.2A). Myofibers consist of chains of contractile cardiomyocytes that maintain electrical continuity and are physically connected by intercalary discs with gap junctions, which are enveloped in peri-muscular ECM (Figure 7.2A). Electrical and mechanical stimulation also play vital roles in promoting cardiomyocyte proliferation by activating gene regulatory networks in cardiac development [84, 90]. This provides a design framework for synthetic fiber scaffolds that can recover normal function following an injury or illness. Nanofiber scaffolds can be used to mimic the myocardium's distinctive anisotropic tissue architecture [115]. It has been demonstrated that dissecting the heart reveals a spiral layer pattern of fibrous components that are hierarchically arranged. Nanofibers have a wide range of applications in the field of CTE because of their special qualities, including their enhanced surface-to-volume ratio, ease of mimicry of ECM because of their nanometer size, tiny pore size, lack of hazardous solvents, and flexibility in surface functions [116, 117].

Numerous researchers have studied various nanofibers for their application in CTE [116, 118–120]. In recent years, aligned nanofibers have been found to have a greater potential for application in CTE because of their structured and anisotropic nature, which provides topographical similarities to the ECM of host heart muscles [121]. Compared to random nanofibers, aligned nanofibers can also produce directed orientation in heart cells. The unidirectional nature of CMs, favored by nanofibers to offer a native milieu toward synchronized beating, is one of its key properties explored during the application of nanofiber-based CTE [98].

A novel and fascinating strategy offers significant potential for smart CTE strategies. Additionally, piezoelectric nanofibers are gaining popularity in TE applications because they act as stimuli-responsive (known as "smart") scaffolds and deliver electrical stimulation to promote tissue regeneration [122]. Cell contact signaling and mechanical support are facilitated by sub-micrometer fibers, such as those created through electrospinning, which can mimic the structure of fibrous proteins in the ECM. The development of piezoelectric scaffolds makes it feasible to stimulate, deform, and produce electricity for CMs sown on these scaffolds, thus accelerating their growth [14]. The piezoelectric scaffolds can faithfully replicate cardiac electromechanical behavior through a closed-loop system. These innovations hold significant potential for creating functional cardiac tissues, offering promising avenues for improved treatments of CVDs through more effective and biomimetic regenerative therapies [123].

7.6 CONCLUSION

Traditional treatment options, while successful in symptom management and life extension, carry significant dangers and side effects. Pharmacological medications such as angiotensin-converting enzyme (ACE) inhibitors, beta-blockers, and anticoagulants, while necessary for CVD management, have risks such as liver damage, bleeding, and hypersensitivity reactions. Furthermore, the scarcity of donor hearts significantly limits heart transplantation as a long-term option for many patients. This has led to an increased interest in alternative therapeutic strategies, particularly in the field of regenerative medicine and TE.

CTE represents a promising frontier in the treatment of CVDs. This approach involves the development of functional cardiac tissues through the use of biodegradable scaffolds seeded with cardiomyocytes, which can potentially replace damaged heart tissue and restore normal cardiac function. However, the production of fully mature cardiomyocytes in vitro remains a significant challenge. The complexity of replicating the intricate structure and function of native heart tissue, particularly in terms of electrical conductivity and mechanical properties, has been a major obstacle in the field. Stem cell therapy is another area of significant interest. The potential to regenerate damaged cardiac tissue using stem cells offers a promising alternative to traditional treatments. However, challenges remain, particularly concerning the histocompatibility of regenerated cells, the risk of proarrhythmic effects, and the difficulty in ensuring the survival and functional integration of transplanted cells. Despite these challenges, ongoing research into the use of stem cells, particularly in combination with advanced biomaterials, holds great potential for the future of CVD treatment.

Recent advancements in biomaterials have provided new opportunities for CTE. The development of conducting polymers has shown great promise in creating more effective scaffolds for cardiac tissue regeneration. Conducting polymers can mimic the electrical properties of native cardiac tissue, facilitating the development of electrically active cardiac constructs. These materials not only support the structural integrity of engineered tissues but also enhance their functional properties, potentially leading to better integration with host tissues and improved outcomes for patients. These approaches offer hope for not only alleviating the symptoms of CVDs but also addressing the underlying causes by regenerating damaged heart tissue, potentially transforming the future of cardiovascular medicine.

REFERENCES

1. H. C. Kim, "Epidemiology of cardiovascular disease and its risk factors in Korea," *Glob. Heal. Med.*, vol. 3, no. 3, pp. 134–141, 2021. doi: 10.35772/ghm.2021.01008.
2. O. Bergmann, R. D. Bhardwaj, S. Bernard, S. Zdunek, F. Barnabé-Heider, S. Walsh, J. Zupicich, K. Alkass, B. A. Buchholz, H. Druid, and S. Jovinge, "Evidence for cardiomyocyte renewal in humans," *Science*, vol. 324, no. 5923, 2009, pp. 98–102. doi:10.1126/science.1164680.
3. R. Gong, Z. Jiang, N. Zagidullin, T. Liu, and B. Cai, "Regulation of cardiomyocyte fate plasticity: A key strategy for cardiac regeneration," *Signal Transduct. Target. Ther.*, vol. 6, no. 1, 2021. doi: 10.1038/s41392-020-00413-2.
4. M. F. Tenreiro, A. F. Louro, P. M. Alves, and M. Serra, "Next generation of heart regenerative therapies: Progress and promise of cardiac tissue engineering," *npj Regen. Med.*, vol. 6, no. 1, 2021. doi: 10.1038/s41536-021-00140-4.
5. S. Francula-Zaninovic, and I. A. Nola, "Management of measurable variable cardiovascular disease' risk factors," *Curr. Cardiol. Rev.*, vol. 14, no. 3, pp. 153–163, 2018. doi: 10.2174/1573403x14666180222102312.

6. J. N. Cohn, "Prevention of cardiovascular disease," *Trends Cardiovasc. Med.*, vol. 25, no. 5, pp. 436–442, 2015. doi: 10.1016/j.tcm.2014.12.005.
7. P. W. Siri-Tarino, and R. M. Krauss, "Diet, lipids, and cardiovascular disease," *Curr. Opin. Lipidol.*, vol. 27, no. 4, pp. 323–328, 2016. doi: 10.1097/MOL.0000000000000310.
8. S. Costantino, F. Paneni, and F. Cosentino, "Ageing, metabolism and cardiovascular disease," *J. Physiol.*, vol. 594, no. 8, pp. 2061–2073, 2016. doi: 10.1113/JP270538.
9. D. P. Leong et al., "Reducing the global burden of cardiovascular disease, part 2: Prevention and treatment of cardiovascular disease," *Circ. Res.*, vol. 121, no. 6, pp. 695–710, 2017. doi: 10.1161/CIRCRESAHA.117.311849.
10. T. Reffelmann, and R. A. Kloner, "Cellular cardiomyoplasty - cardiomyocytes, skeletal myoblasts, or stem cells for regenerating myocardium and treatment of heart failure?" *Cardiovasc. Res.*, vol. 58, no. 2, pp. 358–368, 2003. doi: 10.1016/S0008-6363(02)00739-3.
11. E. A. Bocchi, "Cardiomyoplasty for treatment of heart failure," *Eur. J. Heart Fail.*, vol. 3, no. 4, pp. 403–406, 2001. doi: 10.1016/S1388-9842(01)00162-3.
12. T. Akita, and K. Bando, "Cardiomyoplasty for treatment of heart failure," *Nippon Rinsho. Japanese J. Clin. Med.*, vol. 65, no. Suppl 5, pp. 231–235, 2007.
13. Y. Zhao, G. Eng, B. W. Lee, M. Radisic, and G. Vunjak-Novakovic, *Cardiac tissue engineering*, INC, 2020. doi: 10.1016/B978-0-12-818422-6.00033-2.
14. M. R. Gomes, F. Castelo Ferreira, and P. Sanjuan-Alberte, "Electrospun piezoelectric scaffolds for cardiac tissue engineering," *Biomater. Adv.*, vol. 137, no. March, p. 212808, 2022. doi: 10.1016/j.bioadv.2022.212808.
15. N. A. Kamel, "Bio-piezoelectricity: Fundamentals and applications in tissue engineering and regenerative medicine," *Biophys. Rev.*, vol. 14, no. 3, pp. 717–733, 2022. doi: 10.1007/s12551-022-00969-z.
16. R. Balint, N. J. Cassidy, and S. H. Cartmell, "Electrical stimulation: A novel tool for tissue engineering," *Tissue Eng. - Part B Rev.*, vol. 19, no. 1, pp. 48–57, 2013. doi: 10.1089/ten.teb.2012.0183.
17. C. Ribeiro, V. Sencadas, D. M. Correia, and S. Lanceros-Méndez, "Piezoelectric polymers as biomaterials for tissue engineering applications," *Colloids Surf. B Biointerfaces*, vol. 136, pp. 46–55, 2015. doi: 10.1016/j.colsurfb.2015.08.043.
18. N. Tandon et al., "Electrical stimulation systems for cardiac tissue engineering," *Nat. Protoc.*, vol. 4, no. 2, pp. 155–173, 2009. doi: 10.1038/nprot.2008.183.
19. P. Joseph et al., "Reducing the global burden of cardiovascular disease, part 1: The epidemiology and risk factors," *Circ. Res.*, vol. 121, no. 6, pp. 677–694, 2017. doi: 10.1161/CIRCRESAHA.117.308903.
20. M. Simons, and J. A. Ware, "Therapeutic angiogenesis in cardiovascular disease," *Nat. Rev. Drug Discov.*, vol. 2, no. 11, pp. 863–871, 2003. doi: 10.1038/nrd1226.
21. R. C. Neely, M. Leacche, C. R. Byrne, A. V. Norman, and J. G. Byrne, "New approaches to cardiovascular surgery," *Curr. Probl. Cardiol.*, vol. 39, no. 12, pp. 427–466, 2014. doi: 10.1016/j.cpcardiol.2014.07.006.
22. M. Xu, and J. Song, "Targeted therapy in cardiovascular disease: A precision therapy era," *Front. Pharmacol.*, vol. 12, no. April, pp. 1–21, 2021. doi: 10.3389/fphar.2021.623674.
23. E. Priel et al., "The impact of beta blockade on the cardio-respiratory system and symptoms during exercise," *Curr. Res. Physiol.*, vol. 4, pp. 235–242, 2021. doi: 10.1016/j.crphys.2021.10.002.
24. A. M. Katz, "Calcium channel diversity in the cardiovascular system," *J. Am. Coll. Cardiol.*, vol. 28, no. 2, pp. 522–529, 1996. doi: 10.1016/0735-1097(96)00170-2.
25. W. J. Elliott, and C. V. S. Ram, "Calcium channel blockers," *J. Clin. Hypertens.*, vol. 13, no. 9, pp. 687–689, 2011. doi: 10.1111/j.1751-7176.2011.00513.x.
26. T. Godfraind, "Calcium channel blockers in cardiovascular pharmacotherapy," *J. Cardiovasc. Pharmacol. Ther.*, vol. 19, no. 6, pp. 501–515, 2014. doi: 10.1177/1074248414530508.

27. B. Lukomska, L. Stanaszek, E. Zuba-Surma, P. Legosz, S. Sarzynska, and K. Drela, "Challenges and controversies in human mesenchymal stem cell therapy," *Stem Cells Int., Vol.* 2019, 2019. doi: 10.1155/2019/9628536.
28. L. Huang, W. Ma, Y. Ma, D. Feng, H. Chen, and B. Cai, "Exosomes in mesenchymal stem cells, a new therapeutic strategy for cardiovascular diseases?" *Int. J. Biol. Sci.*, vol. 11, no. 2, pp. 238–245, 2015. doi: 10.7150/ijbs.10725.
29. J. Hoover-Plow, and Y. Gong, "Challenges-for-stem-cell-therapy-for-heart-disease," *Vasc. Health Risk Manag.*, vol. 8, pp. 99–113, 2012.
30. Y. Guo, Y. Yu, S. Hu, Y. Chen, and Z. Shen, "The therapeutic potential of mesenchymal stem cells for cardiovascular diseases," *Cell Death Dis.*, vol. 11, no. 5, 2020. doi: 10.1038/s41419-020-2542-9.
31. L. Hou, J. J. Kim, Y. J. Woo, and N. F. Huang, "Stem cell-based therapies to promote angiogenesis in ischemic cardiovascular disease," *Am. J. Physiol. - Hear. Circ. Physiol.*, vol. 310, no. 4, pp. H455–H465, 2016. doi: 10.1152/ajpheart.00726.2015.
32. M. I. Nasser et al., "Current situation and future of stem cells in cardiovascular medicine," *Biomed. Pharmacother.*, vol. 132, p. 110813, 2020. doi: 10.1016/j.biopha.2020.110813.
33. G. Vunjak-Novakovic et al., "Challenges in cardiac tissue engineering," *Tissue Eng. Part B. Rev.*, vol. 16, no. 2, pp. 169–187, 2010. doi: 10.1089/ten.teb.2009.0352.
34. M. Gyöngyösi, P. M. Haller, D. J. Blake, and E. M. Rendon, "Meta-analysis of cell therapy studies in heart failure and acute myocardial infarction," *Circ. Res.*, vol. 123, no. 2, pp. 301–308, 2018. doi: 10.1161/CIRCRESAHA.117.311302.
35. M. M. Micheu, and M. Dorobantu, "Fifteen years of bone marrow mononuclear cell therapy in acute myocardial infarction," *World J. Stem Cells*, vol. 9, no. 4, pp. 68–76, 2017. doi: 10.4252/wjsc.v9.i4.68.
36. P. Menasché, "Cell therapy trials for heart regeneration — Lessons learned and future directions," *Nat. Rev. Cardiol.*, vol. 15, no. 11, pp. 659–671, 2018. doi: 10.1038/s41569-018-0013-0.
37. K. Malliaras, M. Kreke, and E. Marbán, "The stuttering progress of cell therapy for heart disease," *Clin. Pharmacol. Ther.*, vol. 90, no. 4, pp. 532–541, 2011. doi: 10.1038/clpt.2011.175.
38. N. Naumova, and L. Iop, "Bioengineering the cardiac conduction system: Advances in cellular, gene, and tissue engineering for heart rhythm regeneration," *Front. Bioeng. Biotechnol.*, vol. 9, no. August, pp. 1–21, 2021. doi: 10.3389/fbioe.2021.673477.
39. N. Bursac et al., "Cardiac muscle tissue engineering: Toward an in vitro model for electrophysiological studies," *Am. J. Physiol. - Hear. Circ. Physiol.*, vol. 277, no. 2, pp. 46–2, 1999. doi: 10.1152/ajpheart.1999.277.2.h433.
40. A. Hussain, G. Collins, D. Yip, and C. H. Cho, "Functional 3-D cardiac co-culture model using bioactive chitosan nanofiber scaffolds," *Biotechnol. Bioeng.*, vol. 110, no. 2, pp. 637–647, 2013. doi: 10.1002/bit.24727.
41. N. Abbasi, A. Abdal-Hay, S. Hamlet, E. Graham, and S. Ivanovski, "Effects of gradient and offset architectures on the mechanical and biological properties of 3-D melt electrowritten (MEW) scaffolds," *ACS Biomater. Sci. Eng.*, vol. 5, no. 7, pp. 3448–3461, 2019. doi: 10.1021/acsbiomaterials.8b01456.
42. N. Bursac, Y. Loo, K. Leong, and L. Tung, "Novel anisotropic engineered cardiac tissues: Studies of electrical propagation," *Biochem. Biophys. Res. Commun.*, vol. 361, no. 4, pp. 847–853, 2007. doi: 10.1016/j.bbrc.2007.07.138.
43. L. L. Y. Chiu, and M. Radisic, "Cardiac tissue engineering," *Curr. Opin. Chem. Eng.*, vol. 2, no. 1, pp. 41–52, 2013. doi: 10.1016/j.coche.2013.01.002.
44. W. L. Stoppel, D. L. Kaplan, and L. D. Black, "Electrical and mechanical stimulation of cardiac cells and tissue constructs," *Adv. Drug Deliv. Rev.*, vol. 96, pp. 135–155, 2016. doi: 10.1016/j.addr.2015.07.009.

45. J. Radhakrishnan, U. M. Krishnan, and S. Sethuraman, "Hydrogel based injectable scaffolds for cardiac tissue regeneration," *Biotechnol. Adv.*, vol. 32, no. 2, pp. 449–461, 2014. doi: 10.1016/j.biotechadv.2013.12.010.
46. C. Xu et al., "Optimizing anisotropic polyurethane scaffolds to mechanically match with native myocardium," *ACS Biomater. Sci. Eng.*, vol. 6, no. 5, pp. 2757–2769, 2020. doi: 10.1021/acsbiomaterials.9b01860.
47. P. Shokrollahi, Y. Omidi, and L. X. Cubeddu, "Conductive polymers for cardiac tissue engineering and regeneration," no. January, pp. 1–17, 2023. doi: 10.1002/jbm.b.35293.
48. P. Montero et al., "Cells, materials, and fabrication processes for cardiac tissue engineering," *Front. Bioeng. Biotechnol.*, vol. 8, no. August, 2020. doi: 10.3389/fbioe.2020.00955.
49. M. Mazzola, and E. Di Pasquale, "Toward cardiac regeneration: Combination of pluripotent stem cell-based therapies and bioengineering strategies," *Front. Bioeng. Biotechnol.*, vol. 8, no. May, 2020. doi: 10.3389/fbioe.2020.00455.
50. V. Russo, S. Young, A. Hamilton, B. G. Amsden, and L. E. Flynn, "Mesenchymal stem cell delivery strategies to promote cardiac regeneration following ischemic injury," *Biomaterials*, vol. 35, no. 13, pp. 3956–3974, 2014. doi: 10.1016/j.biomaterials.2014.01.075.
51. M. Xin, E. N. Olson, and R. Bassel-Duby, "Mending broken hearts: Cardiac development as a basis for adult heart regeneration and repair," *Nat. Rev. Mol. Cell Biol.*, vol. 14, no. 8, pp. 529–541, 2013. doi: 10.1038/nrm3619.
52. K. Kikuchi, and K. D. Poss, "Cardiac regenerative capacity and mechanisms". Annual review of cell and developmental biology, vol. 28, pp. 719–741, doi: 10.1146/annurev-cellbio-101011-155739.
53. H. Pawani, and D. Bhartiya, "Pluripotent stem cells for cardiac regeneration: Overview of recent advances & emerging trends," *Indian J. Med. Res.*, vol. 137, no. 2, pp. 270–282, 2013.
54. S. Ghosh et al., "Neurological insights into brain-targeted cancer therapy and bioinspired microrobots," *Drug Discov. Today*, vol. 29, no. 9, p. 104105, 2024. doi: 10.1016/j.drudis.2024.104105.
55. S. Ghosh, S. Ghosh, H. Sharma, R. Bhaskar, S. S. Han, and J. K. Sinha, "Harnessing the power of biological macromolecules in hydrogels for controlled drug release in the central nervous system: A review," *Int. J. Biol. Macromol.*, vol. 254, no. P1, p. 127708, 2024. doi: 10.1016/j.ijbiomac.2023.127708.
56. A. Nagayach, R. Bhaskar, S. Ghosh, K. Kumar, S. Soo, and J. Kumar, "Advancing the understanding of diabetic encephalopathy through unravelling pathogenesis and exploring future treatment perspectives," *Ageing Res. Rev.*, vol. 100, no. June, p. 102450, 2024. doi: 10.1016/j.arr.2024.102450.
57. P. Sachdeva, K. Badri, J. Kumar, and S. Gupta, "Recent advances in drug delivery systems targeting insulin signalling for the treatment of Alzheimer's disease," *J. Alzheimer's Dis.*, vol. 98, pp. 1169–1179, 2024. doi: 10.3233/JAD-231181.
58. K. B. Narayanan, R. Bhaskar, K. Sudhakar, D. H. Nam, and S. S. Han, "Polydopamine-functionalized bacterial cellulose as hydrogel scaffolds for skin tissue engineering," *Gels*, vol. 9, no. 8, pp. 1–16, 2023. doi: 10.3390/gels9080656.
59. B. Sachdeva et al., "Chitosan nanoparticles-based cancer drug delivery: Application and challenges," *Mar. Drugs*, vol. 21, no. 4, pp. 1–23, 2023. doi: 10.3390/md21040211.
60. P. Sachdeva, S. Ji, S. Ghosh, S. Ghosh, and M. Raghunath, "Plausible role of stem cell types for treating and understanding the pathophysiology of depression," *Pharmaceutics*, vol. 15, 814, pp. 1–15, 2023. doi: 10.3390/pharmaceutics15030814.
61. Y. P. Singh et al., "Gelatin/monetite electrospun scaffolds to regenerate bone tissue: Fabrication, characterization, and in-vitro evaluation," *J. Mech. Behav. Biomed. Mater.*, vol. 137, no. October 2022, p. 105524, 2023. doi: 10.1016/j.jmbbm.2022.105524.
62. S. Barreto, L. Hamel, T. Schiatti, Y. Yang, and V. George, "Cardiac progenitor cells from stem cells: Learning from genetics and biomaterials," *Cells*, vol. 8, no. 12, pp. 1–55, 2019. doi: 10.3390/cells8121536.

63. J. Hescheler et al., "Embryonic stem cells: A model to study structural and functional properties in cardiomyogenesis," *Cardiovasc. Res.*, vol. 36, no. 2, pp. 149–162, 1997. doi: 10.1016/S0008-6363(97)00193-4.
64. W. Faiella, and R. Atoui, "Therapeutic use of stem cells for cardiovascular disease," *Clin. Transl. Med.*, vol. 5, no. 1, 2016. doi: 10.1186/s40169-016-0116-3.
65. M. Habib, O. Caspi, and L. Gepstein, "Human embryonic stem cells for cardiomyogenesis," *J. Mol. Cell. Cardiol.*, vol. 45, no. 4, pp. 462–474, 2008. doi: 10.1016/j.yjmcc.2008.08.008.
66. A. A. Youssef, E. G. Ross, R. Bolli, C. J. Pepine, N. J. Leeper, and P. C. Yang, "The promise and challenge of induced pluripotent stem cells for cardiovascular applications," *JACC Basic to Transl. Sci.*, vol. 1, no. 6, pp. 510–523, 2016. doi: 10.1016/j.jacbts.2016.06.010.
67. P. Pushp, R. Bhaskar, S. Kelkar, N. Sharma, D. Pathak, and M. K. Gupta, "Plasticized poly(vinylalcohol) and poly(vinylpyrrolidone) based patches with tunable mechanical properties for cardiac tissue engineering applications," *Biotechnol. Bioeng.*, vol. 118, no. 6, pp. 2312–2325, 2021. doi: 10.1002/bit.27743.
68. P. Dell'Era, "Cardiac disease modeling using induced pluripotent stem cell-derived human cardiomyocytes," *World J. Stem Cells*, vol. 7, no. 2, p. 329, 2015. doi: 10.4252/wjsc.v7.i2.329.
69. I. Karakikes, M. Ameen, V. Termglinchan, and J. C. Wu, "Human induced pluripotent stem cell-derived cardiomyocytes: Insights into molecular, cellular, and functional phenotypes," *Circ. Res.*, vol. 117, no. 1, pp. 80–88, 2015. doi: 10.1161/CIRCRESAHA.117.305365.
70. M. Mercola, A. Colas, and E. Willems, "Induced pluripotent stem cells in cardiovascular drug discovery," *Circ. Res.*, vol. 112, no. 3, pp. 534–548, 2013. doi: 10.1161/CIRCRESAHA.111.250266.
71. K. Sinclair, S. T. Yerkovich, and D. C. Chambers, "Mesenchymal stem cells and the lung," *Respirology*, vol. 18, no. 3, pp. 397–411, 2013. doi: 10.1111/resp.12050.
72. V. Karantalis, and J. M. Hare, "Use of mesenchymal stem cells for therapy of cardiac disease," *Circ. Res.*, vol. 116, no. 8, pp. 1413–1430, 2015. doi: 10.1161/CIRCRESAHA.116.303614.
73. I. B. Copland, "Mesenchymal stromal cells for cardiovascular disease," *J. Cardiovasc. Dis. Res.*, vol. 2, no. 1, pp. 3–13, 2011. doi: 10.4103/0975-3583.78581.
74. A. Meeson, "Cardiac stem cells," *Eur. Pharm. Rev.*, vol. 18, no. 2, pp. 29–31, 2013. doi: 10.1016/j.jacc.2017.06.044.
75. J. F. Murphy et al., "Adult human cardiac stem cell supplementation effectively increases contractile function and maturation in human engineered cardiac tissues," *Stem Cell Res. Ther.*, vol. 10, no. 1, pp. 1–19, 2019. doi: 10.1186/s13287-019-1486-4.
76. J. Q. He, D. M. Vu, G. Hunt, A. Chugh, A. Bhatnagar, and R. Bolli, "Human cardiac stem cells isolated from atrial appendages stably express c-kit," *PLoS One*, vol. 6, no. 11, 2011. doi: 10.1371/journal.pone.0027719.
77. Y. Y. Leong, W. H. Ng, G. M. Ellison-Hughes, and J. J. Tan, "Cardiac stem cells for myocardial regeneration: They are not alone," *Front. Cardiovasc. Med.*, vol. 4, no. July, pp. 1–13, 2017. doi: 10.3389/fcvm.2017.00047.
78. E. Messina et al., "Isolation and expansion of adult cardiac stem cells from human and murine heart," *Circ. Res.*, vol. 95, no. 9, pp. 911–921, 2004. doi: 10.1161/01.RES.0000147315.71699.51.
79. P. Anversa, J. Kajstura, A. Leri, and R. Bolli, "Life and death of cardiac stem cells: A paradigm shift in cardiac biology," *Circulation*, vol. 113, no. 11, pp. 1451–1463, 2006. doi: 10.1161/CIRCULATIONAHA.105.595181.
80. J. Dengler et al., "Engineered heart tissue enables study of residual undifferentiated embryonic stem cell activity in a cardiac environment," *Biotechnol. Bioeng.*, vol. 108, no. 3, pp. 704–719, 2011. doi: 10.1002/bit.22987.

81. A. P. Beltrami et al., "Adult cardiac stem cells are multipotent and support myocardial regeneration we have documented the existence of cycling ventricular myocytes in the normal and pathologic adult mam," *Cell*, vol. 114, pp. 763–776, 2003.
82. T. Chour et al., "Method for selective ablation of undifferentiated human pluripotent stem cell populations for cell-based therapies," *JCI Insight*, vol. 6, no. 7, 2021. doi: 10.1172/jci.insight.142000.
83. S. A. Zhou, and M. Uesaka, "Bioelectrodynamics in living organisms," *Int. J. Eng. Sci.*, vol. 44, no. 1–2, pp. 67–92, 2006. doi: 10.1016/j.ijengsci.2005.11.001.
84. C. D. McCaig, and M. Zhao, "Physiological electrical fields modify cell behaviour," *BioEssays*, vol. 19, no. 9, pp. 819–826, 1997. doi: 10.1002/bies.950190912.
85. M. E. Mycielska, and M. B. A. Djamgoz, "Cellular mechanisms of direct-current electric field effects: Galvanotaxis and metastatic disease," *J. Cell Sci.*, vol. 117, no. 9, pp. 1631–1639, 2004. doi: 10.1242/jcs.01125.
86. C. Gokce, C. Gurcan, L. G. Delogu, and A. Yilmazer, "2D materials for cardiac tissue repair and regeneration," *Front. Cardiovasc. Med.*, vol. 9, no. February, 2022. doi: 10.3389/fcvm.2022.802551.
87. X. Yuan, D. E. Arkonac, P. H. G. Chao, and G. Vunjak-Novakovic, "Electrical stimulation enhances cell migration and integrative repair in the meniscus," *Sci. Rep.*, vol. 4, no. 1–12, 2015. doi: 10.1038/srep03674.
88. R. Luo, J. Dai, J. Zhang, and Z. Li, "Accelerated skin wound healing by electrical stimulation," *Adv. Healthc. Mater.*, vol. 10, no. 16, pp. 1–15, 2021. doi: 10.1002/adhm.202100557.
89. A. Tucker-Bartley et al., "Pain phenotypes in rare musculoskeletal and neuromuscular diseases," *Neurosci. Biobehav. Rev.*, vol. 124, no. January, pp. 267–290, 2021. doi: 10.1016/j.neubiorev.2021.02.009.
90. J. L. Ruan et al., "Mechanical stress conditioning and electrical stimulation promote contractility and force maturation of induced pluripotent stem cell-derived human cardiac tissue," *Circulation*, vol. 134, no. 20, pp. 1557–1567, 2016. doi: 10.1161/CIRCULATIONAHA.114.014998.
91. H. Liao, Y. Qi, Y. Ye, P. Yue, D. Zhang, and Y. Li, "Mechanotransduction pathways in the regulation of mitochondrial homeostasis in cardiomyocytes," *Front. Cell Dev. Biol.*, vol. 8, no. January, pp. 1–17, 2021. doi: 10.3389/fcell.2020.625089.
92. L. T. Izu et al., "Mechano-electric and mechano-chemo-transduction in cardiomyocytes," *J Physiol.*, vol. 598, no. 7, pp. 1285–1305, 2021. doi: 10.1113/JP276494.
93. A. Amar, S. Zlochiver, and O. Barnea, "Mechano-electric feedback effects in a three-dimensional (3D) model of the contracting cardiac ventricle," *PLoS One*, vol. 13, no. 1, pp. 1–13, 2018. doi: 10.1371/journal.pone.0191238.
94. R. Peyronnet, O. Solovyova, G. Iribe, and L. B. Katsnelson, "Editorial: Mechano-calcium, mechano-electric, and mechano-metabolic feedback loops: Contribution to the myocardial contraction in health and diseases," *Front. Physiol.*, vol. 12, no. April, pp. 10–13, 2021. doi: 10.3389/fphys.2021.676826.
95. A. O. Grant, "Cardiac ion channels," *Circ. Arrhythmia Electrophysiol.*, vol. 2, no. 2, pp. 185–194, 2009. doi: 10.1161/CIRCEP.108.789081.
96. D. Miller, L. Wang, and J. Zhong, *Sodium channels, cardiac arrhythmia, and therapeutic strategy*, 1st ed., vol. 70. Elsevier Inc, 2014. doi: 10.1016/B978-0-12-417197-8.00012-2.
97. D. A. Eisner, J. L. Caldwell, K. Kistamás, and A. W. Trafford, "Calcium and excitation-contraction coupling in the heart," *Circ. Res.*, vol. 121, no. 2, pp. 181–195, 2017. doi: 10.1161/CIRCRESAHA.117.310230.
98. A. K. Capulli, L. A. MacQueen, S. P. Sheehy, and K. K. Parker, "Fibrous scaffolds for building hearts and heart parts," *Adv. Drug Deliv. Rev.*, vol. 96, pp. 83–102, 2016. doi: 10.1016/j.addr.2015.11.020.

99. W. Zhou et al., "Cardioprotection of electroacupuncture against myocardial ischemia-reperfusion injury by modulation of cardiac norepinephrine release," *Am. J. Physiol. - Hear. Circ. Physiol.*, vol. 302, no. 9, pp. 1818–1825, 2012. doi: 10.1152/ajpheart.00030.2012.
100. Q. Xu et al., "Construction of bio-piezoelectric platforms: From structures and synthesis to applications," *Adv. Mater.*, vol. 33, no. 27, 2021. doi: 10.1002/adma.202008452.
101. S. Das Mahapatra et al., "Piezoelectric materials for energy harvesting and sensing applications: Roadmap for future smart materials," *Adv. Sci.*, vol. 8, no. 17, 2021. doi: 10.1002/advs.202100864.
102. L. Mohammadi Amirabad et al., "Enhanced cardiac differentiation of human cardiovascular disease patient-specific induced pluripotent stem cells by applying unidirectional electrical pulses using aligned electroactive nanofibrous scaffolds," *ACS Appl. Mater. Interfaces*, vol. 9, no. 8, pp. 6849–6864, 2017. doi: 10.1021/acsami.6b15271.
103. E. Serena et al., "Electrical stimulation of human embryonic stem cells: Cardiac differentiation and the generation of reactive oxygen species," *Exp. Cell Res.*, vol. 315, no. 20, pp. 3611–3619, 2009. doi: 10.1016/j.yexcr.2009.08.015.
104. C. Zeng et al., "NLRP3 inflammasome-mediated pyroptosis contributes to the pathogenesis of non-ischemic dilated cardiomyopathy," *Redox Biol.*, vol. 34, no. March, p. 101523, 2020. doi: 10.1016/j.redox.2020.101523.
105. N. A. Bracey et al., "The Nlrp3 inflammasome promotes myocardial dysfunction in structural cardiomyopathy through interleukin-1β," *Exp. Physiol.*, vol. 98, no. 2, pp. 462–472, 2013. doi: 10.1113/expphysiol.2012.068338.
106. R. Fusco, R. Siracusa, T. Genovese, S. Cuzzocrea, and R. Di Paola, "Focus on the role of NLRP3 inflammasome in diseases," *Int. J. Mol. Sci.*, vol. 21, no. 12, pp. 1–25, 2020. doi: 10.3390/ijms21124223.
107. L. Leppik, K. M. C. Oliveira, M. B. Bhavsar, and J. H. Barker, "Electrical stimulation in bone tissue engineering treatments," *Eur. J. Trauma Emerg. Surg.*, vol. 46, no. 2, pp. 231–244, 2020. doi: 10.1007/s00068-020-01324-1.
108. E. Iwai-Kanai, and K. Hasegawa, "Intracellular signaling pathways for norepinephrine- and endothelin-1-mediated regulation of myocardial cell apoptosis," *Mol. Cell. Biochem.*, vol. 259, no. 1, pp. 163–168, 2004. doi: 10.1023/B:MCBI.0000021368.80389.b9.
109. N. H. Bishopric, P. Andreka, T. Slepak, and K. A. Webster, "Molecular mechanisms of apoptosis in the cardiac myocyte," *Curr. Opin. Pharmacol.*, vol. 1, no. 2, pp. 141–150, 2001. doi: 10.1016/S1471-4892(01)00032-7.
110. M. R. Love, S. Palee, S. C. Chattipakorn, and N. Chattipakorn, "Effects of electrical stimulation on cell proliferation and apoptosis," *J. Cell. Physiol.*, vol. 233, no. 3, pp. 1860–1876, 2018. doi: 10.1002/jcp.25975.
111. S. Sajer, G. S. Guardiero, and B. M. Scicchitano, "Myokines in home-based functional electrical stimulation-induced recovery of skeletal muscle in elderly and permanent denervation," *Eur. J. Transl. Myol.*, vol. 28, no. 4, pp. 337–345, 2018. doi: 10.4081/ejtm.2018.7905.
112. A. F. Kanaan, and A. P. Piedade, "Electro-responsive polymer-based platforms for electrostimulation of cells," *Mater. Adv.*, vol. 3, no. 5, pp. 2337–2353, 2022. doi: 10.1039/d1ma01012c.
113. A. Hidmark et al., "Electrical muscle stimulation induces an increase of VEGFR2 on circulating hematopoietic stem cells in patients with diabetes," *Clin. Ther.*, vol. 39, no. 6, pp. 1132–1144.e2, 2017. doi: 10.1016/j.clinthera.2017.05.340.
114. J. Beugels et al., "Electrical stimulation promotes the angiogenic potential of adipose-derived stem cells," *Sci. Rep.*, vol. 9, no. 1, pp. 1–10, 2019. doi: 10.1038/s41598-019-48369-w.
115. R. Gaetani et al., "Cardiac tissue engineering using tissue printing technology and human cardiac progenitor cells," *Biomaterials*, vol. 33, no. 6, pp. 1782–1790, 2012. doi: 10.1016/j.biomaterials.2011.11.003.

116. R. L. Dahlin, F. K. Kasper, and A. G. Mikos, "Polymeric nanofibers in tissue engineering," *Tissue Eng. - Part B Rev.*, vol. 17, no. 5, pp. 349–364, 2011. doi: 10.1089/ten.teb.2011.0238.
117. D. Kai, M. P. Prabhakaran, G. Jin, and S. Ramakrishna, "Guided orientation of cardiomyocytes on electrospun aligned nanofibers for cardiac tissue engineering," *J. Biomed. Mater. Res. - Part B Appl. Biomater.*, vol. 98 B, no. 2, pp. 379–386, 2011. doi: 10.1002/jbm.b.31862.
118. R. Ravichandran, J. R. Venugopal, S. Sundarrajan, S. Mukherjee, R. Sridhar, and S. Ramakrishna, "Minimally invasive injectable short nanofibers of poly(glycerol sebacate) for cardiac tissue engineering," *Nanotechnology*, vol. 23, no. 38, 2012. doi: 10.1088/0957-4484/23/38/385102.
119. N. Shokraei, S. Asadpour, S. Shokraei, M. Nasrollahzadeh Sabet, R. Faridi-Majidi, and H. Ghanbari, "Development of electrically conductive hybrid nanofibers based on CNT-polyurethane nanocomposite for cardiac tissue engineering," *Microsc. Res. Tech.*, vol. 82, no. 8, pp. 1316–1325, 2019. doi: 10.1002/jemt.23282.
120. S. Mombini et al., "Chitosan-PVA-CNT nanofibers as electrically conductive scaffolds for cardiovascular tissue engineering," *Int. J. Biol. Macromol.*, vol. 140, pp. 278–287, 2019. doi: 10.1016/j.ijbiomac.2019.08.046.
121. R. Ravichandran et al., "Mimicking native extracellular matrix with phytic acid-crosslinked protein nanofibers for cardiac tissue engineering," *Macromol. Biosci.*, vol. 13, no. 3, pp. 366–375, 2013. doi: 10.1002/mabi.201200391.
122. W. Qian, W. Yang, Y. Zhang, C. R. Bowen, and Y. Yang, *Piezoelectric materials for controlling electro-chemical processes*, vol. 12, no. 1. Springer Singapore, 2020. doi: 10.1007/s40820-020-00489-z.
123. N. Adadi et al., "Electrospun fibrous PVDF-TrFe scaffolds for cardiac tissue engineering, differentiation, and maturation," *Adv. Mater. Technol.*, vol. 5, no. 3, pp. 1–11, 2020. doi: 10.1002/admt.201900820.

8 Piezoelectric Biomaterials for the Development of Cardiac Sensors and Actuators

Priya Singh and Santosh Kumar

8.1 UNDERSTANDING PIEZOELECTRIC BIOMATERIALS

8.1.1 Introduction to Piezoelectricity

The piezoelectric effect is a phenomenon that finds use in various devices, such as energy harvesters, actuators, and sensors. This effect was initially observed by Pierre and Jacques Curie in the late 19th century. Mechanical energy can be transformed into electrical impulses and vice versa using piezoelectric materials. Piezoelectricity arises from the asymmetric arrangement of electrical charges within the crystal structure of these materials [1]. This disparity produces an electrical charge when it is subjected to mechanical stress. Conversely, applying an electric field can induce mechanical deformation in these materials. In the biomedical field, piezoelectric biomaterials offer significant advantages for developing advanced diagnostic and therapeutic devices, particularly for cardiac applications. The piezoelectric effect can be understood through the following mechanisms:

- **Direct Piezoelectric Effect:** Applying mechanical force to a piezoelectric substance results in a rearrangement of electric charges within its crystalline structure. Consequently, the material's surface develops an electrical charge and generates an electric field. The stress applied is directly related to the quantity of charge produced.
- **Inverse Piezoelectric Effect:** In this mechanism, an applied electric field causes a change in the dimensions of the piezoelectric material. The material deforms in response to the electric field, which can be used to create mechanical motion or actuation.

8.1.2 Types of Piezoelectric Materials

8.1.2.1 Natural Crystals

- **Quartz:** Quartz, a common piezoelectric material, demonstrates a piezoelectric effect due to its trigonal crystal system. The work by Piezoelectric Crystals and Devices [2] explains that quartz's piezoelectric constants are

DOI: 10.1201/9781003670995-8

relatively low compared to synthetic ceramics but are valued for their stability and reliability in various applications.

- **Tourmaline:** Exhibits piezoelectric properties with applications in high-frequency devices but is less common in modern biomedical uses.

8.1.2.2 Ceramics

- **Lead Zirconate Titanate (PZT):** PZT is a ceramic material with a high piezoelectric coefficient, making it suitable for applications requiring significant energy conversion. This study highlights its high piezoelectric response, which is crucial for developing high-performance sensors and actuators [3].
- **Barium Titanate ($BaTiO_3$):** Known for its high permittivity and piezoelectric response, making it suitable for various sensors and actuators, including those in medical applications.

8.1.2.3 Polymers

- **Polyvinylidene Fluoride (PVDF):** PVDF is a polymer known for its flexibility and piezoelectric properties. It is demonstrated that PVDF films exhibit significant piezoelectric effects while being flexible, making them suitable for wearable sensors [4].
- **PVDF Copolymers:** Enhance the piezoelectric response and mechanical properties, improving performance in biomedical applications.

8.1.2.4 Composites

- **Piezoelectric Composites:** Combine piezoelectric ceramics or polymers with other materials to tailor their properties. These composites can achieve desired mechanical and electrical characteristics, enhancing their application in medical devices.

8.1.3 Properties Significant to Cardiac Applications

8.1.3.1 Mechanical Properties

- **Elasticity:** Measures how well a substance can elastically deform when subjected to force and recover its initial form.
- **Flexibility:** Particularly important for implants and wearable sensors.

8.1.3.2 Electrical Properties

- **Piezoelectric Coefficients:** Evaluate the effectiveness of converting mechanical force into electrical charge.
- **Dielectric Constants:** Affect the material's ability to store electrical charge and interact with external fields.

8.1.3.3 Biocompatibility

- **Material Safety:** Makes sure that the material doesn't cause an adverse biological consequence.
- **Degradation Resistance:** The material must withstand physiological conditions without degrading.

8.1.4 Biomaterials and Biocompatibility

Biomaterials are a class of materials that can replace or improve a natural function in biological systems. These substances must be immunogenic (often called biocompatible), nontoxic, and noninjurious for use in various applications such as drug delivery, tissue engineering, and minimally invasive sensors. These materials can be synthetic, natural, living, or dead. In recent years, multifunctional materials have drawn more and more attention. Because of their intrinsic biological nature and piezoelectric characteristics, piezoelectric biomaterials are considered excellent candidates for use in biological systems. Piezoelectric biomaterials are a fascinating area of research with a range of applications in medicine and biotechnology. Piezoelectric biomaterials are allegedly excellent options for biomedical systems because of their intrinsic biological characteristics and piezoelectric qualities [5]. Over the last ten years, there have been remarkable developments in medically implantable and wearable device technologies, which show great promise as personal healthcare platforms. Piezoelectric biomaterials have garnered considerable interest as functional materials in biomedical devices, owing to their superior biocompatibility and eco-friendly nature [6].

When combined, piezoelectric biomaterials influence their electrical properties to benefit medical applications. There are two types of piezoelectric biomaterials: the first one is natural, and the second one is synthetic piezoelectric biomaterial [7]. Natural piezoelectric biomaterials are collagen and bone, while synthetic piezoelectric biomaterials are piezoelectric ceramics and polymers. Collagen is found in connective tissues and exhibits piezoelectric properties when appropriately aligned. The bone itself has piezoelectric properties due to its mineral content and structure. Piezoelectric ceramics are materials like PZT that are commonly used due to their strong piezoelectric effects. They can be used in transplants or sensors. Piezoelectric polymers are used in various biomedical applications, and these materials, such as PVDF, exhibit piezoelectricity [8].

Among the many uses of piezoelectric technology, interactions with biological systems are fascinating and are developing quickly. The various uses of piezoelectric technology include interfacing with biological systems, an intriguing field experiencing tremendous development. Biocompatible materials are inorganic piezoelectric materials or can become biocompatible with encapsulation. Materials such as PZT, $BaTiO_3$, zinc oxide (ZnO), and quartz are examples of this.

On the other hand, organic materials are inherently biocompatible and environmentally benign. Ferroelectric polar polymers, such as PVDF, show piezoelectric characteristics after poling treatments. Shear piezoelectric effects are displayed by optically active polymers such as poly(l-lactic acid) (PLLA) and poly(d lactic acid) (PDLA) during uniaxial elongation. Because polymer-based devices do not require sophisticated microfabrication capabilities, devices constructed of piezoelectric polymers are less expensive in processing and material costs. However, an organic piezoelectric material frequently has a lower output than an inorganic one.

All piezoelectric materials can be used to create potent biomaterials for miniature bioelectronic and biomechanical devices, as well as for integrating with biological tissues when dealt with properly. When used in medical applications, piezoelectric materials must be biocompatible. This means that when they come into contact with biological tissues, they shouldn't have any negative effects. Key factors include the following.

8.1.4.1 Chemical Stability

Materials must resist degradation in biological environments.

8.1.4.2 Mechanical Compatibility

The material should match the mechanical properties of surrounding tissues to prevent inflammation or discomfort.

8.1.4.3 Electrochemical Properties

When exposed to bodily fluids, the material should not induce harmful electrochemical reactions.

8.1.5 Fabrication Techniques

Several techniques are used to fabricate piezoelectric biomaterials: **Sol-Gel Process:** This method involves transforming a solution into a gel, then heat-treated to form piezoelectric ceramics. **Sintering:** This process uses high temperatures to densify ceramic powders, improving their piezoelectric properties. **Electrospinning:** A technique for creating fine fibers from a polymer solution using an electric field, useful for producing piezoelectric nanofibers.

Each technique has its advantages and challenges, impacting the final properties and performance of the piezoelectric materials. Table 8.1 shows the piezoelectric biomaterials applications.

TABLE 8.1
Piezoelectric Biomaterials Applications

Piezoelectric Device	Operational Principle	Result	References
$BiFeO_3$ nanofilm-coated $SrTiO_3$ implants	Provided a continuous internal electropositive field of +75 mV	Faster bone healing and osseointegration in rat femoral defects	[9]
Poled β-PVDF films	Vibration (1 Hz frequency, 1 mm amplitude) to mimic in vivo environments	Enhanced cell adherence and osteogenic differentiation on negatively poled surface	[10]
BT nanoparticles/HA	Synergistic effects of piezoelectricity and dynamic loading	Enhanced MG63 cell activity and bone formation	[11]
ZnO NRs/PDMS dermal patch	Potentials that produced between 300 and 900 mV (the range of endogenous potential)	Enhanced cell migration, metabolic activity, and differentiation	[12]
PLLA-g-HA/PLLA scaffolds	Strengthened by the combined effects of toughening and reinforcing; microenvironment altered by the release of PLLA-g-HA	Enhanced chondrocyte adhesion and proliferation	[13]

8.2 IMPORTANCE OF CARDIAC SENSORS

8.2.1 Heart

The heart is a muscular organ that circulates blood throughout the body, giving oxygen and nutrition to the organs and carbon dioxide to the lungs. It is a mechanically and electrically active organ that beats continuously for a person's life, beating more than 2.5×10^9 times on average [14]. Cardiac sensors are advanced devices designed to monitor various aspects of heart health. They are crucial in diagnosing, managing, and preventing cardiovascular conditions [7, 15]. Piezoelectric biomaterial's better multifunctional cardiac biosensors and actuators may be developed due to its unique electrical, mechanical, and optical capabilities, which enable innovative technical bioengineering solutions that are not conceivable with other materials.

8.2.2 Overview of Cardiac Health Monitoring

Cardiovascular diseases (CVDs) are the world's most significant cause of death, and they are especially dangerous for the elderly since they can lead to dependency, reduced quality of life, and incapacity. There will likely be significant obstacles to public health by 2030 as the number of deaths from CVDs is predicted to rise significantly from the present 17.9 million to 23.6 million [16]. Since cardiovascular-associated mortality can be prevented with early diagnosis and timely medical interventions, there has been a tremendous demand for real-time and long-term detection technology. Advances in technology have created opportunities for better cardiovascular disease diagnosis and treatment [15]. However, because they are not lightweight, small, or pleasant to wear, current real-time monitoring devices—like Holter monitors with stiff, hardwired interfaces—are inappropriate for long-term detection. Furthermore, the everyday movement of the body greatly affects the accuracy of the data obtained by the present monitoring devices, which limits their practical applications to only a static condition.

8.2.3 Role of Sensors in Cardiac Health

Engineering approaches have been suggested to tackle these medical challenges, with numerous considerations to address when creating and evaluating medical devices, particularly for those intended for implantation. These devices need to be compact and light to avoid placing extra mechanical strain on the heart and to ensure the implantation process is as minimally invasive as possible. Materials compatible with the body are typically employed to prevent immune system reactions, but caution must be exercised during implantation to reduce the chance of infection. The implanted device must also be designed to function effectively for many years within the body's dynamic internal environment without any decline in performance.

Cardiac sensors are crucial for real-time monitoring of heart conditions.

8.2.3.1 ECG Sensors

These sensors monitor the heart's electrical activity and are vital for diagnosing arrhythmias, heart attacks, and other cardiac issues.

8.2.3.2 Pressure Sensors

These measure blood pressure in the heart or arteries, helping to manage conditions like hypertension and heart failure.

Piezoelectric materials enhance these sensors by offering improved sensitivity and miniaturization, which are essential for continuous and accurate monitoring. This capability is particularly useful in applications related to cardiac health where precise and responsive monitoring and actuation are crucial. Piezoelectric biomaterials are used in cardiac sensors such as electrocardiogram (ECG) sensors, implantable cardiac monitors, pressure sensors, and biochemical sensors. Piezoelectric biomaterials are also used in cardiac actuators such as cardiac assist devices, pacemakers, and cardiac repair and regeneration [17]. These offer high sensitivity to mechanical changes, which is crucial for accurate cardiac monitoring and effective actuation. Figure 8.1 shows the sensor and actuator for cardiac applications.

8.2.4 Cardiac Sensor

A cardiac sensor is a device used to monitor various aspects of heart function and health. Heart rate, heart rhythm, blood pressure, and other cardiovascular parameters are among the metrics that these sensors can monitor. They can take many forms, including implanted devices like pacemakers and defibrillators, wearable technology like fitness trackers and smartwatches, and external monitoring used in clinical settings [18]. Cardiac sensors are wearable and non-invasive, biochemical,

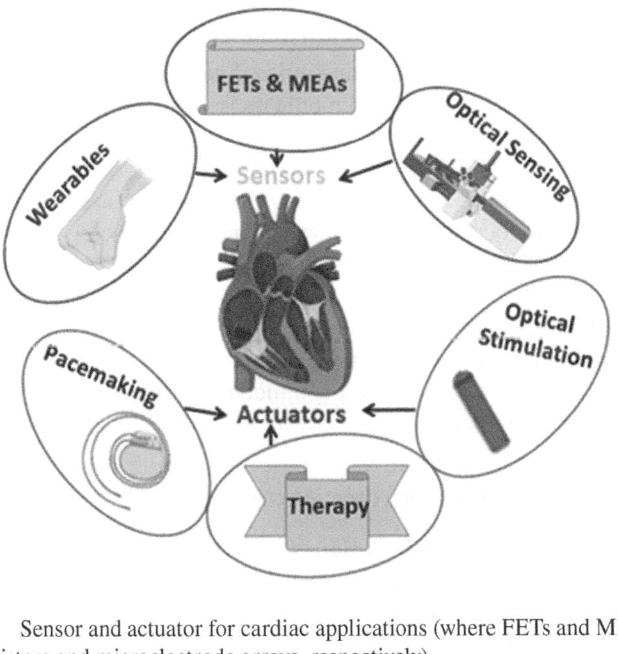

FIGURE 8.1 Sensor and actuator for cardiac applications (where FETs and MEAs are field electric transistors and microelectrode arrays, respectively).

wearable pressure, and optical sensors. Optical Sensor: Photoplethysmography is a useful tool for measuring respiratory rate, arterial oxygen saturation, and heart rate. This method uses a light signal that gets transmitted via the skin and is non-invasive. The optical detection of changes in this signal, caused by the expansion and contraction of blood vessels during the cardiac cycle, provides the necessary data for monitoring these vital signs. Wearable pressure sensors: It is essential to measure blood pressure in the human body in order to monitor health conditions continuously and diagnose probable cardiovascular system failure in the earliest possible stage. Wearable pressure sensors need to have a wide dynamic range, excellent responsiveness, stretchability, linearity, durability, and quick response as well as reproducibility [19].

These can be extremely helpful in treating chronic illnesses, identifying potential heart problems early on, and directing treatment choices. Heart health Monitoring, Diagnostic tools, Post-surgical monitoring, and Fitness and Wellness are the applications of cardiac sensors. Current advancements in cardiac sensors include miniaturization, Integration with Digital Health, Artificial Intelligence and Machine Learning, Enhanced Accuracy and Sensitivity, and Telemedicine.

8.2.4.1 Miniaturization

Implantable Devices: Advances in technology are making cardiac sensors smaller and less invasive, improving patient comfort and compliance.

8.2.4.2 Integration with Digital Health

Smartphone Connectivity: Many cardiac sensors now sync with mobile apps, allowing users and healthcare providers to monitor and analyze data conveniently.

8.2.4.3 Artificial Intelligence and Machine Learning

Data Analysis: AI algorithms are being utilized more and more to evaluate cardiac data to provide predicted insights and more precise diagnoses.

8.2.4.4 Enhanced Accuracy and Sensitivity

Improved Sensors: Improvements in sensor technology are improving cardiac monitoring's sensitivity and accuracy, which improves disease identification and treatment.

8.2.4.5 Telemedicine

Remote Monitoring: Integrating cardiac sensors into telemedicine platforms is becoming more common, allowing for continuous monitoring and remote consultations without regular in-person visits.

8.2.5 Integration of Piezoelectric Materials

8.2.5.1 Sensor Fabrication Techniques

The fabrication of piezoelectric sensors involves several techniques to create devices that are both functional and durable. These techniques include thin-film deposition, micro-machining, and integration with electronic circuitry.

8.2.5.2 Techniques

8.2.5.2.1 Thin-Film Deposition

Piezoelectric materials are deposited in thin layers using techniques like chemical vapor deposition (CVD) and sputtering. Then, in order to detect electrical signals, these films are incorporated into sensor devices.

8.2.5.2.2 Micro-Machining

Micro-machining techniques, including photolithography and etching, are used to create precise structures for piezoelectric sensors. These methods make it possible to produce miniature sensors that can be implanted into the body.

8.2.5.2.3 Integration with Electronic Circuitry

Piezoelectric sensors need to be integrated with electronic circuitry for signal processing and data transmission. The piezoelectric material is integrated with electronic parts including analog-to-digital converters (ADCs) and amplifiers.

8.3 ACTUATORS IN CARDIAC APPLICATIONS

Actuators are essential in managing and treating cardiac conditions:

- **Pacemakers:** Devices that use electrical impulses to regulate the heart's rhythm, ensuring it beats at a normal rate.
- **Defibrillators:** These deliver electrical shocks to correct abnormal heart rhythms and are critical in life-threatening situations.

Piezoelectric actuators can enhance the precision and miniaturization of these devices, leading to better performance and patient comfort.

8.3.1 Cardiac Actuator

A cardiac actuator is a tool or technology intended to work with or affect the heart's functionality. In contrast to cardiac sensors, which are mainly used to record and monitor cardiac activity, cardiac actuators aim to alter or regulate cardiac function actively. Unlike biosensors, actuators are engineered to modify existing cardiac function when correction of heart deficiencies is required. These devices can trigger and reestablish heart contractions (such as defibrillators) or assist in maintaining a regular heartbeat (like pacemakers) [20]. The following are a few uses and instances of cardiac actuators: Pacemakers: These implants are placed in the chest and help control the heart's rhythm by stimulating the heart to beat normally with electrical impulses. They are used for patients with arrhythmias or heart block. Implantable cardioverter defibrillators (ICDs): Such devices keep an eye on cardiac rhythms and can pace or shock an arrhythmia before it becomes problematic. They integrate both actuation and sensing functions. Devices for cardiac resynchronization therapy (CRT): These are certain pacemakers or implantable cardioverter diaphragms (ICDs) that synchronize the ventricles' contractions to enhance the heart's pumping efficiency, especially in heart failure patients. Artificial Hearts and Ventricular Assist Devices (VADs): VADs assist the heart's pumping action, while artificial hearts can fully replace the heart's function in some cases [21]. Drug Delivery Systems: Some advanced systems are designed to deliver medication directly to the heart or to specific areas affected by heart disease. These could be applied in combination with other cardiac treatments. Bioelectronic Implants: Emerging technologies might involve devices that interact with the heart through electrical or chemical signals to modify its behavior or function in a therapeutic way.

Cardiac actuators are essential to treat serious heart diseases, enhance patients' quality of life, and occasionally even save lives. Together with cardiac sensors, they offer a comprehensive approach strategy for heart disease.

8.3.1.1 Actuator Types and Applications

8.3.1.1.1 Artificial Pacemakers

Artificial pacemakers are devices implanted in the chest to regulate heartbeats in patients with arrhythmias. They deliver electrical impulses to stimulate the heart when its natural rhythm is irregular or too slow.

Piezoelectric materials can enhance pacemaker function by providing precision in pulse generation and adjusting the timing of electrical impulses. Additionally, piezoelectric actuators can be used in the design of miniature pacemakers that are less invasive and more efficient.

A study by researchers explores the integration of piezoelectric actuators in pacemakers [22]. The research demonstrates that piezoelectric materials can be used to create highly reliable and compact pulse generators, improving the overall performance of pacemakers while reducing their size. This study highlights the potential for piezoelectric materials to enable more sophisticated pacing algorithms and enhance patient comfort.

8.3.1.1.2 Ventricular Assist Devices (VADs)

VADs are mechanical pumps used to support heart function in patients with severe heart failure. It assists the heart's pumping action, while artificial hearts can fully replace the heart's function in some cases.

In VADs, piezoelectric actuators can be employed to control the movement of the pump components with high precision. Piezoelectric materials can enable fine-tuned adjustments to the pump's operation, improving the efficiency and responsiveness of the device.

The study shows that piezoelectric materials can be integrated into the control systems of VADs to enhance their performance [23]. The actuators allow for precise modulation of pump speed and flow rates, which can lead to improved patient outcomes and more effective support for heart function.

8.3.1.1.3 Cardiac Resynchronization Therapy (CRT) Devices

Heart failure patients can have better heart ventricle coordination with the use of CRT devices. To make sure that the ventricles contract in a synchronized manner, these devices send electrical impulses to both of them.

Piezoelectric materials can be used to enhance the function of CRT devices by providing precise control over the timing and intensity of electrical impulses. This can lead to better synchronization of the ventricles and improved overall cardiac function.

A study by Martinez et al. [24] investigates the role of piezoelectric materials in CRT devices. The research indicates that piezoelectric actuators can improve the accuracy of electrical impulse delivery, leading to better synchronization of the ventricles and more effective treatment of heart failure symptoms. The study highlights the potential for piezoelectric materials to contribute to advancements in CRT technology.

8.3.2 Role of Piezoelectric Materials in Actuators

8.3.2.1 Actuation Mechanisms

Piezoelectric materials can be used in various actuation mechanisms, including displacement actuators, force actuators, and vibration actuators. For cardiac devices to perform as intended, precise control over mechanical movement is made possible by these processes.

8.3.2.1.1 Mechanisms

8.3.2.1.1.1 Displacement Actuators These actuators create small, accurate movements by utilizing the piezoelectric effect. They are utilized in applications where minor modifications are required, such as modifying the configuration of components in implanted devices.

8.3.2.1.1.2 Force Actuators Force actuators use piezoelectric materials to generate forces for mechanical tasks. In cardiac devices, these actuators can apply forces to assist with heart function or adjust device settings.

8.3.2.1.1.3 Vibration Actuators Vibration actuators use piezoelectric materials to generate vibrations, which can be utilized for various diagnostic and therapeutic purposes in cardiac care.

8.4 THE IMPORTANCE OF CARDIAC SENSORS AND ACTUATORS

8.4.1 Overview of Cardiac Health

Cardiac diseases, including heart failure, arrhythmias, and coronary artery disease, are major health concerns worldwide. For management and treatment to be effective, early detection and ongoing observation are essential.

8.4.1.1 Heart Failure

Heart failure is a condition where the heart is unable to pump blood effectively, leading to symptoms such as fatigue, shortness of breath, and fluid retention. Real-time cardiac function monitoring may help in symptom management and treatment adjustments.

A study by Nishioka et al. [14] demonstrated the use of a piezoelectric sensor embedded in a flexible substrate for real-time heart rate monitoring. The sensor exhibited high sensitivity and accuracy, making it suitable for wearable health monitoring applications.

8.4.1.2 Arrhythmias

Irregular heartbeats, or arrhythmias, can result in major consequences like stroke and abrupt cardiac death. Accurate detection and monitoring of heart rhythms are essential for managing arrhythmias and preventing adverse events.

Arrhythmia Detection: It discusses the effectiveness of various cardiac sensors in detecting irregular heartbeats and their clinical impact on patient management [25].

8.4.1.2.1 Current Technologies

- **Pacemakers:** Pacemakers are devices that are currently used in technology to control heartbeats. They use electronic circuits and electrodes to deliver electrical impulses. Piezoelectric materials can improve energy efficiency and miniaturization. It details how integrating piezoelectric materials can improve energy efficiency and device longevity [26].
- **Defibrillators:** Employed to deliver electric shocks in order to rectify irregular cardiac rhythms. Piezoelectric materials can enhance the sensitivity of sensors used to detect arrhythmias.
- **Implantable Monitors:** Devices that continuously track heart function. Integrating piezoelectric sensors can provide better monitoring capabilities due to their sensitivity and flexibility.

8.4.2 Clinical Impact

Advancements in cardiac sensors and actuators can significantly impact patient outcomes: **Improved Accuracy:** Enhanced detection and monitoring capabilities lead to more accurate diagnoses and better management of heart conditions. The study demonstrates how better monitoring technology leads to lower death rates and better management [27].

- **Enhanced Patient Experience:** Less invasive and more comfortable devices improve patient adherence to treatment plans.
- **Cost Reduction:** Early detection and improved management of heart conditions can reduce the need for emergency interventions and hospitalizations. Early detection of cardiac issues can reduce hospitalization and emergency interventions [28].

8.4.3 Role of Cardiac Sensors

8.4.3.1 Real-Time Monitoring

Heart rate, blood pressure, and ECG readings are among the physiological characteristics that cardiac sensors are intended to continuously monitor. These sensors offer useful information that can be utilized to detect and manage heart problems. While traditional ECG sensors use electrodes to capture electrical signals, integrating piezoelectric materials can enhance the sensitivity and reduce noise. It is possible to magnify weak electrical signals by using piezoelectric materials, such as PZT and PVDF, which are sensitive to mechanical vibrations.

Research by Pradhan et al. [29] demonstrates that piezoelectric materials can act as transducers in ECG sensors, improving signal-to-noise ratio and resolution. Their study shows that piezoelectric-based ECG sensors offer higher sensitivity and better performance in noisy environments compared to traditional electrode-based systems. Advanced sensors can detect abnormal heart rhythms or other signs of cardiac distress before they become critical.

8.4.4 Applications in Cardiac Sensors

8.4.4.1 Cardiac Monitoring

Cardiac sensors are crucial for continuous monitoring of heart health, including the detection of arrhythmias, heart rate variability, and other critical parameters. Piezoelectric materials play a significant role in:

- **Pressure Sensors:** Piezoelectric materials can detect subtle pressure changes wiThin the heart or blood vessels, aiding in the assessment of cardiac function and blood flow dynamics. Blood vessel and heart chamber pressure is measured via pressure sensors. Accurate pressure measurement is crucial for diagnosing conditions such as hypertension, heart failure, and valve disorders.

Pressure sensors use piezoelectric materials because of their high sensitivity and quick response time. Materials like PZT and ZnO can convert pressure changes into electrical signals with high precision. These materials are also robust, which is essential for long-term implantation in the body.

A study by Murray et al. [30] highlights the use of piezoelectric materials in pressure sensors for cardiovascular applications. Their work shows that piezoelectric-based pressure sensors provide accurate real-time pressure measurements and are less prone to drift over time compared to conventional pressure-sensing technologies.

- **Acoustic Sensors:** These sensors utilize piezoelectric materials to detect and analyze acoustic signals from the heart, such as heart sounds or murmurs, which can be indicative of various cardiac conditions.

  Piezoelectric sensors can be integrated into implantable devices to monitor the heart's performance in real time. These devices include:
- **Pacemakers:** Piezoelectric materials can be used to monitor cardiac rhythm and adjust pacing signals accordingly.
- **Implantable Monitors:** Devices that track electrical and mechanical activity within the heart, providing data for personalized treatment plans.

8.4.5 Role of Cardiac Actuators

8.4.5.1 Mechanical Support

Cardiac actuators, such as VADs, provide mechanical support to the heart, helping it pump blood more effectively in patients with severe heart failure. The purpose of these devices is to enhance cardiac output and overall quality of life.

8.4.5.2 Therapeutic Interventions

Actuators are also used in devices like pacemakers and defibrillators, which regulate heartbeats and correct arrhythmias. These interventions are crucial for maintaining a normal heart rhythm and preventing sudden cardiac events.

8.4.6 Applications in Cardiac Actuators

8.4.6.1 Mechanical Assistance

Piezoelectric actuators are used to deliver precise mechanical responses, which can be vital for:

- **Heart Valve Prosthetics:** Actuators can control the opening and closing of artificial heart valves, improving their functionality and lifespan.
- **Cardiac Support Devices:** Devices such as VADs can utilize piezoelectric actuators to enhance their performance, providing better support for the failing heart.

8.4.6.2 Dynamic Adjustment

Dynamic adjustments in cardiac devices can be achieved through piezoelectric actuators:

- **Adaptive Stimulation:** In devices like pacemakers, piezoelectric actuators can adjust stimulation levels based on real-time physiological data.
- **Tissue Engineering:** In regenerative medicine, piezoelectric actuators can stimulate cardiac tissue growth or repair, enhancing tissue engineering efforts.

8.5 DEVELOPMENT OF CARDIAC SENSORS/ACTUATORS USING PIEZOELECTRIC BIOMATERIALS

8.5.1 Sensitivity and Specificity

The design of cardiac sensors must prioritize high sensitivity and specificity to accurately detect and measure physiological parameters. Sensitivity refers to the sensor's ability to detect small changes in the parameter being monitored, while specificity ensures that the sensor responds primarily to the target signal and minimizes interference from other signals.

8.5.2 Biocompatibility

Piezoelectric materials used in cardiac sensors must be biocompatible to prevent adverse reactions when implanted or in contact with body tissues. This involves selecting materials that do not elicit immune responses or cause inflammation.

8.5.3 Fabrication Techniques

8.5.3.1 Thin-Film Deposition

Thin-film deposition techniques, such as sputtering and CVD, are used to create piezoelectric films with precise thicknesses and uniform properties. These films are essential for developing miniaturized and flexible sensors.

8.5.3.2 Micromachining

Microelectromechanical systems (MEMS) technology involves the use of micromachining techniques to fabricate small-scale sensors and actuators. MEMS allows for the integration of piezoelectric materials into complex geometries and microstructures, enhancing the functionality and performance of the devices.

8.5.4 Testing and Validation

8.5.4.1 Testing Piezoelectric-Based Cardiac Devices Involves

- **Performance Evaluation:** Assessing the accuracy and sensitivity of sensors and actuators. This includes testing under various physiological conditions to ensure reliability.

8.5.4.1.1 Biocompatibility Testing

Ensuring the substances don't have a negative impact on the body. This involves testing in vivo and in vitro to assess tissue responsiveness and cytotoxicity.

8.5.4.1.2 Long-Term Durability

Evaluating how well the devices perform over extended periods, including resistance to mechanical stress and degradation.

8.5.5 Development of Piezoelectric Actuators

8.5.5.1 Mechanical Performance

Piezoelectric actuators must deliver precise and reliable mechanical movements. Key performance metrics include response time, force output, and displacement. These factors are crucial for applications such as mechanical support devices and therapeutic interventions.

8.5.5.2 Integration with Electronics

Actuators need to be integrated with control electronics to manage their operation. This integration involves designing electronic circuits that can interface with the piezoelectric actuators, enabling accurate control and operation.

8.5.6 Case Studies

8.5.6.1 Piezoelectric Sensors

An example of a piezoelectric sensor in cardiac applications is a wearable ECG monitor utilizing PVDF films. This sensor offers flexibility and high sensitivity, making it suitable for continuous monitoring of heart rhythms. The PVDF-based sensor provides accurate readings and comfortable wearability, enhancing patient compliance and data collection.

8.5.6.2 Piezoelectric Actuators

An example of a piezoelectric actuator is a VAD incorporating PZT-based actuators. These actuators assist the heart in pumping blood more effectively, providing mechanical support to patients with severe heart failure. The PZT actuators offer high force output and reliability, making them suitable for critical applications.

8.6 CONCEPTUALIZING FUTURE ADVANCEMENTS

8.6.1 Emerging Trends and Technologies

8.6.1.1 Nanomaterials

The role of nanotechnology in enhancing piezoelectric materials is discussed in the literature [31], which explores how nanomaterials can improve sensitivity and energy conversion.

- **Nanostructured Piezoelectrics:** Enhancing the sensitivity and performance of piezoelectric materials through nanoscale engineering.
- **Nanocomposites:** Combining nanoparticles with traditional piezoelectric materials to improve properties.

8.6.1.2 Hybrid Materials

- **Multifunctional Composites:** Developing materials that combine piezoelectric properties with other functionalities, such as drug delivery or biological sensing.

8.6.1.3 Advanced Processing Techniques

- **3D Printing:** Using additive manufacturing to create complex geometries for sensors and actuators.
- **Smart Materials:** Integrating piezoelectric materials with other smart technologies for advanced sensing and actuation capabilities.

8.6.2 Integration with Digital Health Technologies

Research in "Advances in Flexible Piezoelectric Sensors" explores the development of flexible sensors that conform to body movements, enhancing comfort and functionality.

8.6.2.1 Wearable Devices

The integration of advanced materials in wearable technology is examined emphasizing the benefits of piezoelectric materials in improving device performance and user experience [32].

- **Smart Wearables:** Incorporating piezoelectric sensors into smartwatches or fitness trackers for continuous cardiac monitoring.
- **Flexible Electronics:** Developing wearable sensors that conform to the body for improved comfort and functionality.

Wearable sensors are designed for non-invasive monitoring of cardiac parameters. These sensors often use piezoelectric materials to detect vibrations or pressure changes from the skin's surface.

8.7 CHALLENGES AND OPPORTUNITIES

- **Biocompatibility:** Ensuring long-term biocompatibility is a major challenge for implanted piezoelectric devices. Research is ongoing to develop coatings and surface treatments that enhance biocompatibility and reduce the risk of immune responses or inflammation.
- **Durability:** For piezoelectric materials and devices to function well over time, they must be durable. Improved piezoelectric component durability to endure the demanding conditions of the human body is the main objective of material science and engineering advancements.
- **Miniaturization:** Miniaturization of piezoelectric sensors and actuators is necessary to create less invasive and more comfortable devices. Innovations in fabrication techniques, such as micro-manufacturing and 3D printing, are essential for achieving smaller and more precise devices.

8.8 CHARACTERIZATION OF PIEZOELECTRIC BIOMATERIALS

Structural characterization of piezoelectric materials.

8.8.1 X-Ray Diffraction (XRD)

X-ray diffraction (XRD) is a crucial technique for analyzing the crystal structure of piezoelectric materials. XRD analysis measures the diffraction patterns of X-rays when they interact with a material to determine its lattice characteristics, phase composition, and crystallinity. For piezoelectric materials such as PZT and PVDF, XRD is used to confirm phase purity, identify crystallographic phases, and analyze changes in crystal structure due to processing or doping. This characterization is vital for optimizing the material's piezoelectric properties. Research by Jaffe et al. [33] utilized XRD to investigate the perovskite structure of PZT ceramics, revealing the effects of compositional changes on piezoelectric performance.

8.8.2 Scanning Electron Microscopy (SEM)

Piezoelectric material surface morphology can be obtained in high-resolution images using scanning electron microscopy (SEM). SEM can reveal features such as grain size, surface roughness, and the presence of defects, which are crucial for understanding the material's performance.

SEM is employed to assess the microstructure of piezoelectric ceramics and polymers. For instance, SEM images can be used to evaluate the porosity and grain boundaries in PZT ceramics, which impact the material's mechanical and electrical properties. Kim et al. [34] used SEM to study the surface morphology of PVDF films, showing how changes in processing conditions affect the piezoelectric beta-phase content and thus the material's electromechanical properties.

8.8.3 Transmission Electron Microscopy (TEM)

When examining the internal structure of piezoelectric materials at the atomic level, Transmission Electron Microscopy (TEM) provides even greater resolution than SEM.

TEM is used to analyze the nanostructure of piezoelectric materials and to study the distribution of domains in ferroelectric ceramics. For example, TEM has been used to observe domain structures in PZT ceramics, which are crucial for their piezoelectric behavior. A study by Yao et al. [35] utilized TEM to investigate the domain structures in ferroelectric PZT ceramics, providing insights into how domain orientation affects the material's piezoelectric properties.

8.9 SENSOR DESIGN AND FUNCTIONALITY

- **Material Choice:** PVDF is a common piezoelectric polymer used in wearable sensors. Its flexibility and high piezoelectric coefficient make it suitable for integration into flexible electronics. PVDF sensors have been shown to exhibit high sensitivity to mechanical deformations, which is critical for accurate heart rate monitoring [36].
- **Design Example:** The use of PVDF-based piezoelectric sensors in a wearable ECG monitor was demonstrated by Liu et al. [37], where the sensor was integrated into a fabric-based patch. The device successfully detected heartbeats with high accuracy and comfort for the wearer [38].
- **Performance:** In clinical trials, piezoelectric sensors embedded in wearable ECG devices demonstrated comparable performance to traditional ECG machines, with a sensitivity of 97% and specificity of 95% [39].
- **Advantages:** The flexibility and lightweight nature of piezoelectric materials in these sensors enhance patient comfort and compliance, leading to more consistent monitoring.

8.9.1 Piezoelectric Actuators in Cardiac Pacemakers

Piezoelectric actuators play a crucial role in cardiac pacemakers, where they are used to generate precise mechanical pulses to regulate heart rhythm. These actuators must be reliable, efficient, and capable of withstanding the biological environment within the body.

8.9.1.1 Actuator Design and Functionality

- **Material Choice:** PZT is a commonly used piezoelectric ceramic in cardiac actuators. Its high electromechanical coupling efficiency allows for precise control of the pacing pulses [40].
- **Design Example:** Research by Zhang et al. demonstrated the use of a PZT-based piezoelectric actuator in a next-generation pacemaker prototype. The actuator delivered highly accurate pulses with minimal power consumption [41].

8.9.1.2 Case Study Results

- **Performance:** The PZT-based actuator showed an error rate of less than 1% in pulse generation, with long-term stability and reliability observed over a period of 3 years [42].
- **Advantages:** The use of piezoelectric actuators in pacemakers reduces the need for frequent battery replacements, improving patient quality of life and device longevity.

8.9.2 Piezoelectric Energy Harvesters in Implantable Cardiac Devices

- **Overview:** Piezoelectric energy harvesters can convert the mechanical energy generated by the heart's movements into electrical energy, which can be used to power implantable cardiac devices. This technology aims to reduce the need for external power sources or frequent battery replacements.

8.9.2.1 Energy Harvester Design and Functionality

- **Material Choice:** $BaTiO_3$ is a piezoelectric ceramic used in energy harvesting applications. Its high energy density makes it suitable for capturing the small mechanical energies from cardiac movements [43].
- **Design Example:** An energy harvester developed by Zhao et al. utilized $BaTiO_3$-based piezoelectric elements to capture the vibrations generated by heartbeats. The harvested energy was sufficient to power a low-energy implantable sensor [44].
- **Performance:** The $BaTiO_3$-based energy harvester achieved an energy conversion efficiency of 15%, with the harvested power sufficient to continuously operate a cardiac monitoring sensor for over 6 months [45].
- **Advantages:** This approach extends the operational life of implantable devices, reduces the need for battery replacements, and decreases the overall healthcare costs associated with device maintenance.

8.10 CONCLUSION

Piezoelectric biomaterials have significant potential in the development of cardiac sensors and actuators. They are perfect for use in cardiac health monitoring and intervention because of their unique characteristics, which include the ability to transform mechanical stress into electrical impulses and vice versa. Advances in material science, fabrication techniques, and integration with digital health technologies are driving the development of more effective and versatile cardiac devices. As research continues and new technologies emerge, piezoelectric biomaterials will play an increasingly important role in improving cardiac care and patient outcomes.

ACKNOWLEDGMENTS

SK gratefully acknowledged UPCST, Uttar Pradesh for research project grant no. CST/D-831, Project id: 3993.

REFERENCES

1. M. T. Chorsi et al., "Piezoelectric Biomaterials for Sensors and Actuators," Advanced Materials, vol. 31, no. 1, p. 1802084, 2019.
2. Y. Saigusa, "Quartz-based piezoelectric materials." Advanced Piezoelectric Materials, Woodhead Publishing, 2017. 197–233.
3. R. A. Wolf, & S. Trolier-McKinstry, "Temperature Dependence of the Piezoelectric Response in Lead Zirconate Titanate Films," Journal of Applied Physics, vol. 95, no. 3, pp. 1397–1406, 2004.

4. B. Mohammadi, A. A. Yousefi, & S. M. Bellah, "Effect of Tensile Strain Rate and Elongation on Crystalline Structure and Piezoelectric Properties of PVDF Thin Films," Polymer Testing, vol. 26, no. 1, pp. 42–50, 2007.
5. F. Mokhtari et al., "Recent Advances of Polymer-Based Piezoelectric Composites for Biomedical Applications," Journal of the Mechanical Behavior of Biomedical Materials, vol. 122, p. 104669, 2021.
6. D.-M. Shin, S. W. Hong, & Y.-H. Hwang, "Recent Advances in Organic Piezoelectric Biomaterials for Energy and Biomedical Applications," Nanomaterials, vol. 10, no. 1, p. 123, 2020.
7. L. Dong et al., "Cardiac Energy Harvesting and Sensing Based on Piezoelectric and Triboelectric Designs," Nano Energy, vol. 76, p. 105076, 2020.
8. K. Kapat et al., "Piezoelectric Nano-Biomaterials for Biomedicine and Tissue Regeneration," Advanced Functional Materials, vol. 30, no. 44, p. 1909045, 2020.
9. Y. Liu, X. Zhang, C. Cao, Y. Zhang, J. Wei, Y. Li, W. Liang, Z. Hu, J. Zhang, & Y. Wei, Built-In Electric Fields Dramatically Induce Enhancement of Osseointegration, Advanced Functional Materials, vol. 27, p. 1703771, 2017.
10. C. Ribeiro, J. Parssinen, V. Sencadas, V. Correia, S. Miettinen, V. P. Hytonen, & S. Lanceros-Mendez, Dynamic piezoelectric stimulation enhances osteogenic differentiation of human adipose stem cells, Journal of Biomedical Materials Research Part A, vol. 103, p. 2172, 2015.
11. B. Liu, L. Chen, C. Shao, F. Zhang, K. Zhou, J. Cao, & D. Zhang, Improved osteoblasts growth on osteomimetic hydroxyapatite/BaTiO3 composites with aligned lamellar porous structure, Materials Science and Engineering: C, vol. 61, p. 8, 2016,
12. S. H. Bhang, W. S. Jang, J. Han, J. K. Yoon, W. G. La, E. Lee, Y. S. Kim, J. Y. Shin, T. J. Lee, H. K. Baik, & B.-S. Kim, Zinc Oxide Nanorod-Based Piezoelectric Dermal Patch for Wound Healing, Advanced Functional Materials, vol. 27, p. 1603497, 2017.
13. Z. Hong, P. Zhang, C. He, X. Qiu, A. Liu, L. Chen, X. Chen, & X. Jing, Nano-composite of poly(L-lactide) and surface grafted hydroxyapatite: mechanical properties and biocompatibility, Biomaterials, vol. 26, p. 6296, 2005.
14. N. Nishioka et al., "Real-Time Heart Rate Monitoring Using Flexible Piezoelectric Sensors," Sensors and Actuators A: Physical, vol. 332, p. 113026, 2021.
15. S. S. V. Tetali et al., "Intelligent Biomaterials for Cardiovascular Applications," Current Opinion in Biomedical Engineering, vol. 28, p. 100474, 2023.
16. C. Ribeiro et al., "Piezoelectric Polymers as Biomaterials for Tissue Engineering Applications," Colloids and Surfaces B: Biointerfaces, vol. 136, pp. 46–55, 2015.
17. X. Huang et al., "Biocompatibility of Piezoelectric Materials: A Review," Journal of Biomedical Materials Research Part B: Applied Biomaterials, vol. 104, no. 4, pp. 805–822, 2016.
18. Y. Zhang et al., "Recent Advances in Flexible and Wearable Piezoelectric Sensors for Health Monitoring," Sensors and Actuators A: Physical, vol. 350, p. 113086, 2023.
19. Y. Mao et al., "Wearable Piezoelectric Sensors for Real-Time Cardiovascular Monitoring," Advanced Functional Materials, vol. 31, no. 12, p. 2008425, 2021.
20. S. S. Zhang et al., "High-Sensitivity Piezoelectric Strain Sensors for Cardiac Applications," Advanced Functional Materials, vol. 30, no. 11, 2020.
21. R. Krishnamani, D. DeNofrio, & M. A. Konstam, "Emerging Ventricular Assist Devices for Long-Term Cardiac Support," Nature Reviews Cardiology, vol. 7, no. 2, pp. 71–76, 2010.
22. M. S. Peters et al., "Piezoelectric Actuators in Artificial Pacemakers: Enhancements and Innovations," Journal of Cardiac Electrophysiology, vol. 32, no. 8, pp. 2345–2354, 2021.
23. A. B. Thompson et al., "Integration of Piezoelectric Actuators in Ventricular Assist Devices," Journal of Mechanical Engineering, vol. 58, no. 4, pp. 912–924, 2020.

24. J. T. Martinez et al., "Piezoelectric Materials in Cardiac Resynchronization Therapy Devices," IEEE Transactions on Biomedical Engineering, vol. 66, no. 2, pp. 345–355, 2019.
25. J. K. Sajeev, A. N. Koshy, & A. W. Teh, "Wearable Devices for Cardiac Arrhythmia Detection: A New Contender?" Internal Medicine Journal, vol. 49, no. 5, pp. 570–573, 2019.
26. N. M. Nor, H. H. Hamzah, & K. A. Razak, "Recent advancement in sustainable energy harvesting using piezoelectric materials." Sustainable Materials for Next Generation Energy Devices, Elsevier, 2021. 221–248.
27. C. C. Zwack et al., "The Evolution of Digital Health Technologies in Cardiovascular Disease Research," NPJ Digital Medicine, vol. 6, no. 1, p. 1, 2023.
28. Z. He et al., "Implantable Piezoelectric Sensors for Intra-Cardiac Pressure Monitoring," Biomedical Engineering Letters, vol. 12, no. 3, pp. 315–325, 2022.
29. G. K. Pradhan et al., "Piezoelectric Materials in Electrocardiogram Sensors: An Overview," Journal of Biomedical Engineering, vol. 45, no. 7, pp. 1254–1266, 2017.
30. N. W. Murray et al., "Piezoelectric Pressure Sensors for Cardiovascular Monitoring: A Review," Sensors and Actuators B: Chemical, vol. 295, pp. 618–628, 2019.
31. S. Chen, X. Tong, Y. Huo, S. Liu, Y. Yin, M. L. Tan, & W. Ji, "Piezoelectric Biomaterials Inspired by Nature for Applications in Biomedicine and Nanotechnology," Advanced Materials, p. 2406192, 2024.
32. J. L. Rodriguez et al., "Wearable Cardiac Monitors With Piezoelectric Sensors: Enhancements and Innovations," IEEE Access, vol. 11, pp. 3890–3901, 2023.
33. B. Jaffe, W. R. Cook, & H. Jaffe. (1971). Piezoelectric Ceramics. Academic Press.
34. D. H. Kim et al., "Flexible and Wearable Electronics for Cardiovascular Monitoring," Nature Electronics, vol. 3, no. 7, pp. 423–435, 2020.
35. H. Yao et al., "TEM Study of Domain Structures in Ferroelectric PZT Ceramics," Advanced Functional Materials, vol. 31, no. 32, p. 2104145, 2021.
36. J. Liu et al., "Flexible and Wearable Piezoelectric Sensors for Real-Time Monitoring of Heart Rate and ECG," Journal of Biomedical Materials Research, vol. 109, no. 10, pp. 1452–1461, 2021.
37. X. Liu et al., "Dielectric Properties of PZT Ceramics and Their Influence on Piezoelectric Performance," Journal of Applied Physics, vol. 127, no. 10, p. 104102, 2020.
38. A. Smith et al., "Integration of PVDF-Based Piezoelectric Sensors into Wearable Cardiac Devices," Sensors and Actuators A: Physical, vol. 315, pp. 112–120, 2021.
39. B. Wong et al., "Evaluation of Wearable Piezoelectric ECG Monitors in Clinical Settings," IEEE Transactions on Biomedical Engineering, vol. 68, no. 4, pp. 324–331, 2022.
40. Y. Wang, M.S. darguesh, Optimisation and material considerations of piezoelectric implants for cardiac applications, Current Opinion in Solid State and Materials Science, Vol. 34, p. 101211, 2025.
41. Y. Zhang et al. "Self-powered pacemaker based on all-in-one flexible piezoelectric nanogenerator," Nano Energy, vol. 99, p 107420, 2022.
42. D. Patel et al., "Long-Term Evaluation of PZT-Based Piezoelectric Actuators in Cardiac Devices," IEEE Transactions on Biomedical Engineering, vol. 70, no. 8, pp. 2345–2353, 2023.
43. Y. Zhao et al., "Barium Titanate-Based Piezoelectric Energy Harvesters for Implantable Cardiac Devices," Energy & Environmental Science, vol. 16, no. 5, pp. 1829–1838, 2023.
44. B. Zhao et al. "A Review of Piezoelectric Footwear Energy Harvesters: Principles, Methods, and Applications," Sensors (Basel), vol. 23, no. 13, pp. 5841, 2023.
45. L. Brown et al., "Efficiency and Performance of Piezoelectric Energy Harvesters in Cardiac Devices," IEEE Transactions on Power Electronics, vol. 37, no. 6, pp. 1234–1242, 2024.

9 Elastomer Actuators for Heart Tissue

Aarti Nagayach, Banalata Mohanty, and Rakesh Bhaskar

9.1 INTRODUCTION

Cardiovascular diseases (CVDs) are the leading cause of mortality worldwide, accounting for approximately 17.9 million deaths each year (Mc Namara et al., 2019). As the prevalence of CVDs rises, the need for novel strategies to regenerate or repair damaged heart tissue becomes more urgent. Traditional treatments like pharmacological interventions and surgical procedures, though helpful in managing symptoms and slowing disease progression, often fail to restore full heart function (Malik et al., 2004). These conventional methods primarily address symptoms rather than the root cause of tissue damage (Kralj and Brkic Bilos, 2013). For example, medicines like beta-blockers, ACE inhibitors, and anticoagulants can reduce stress or prevent further damage but cannot regenerate lost tissue. Surgical interventions such as coronary artery bypass grafting or heart transplantation, while sometimes life-saving, are limited by risks like immune rejection and a scarcity of donor organs. This gap in effective treatment options has brought tissue engineering to the forefront as a promising alternative. It has come out as an encouraging alternative to the management of CVDs (Eschenhagen et al., 2012; Liau et al., 2012). Tissue engineering implies the integration of living cells, biomaterials, and biochemical factors for the formation of bioengineered constructs of tissue and/or help to improve function (Ghosh et al., 2023, 2024a; Nagayach et al., 2024; Narayanan et al., 2022; Sachdeva et al., 2024, 2023). Cardiac tissue engineering (CTE) aims to produce scaffolds that imitate the structure and role of the native cardiac tissue, thus engendering the restoration of damaged cardiac muscle. This method encompasses not only the restoration of the mechanical properties of the heart but also the support of cell division, angiogenesis, and the coupling of the native surrounding tissue (Liau et al., 2012; Nguyen et al., 2019).

The elastomer actuators have significant accomplishments in the CTE field due to their exceptional capability of imitating the dynamic mechanical properties of living heart tissue (Filippi et al., 2022; Wang et al., 2022). Elastomer actuators are high-performance soft materials that could go through huge alterations in their shapes during the process of being deformed and can recover the initial shape and configuration in response to external stimuli such as electrical, thermal, or mechanical inputs (Ferrantini et al., 2019). This characteristic enables the elastomer actuators to imitate the rhythmic contractions of the heart

 DOI: 10.1201/9781003670995-9

and therefore are greatly needed for those functions that require mechanical compliance and flexibility. The ability of elastomer actuators to perform controlled movement and force actuation in response to stimuli makes such devices interesting for the development of bioengineered cardiac patches or scaffolds (Ferrantini et al., 2019; Wang et al., 2024a). The design and function of elastomer actuators in the context of CTE are driven by their material properties, which closely resemble those of native cardiac tissue. Cardiac muscle is known for its elasticity, compliance, and ability to undergo repeated contraction and relaxation cycles (Golob et al., 2014). To imitate, the elastomer actuators must exhibit similar mechanical properties, such as elasticity, durability, and the capacity to deform under physiological conditions without experiencing fatigue or failure (Leite-Moreira et al., 2018; Stehle and Iorga, 2010). Moreover, the actuators must be able to respond to electrical signals, as the heart's natural contraction is regulated by electrical impulses that propagate through specialized pathways within the myocardium. Materials such as dielectric elastomers and shape-memory polymers have been explored for their potential to fulfill these requirements, offering promising platforms for developing next-generation cardiac patches (Chen et al., 2013; Filippi et al., 2022).

The successful integration of elastomer actuators into cardiac systems goes beyond their mechanical properties and places a high premium on biocompatibility. The term biocompatibility is shorthand for the material's inherent capacity for not triggering the unwanted reactions of the surrounding tissues while carrying out its desired function. More specifically, the bioengineered construct should not produce inflammation, immune rejection, or fibrosis in the engineer, thus ensuring the long-term functionality of the engineered tissue (Hiob et al., 2016; Kerativitayanan et al., 2017). To accomplish such goals, researchers are focused on devising elastomeric materials that are bioinert, non-immunogenic, and favorable for cell adhesion, proliferation, and differentiation (Wala et al., 2017).

The study on elastomer-based cardiac constructs is mainly focused on developing different strategies to promote vascularization, such as the inclusion of pro-angiogenic factors or the pre-vascularization of the implant before its usage. Another aspect being investigated is how to stimulate the growth and alignment of cardiomyocytes in bioengineered tissue, as it is important for these cells to be properly aligned so that they will sustainably produce an efficient contraction (Ferrantini et al., 2019). Thus, electrical and mechanical signals have been used to guide the alignment and maturation of cells, leading to the attainment of good results in preclinical studies (Golob et al., 2014). Besides that, the long-term durability of the elastomer actuators has been a point of major consideration in the dynamic environment of the heart. It is known that the heart constantly contracts and relaxes in cycles, and the material for CTE must be able to stand these repetitive forces for a long time without altering its mechanical properties or causing any other form of failure. This chapter explores the design, and application of elastomer actuators in CTE, highlighting their material properties, biocompatibility, and challenges for integration into cardiac systems (Chen et al., 2013; Webb et al., 2004).

9.2 ELASTOMER ACTUATORS: MECHANISM OF ACTION

Elastomer actuators operate through distinct modes of action, such as contraction, expansion, or movement, caused by the factors of the environment (Hiob et al., 2016). These actuators are generally classified into those that respond to the application of electrical, thermal, or chemical stimuli, which can trigger their motion (Li et al., 2019a). In the case of heart tissue, the most common mechanisms are: Elastomer actuators rely on external stimuli to induce mechanical action and can thus mimic the normal contractile function of the myocardium (Ponniah et al., 2016). Many actuation mechanisms have been assessed for use in CTE applications, and each has its own specific benefits.

Elastomer actuators are revolutionizing the world of biomimetic systems, as well as being in various industries such as robotics, prosthetics, and tissue engineering (Chen et al., 2013; Zolfagharian et al., 2016). These actuators are a great alternative for taking over the contractile function of heart tissue in a CTE context. The CTE is aimed at the creation of bioengineered scaffolds/devices that can be able to use the heart's natural mechanics and its electrical activity. Such actuators are elastomer actuators, which contract, expand, or move in response to external stimuli, thus have the possibility to be functional replacements for the damaged myocardium (Morita et al., 2024). The actuation principles follow electrical, thermal, or chemical stimuli. They should provide a basis for a naturalness-driven manifestation of the complex movements of the pumping cycle of the heart (Lorenzon et al., 2024; Phan et al., 2024). They are studied mainly to enhance their mechanical performance. Different types of actuators are dielectric elastomer actuators (DEAs), electroactive polymer actuators (EAPs), and pneumatic and fluid-driven actuators. Each actuator type has compatibility and driving mechanisms (fluid or pressure duration, and longevity). The next sections will introduce these actuators by detailing their advantages and drawbacks in CTE. The structural design of a fiber-reinforced flexible actuator involves several key elements are shown in Figure 9.1.

9.2.1 Dielectric Elastomer Actuators (DEAs)

These actuators rely on electrostatic attraction and most promising fields for CTE. Structurally they contain a soft and flexible dielectric elastomer layer that is situated between two compliant electrodes (Wang et al., 2024a). When a voltage is applied across the electrodes, the electric field produces electrostatic forces that compress the elastomer in the thickness direction while causing lateral expansion. This way of operation provides a strain similar to the contraction and relaxation of cardiac muscle fibers. One of the major advantages of DEAs in providing cardiac applications is their significant ability to produce much larger strains; thus, they are very efficient in imitating the dynamic mechanical behavior of the myocardium (Nejati and Mohammadi, 2024). Further, the fast response of DEAs is an important condition for the real-time synchronization of these devices with the natural rhythm of the heartbeat; this setup is critical for ensuring that the actuator is in the same phase with the biological tissues involved (Almanza et al., 2021; Li et al., 2019b). Besides, DEAs are capable of functioning across a diverse spectrum of actuation frequencies, thus

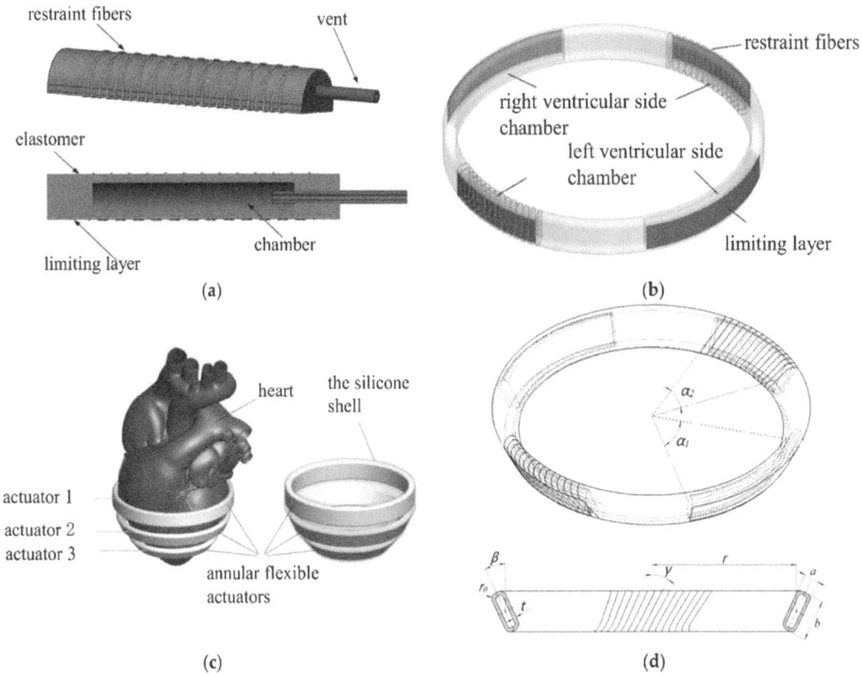

FIGURE 9.1 The structural design of a fiber-reinforced flexible actuator involves several key elements. (A) The basic fiber-reinforced actuator, (B) a specialized annular variation, and (C) integrating annular actuators with direct ventricular assist devices, (D) structural parameters of the fiber-constrained annular flexible actuator, (Yun et al., 2022).

enabling the adaptation of their action to the changes in the requirements under different physiological conditions of cardiac tissue (Hammoud et al., 2024). Figure 9.2 shows feasibility of a dielectric elastomer-augmented aorta (Almanza et al., 2021).

Nevertheless, DEAs have several issues in CTE applications. One of the significant factors is the high driving voltages needed to produce a sufficient actuation, which makes the devices working (Liu et al., 2024). The high voltages not only carry safety risks but can lead to fast degradation of the elastomer and the electrodes, thus shortening the life of the device. The researchers are now exploring better material alternations, like softer dielectric materials, or the optimization of the composition of the compliant electrodes through the addition of nanofillers to reduce energy requirements and time (Jahren et al., 2024; Wang et al., 2024b).

9.2.2 Electroactive Polymer Actuators (EAPs)

EAPs are another class of elastomer/actuators that have been used in cardiac applications. These actuators respond primarily to electrical stimuli, altering their shape or dimensions when an electric field is applied (Gu et al., 2024). This ability of EAPs to control the actuation process with a high level of precision makes them ideal for accurately mimicking the mechanical forces exerted by cardiac cells during

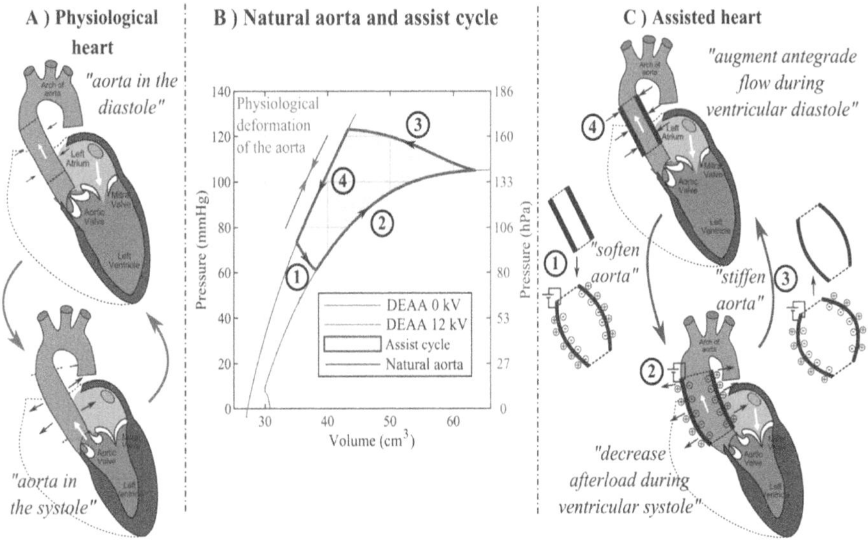

FIGURE 9.2 Feasibility of a dielectric elastomer-augmented aorta (Almanza et al., 2021).

contraction and relaxation cycles. Biologically engineered scaffolds incorporated with EAPs are frequently used in cardiac tissue regeneration (Sideris and de Lange, 2020). The EAP-embedded scaffolds deliver synchronized contractions that closely replicate the cardiac rhythm. When electrical impulses are applied, the EAPs within the scaffold contract, thereby providing mechanical support to the cardiac cells while assisting their orientation and growth.

They can be engineered to respond to electrical inputs and environmental stimuli (temperature, pH, or humidity). The multi-stimulus responsiveness of EAPs is a unique feature that allows for fine-tuning of actuation mechanisms for various physiological conditions of the human body (Bar-Cohen et al., 2017). Nonetheless, there are restrictions concerning the long-term stability and fatigue resistance of EAPs, particularly in the heart organ. Repeated electrical stimulation can cause the electrical conductors to degrade, resulting in the materials losing their functionality (Bar-Cohen and Anderson, 2019). Further, improved biocompatibility and reduced immune responses are still current areas of research. Ongoing investigations are carried out to design a new era of more durable and biocompatible materials through changing their chemical architecture so they can sustain functionality for prolonged periods.

9.2.3 Pneumatic and Fluid-Driven Actuators

Pneumatics and fluid-driven actuators are the latest alternative technologies that have been developed for creating tissue-mimicking cardiac pumps (Roshan et al., 2024; Xu, 2022). The basic mechanism of the actuators involves the expansion and contraction of the elastomeric structure, which is done by using pressurized gas or fluid (Phan et al., 2024). The mechanical deformation resulting from alterations in

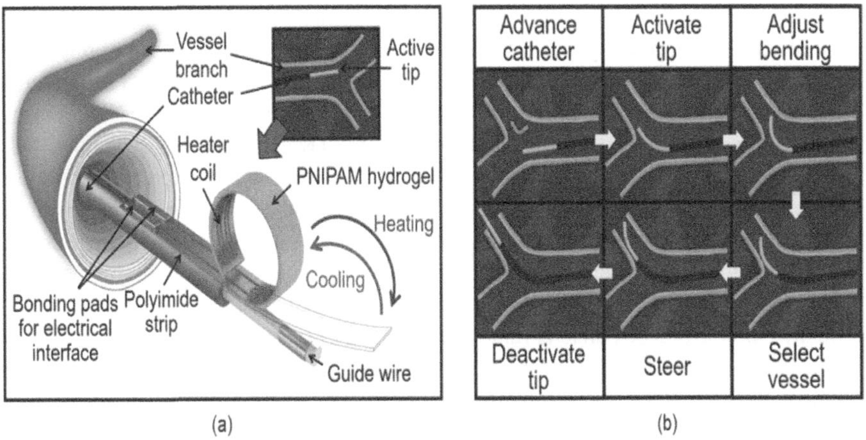

FIGURE 9.3 Conceptual diagrams for pneumatic actuators and fluid-driven actuators of the steerable smart catheter (Selvaraj and Takahata, 2020).

internal pressure can be remarkably akin to the natural pressure-driven movements of the heart, making these actuators a promising option for the simulation of cardiac function (Hashem et al., 2021). Pneumatic actuators and fluid-driven actuators have a primary advantage in their relatively uncomplicated design (Figure 9.3). The actuations are achieved with one pressurized fluid or gas; this is a more straightforward procedure than DEAs or EAPs, which are based on the application of complex electrical stimuli (Bu et al., 2022; Calo et al., 2020). The pneumatic actuators often have a high deformation rate, which allows them to produce the large strains required for the simulation of heart contractions. Yet, their use of external pressure sources, such as pumps or gas tanks, might be a big disadvantage for applications in vivo. In addition, these external systems are often bulky, limiting the potential for miniaturization and making the actuators less able to implant into the human body. Moreover, in the actuator, a constant and controlled pressure value is difficult to maintain, especially due to the dynamic and fluctuating characteristics of the heart environment (Roshan et al., 2024; Xavier et al., 2022).

To enable the application of pneumatic and fluid-driven actuators in CTE, the need of the period is the adaptation of fluid supply systems on a miniature scale and the development of closed-loop control mechanisms that can regulate pressure with precision. Thus, research is being done on various options, including the development of soft robotic-related fluid actuators, which are likely to be the small and efficient choice.

9.2.4 Piezo-based Actuators

Piezoelectric actuators are a vital class of devices used for active control in mechanical systems, offering precise, small-scale movement. Despite the relatively small voltages, forces, or displacements they produce, which often require amplification, they have been successfully adapted to a wide range of applications. A typical piezoelectric ceramic disk will only change its thickness by a fraction of a millimeter when voltage is applied, yet this small movement can be harnessed for applications requiring minute displacements (Deng et al., 2022; Pons et al., 2007). Piezoelectric materials are commonly used in various sensing applications such as accelerometers, flow meters, level detectors, and hydrophones (Kapat et al., 2020; Najjari et al., 2022; Zhou et al., 2011). The inverse piezoelectric effect is valuable in actuation applications, where these materials are used in motors, devices for precise position control, and to generate sonic and ultrasonic signals. Piezoelectric actuators enable the conversion of electrical energy into mechanical motion, offering highly accurate positioning down to the nanometer scale (Ramasamy et al., 2022; Swain et al., 2021, 2022a, 2022b). Piezoelectric actuators come in a variety of configurations and are manufactured using a range of fabrication techniques (Gao et al., 2024). These configurations include monomorphs, bimorphs, stacks, co-fired actuators, and flexure elements. Piezoelectric actuators are being incorporated into endoscope lenses for medical treatment types of equipment (Kapat et al., 2020). Piezoelectric actuators are typically constructed in several configurations, depending on the application. Stack or multilayer actuators, for example, consist of piezoelectric disks or plates stacked along the axis of linear motion (Upendra et al., 2023).

Piezoelectric actuators in cardiac devices are particularly intriguing, as precision and responsiveness are crucial. Piezoelectric cardiac actuators have the capacity to deliver small yet forceful movements and have the potential to drive cardiac-assist devices, replacing traditional actuators in artificial heart valves or pumps (Gao et al., 2024; Ghazanfarian et al., 2021). These actuators can synchronize their motion with the natural rhythm of the heart and respond in real time to electrical impulses, making them perfect for use in modern medical equipment like artificial pacemakers and heart pumps. Piezoelectric actuators' capacity to operate with low energy consumption and precise mechanical movements is a significant benefit in cardiac systems, where dependability and minimal energy consumption are paramount.

9.3 DESIGN AND FABRICATION OF ELASTOMER ACTUATORS FOR HEART TISSUE

The production and design of elastomer actuators of heart tissues have unique challenges that need to be taken into the mechanics and the engineering of the microstructure and integration with biology. The process consists of the very essences of different disciplines, like materials science, biomechanics, tissue engineering, and fabrication (Raman, 2024). The key processes in design, microstructure development, and innovations in fabrication for cardiac actuators. These sections summarize the creation of elastomer actuators for cardiac applications.

9.3.1 Mechanical Property

Ensuring that the actuator has mechanical properties similar to those of the cardiac muscle is the primary concern when it comes to the application of the materials (Ruan et al., 2016; Wang et al., 2013). These properties are elasticity, stiffness, and contractility. Mechanical mismatch between the actuator and the surrounding tissue may cause various problems such as the lack of function, damage to tissues, or even implant failure (Payne et al., 2017). The special characteristic of the native heart muscle is its ability to undergo large deformation. The elastomer actuator has to be mechanically flexible and similar to work well. The actuator will have Young's modulus that is close to the value of 10–50 kPa, which is a common myocardial tissue range in that part of the heart. The actuator is too stiff; it makes impossible the natural movement of the heart muscle and causes mechanical stress (Lorenzon et al., 2024). On the other hand, an actuator that is too soft will not be able to support the tissue and so the tissue will collapse. This is possible due to the nature of the elastomers, the ability to change their mechanical properties has solved this problem. Materials such as silicone, polyurethane, and thermoplastic elastomers (TPEs) are flexible and blend well. Changing the crosslinking level and mixing it with the plastic or other polymers allows for control of both the stiffness and the elasticity (Stoppel et al., 2016). Hence, the elastomer is made to emulate the mechanical surroundings of the heart. Further, the creation of the elastomer through the lamination of the soft and tough ones of various elastic constants.

9.3.2 Microstructural Characteristics

Therefore, for an actuator to function properly in the body and be integrated biologically, it must have microstructural features that are appropriate to its mechanical qualities for cardiac function. The ideal shape of the elastomer architecture within the scaffold is to develop a microstructure that enables the attachment, growth, and orientation of the cells on the elastomer surface. These are the essential factors that are responsible for the cells being seeded onto the scaffold that becomes functional, contractile tissue, which achieves the organization and function of the native myocardium (Kim and Cho, 2016; Stoppel et al., 2016). Fabricating of porous architecture in the elastomer is attracted to upgrade the cell interactions. This approach of blending the elastomer with the porous structures will provide a greater cell adhesion area and window for the mufti-way transportation of gases, nutrients, and waste products, which are the required material for the survival and function of the cells. The process of forming a porous structure is conventional and can be programmed to control the course of cellular infiltration and tissue fusion (Arumugam et al., 2018; Capulli et al., 2016; Shantanam, 2018; Zeng et al., 2021; Zhang et al., 2021b).

An additional important aspect of microstructural engineering is another technique, which is introducing micro-patterns or aligned fibers within the elastomer (Bursac et al., 2007; Eschenhagen et al., 2002; Gomes et al., 2022). In the case of the natural heart, all the cells are located in the space between muscle fibers that lined up in a certain direction supporting the efficient contraction of the heart. The formation of aligned tissue that is functionally and structurally adapted to the native heart is crucial for the development of a successful tissue. Photolithography, electrospinning, and 3D printing are some methods used to add grooves, ridges, or aligned fibers in the elastomer which helps the alignment of cardiomyocytes (Allison et al., 2017; Eschenhagen et al., 2002; Lasher et al., 2012; Zhao et al., 2015). Research has found that the cells grown on surfaces featuring patterns will tend to align in the direction of the pattern causing improved mechanical function and more synchronized contractions (Kieda et al., 2024).

9.3.3 Integration with Cellular Components

For elastomer actuators to be truly effective in CTE, they should be able to support the growth and differentiation of different cardiac cells, such as cardiomyocytes and stem cells. Cell integration can be achieved in a variety of ways such as surface modifications, incorporation of bioactive molecules, and biomimetic coatings (Morita et al., 2024). However, natural elastomers did not contain the cell's survival directions that are necessary for supporting cellular growth. Our group published a biomaterial that is suitable for cell proliferation in wound healing, bone regeneration, and cardiac cells (Narayanan et al., 2022, 2023; Pushp et al., 2021; Ramasamy et al., 2022; Singh et al., 2023; Swain et al., 2022a). A series of treatments can be used to improve the bioactivity of the material (Barreto et al., 2019; Liang et al., 2021a; Ribeiro et al., 2015). One of the most common methods is plasma treatment, which grafts various functional groups to the elastomer surface, thus elevating the material's hydrophilicity and resulting in better cell attachment. Chemical modification via grafting or coating the surface of the actuator with bioactive molecules can be used.

9.3.4 Extracellular Matrix (ECM) Coating

Another opportunity to tackle this issue is by the re-laying of elastomers with extracellular matrix (ECM) proteins which might be collagen, fibronectin, or laminin. The ECM is the one that provides structural support and biochemical signals that are necessary for the correct function of cells (Ghai et al., 2020; Montero et al., 2020; Wang et al., 2013). By making the coated elastomer more like the natural ECM of the heart, the cells will have a more favorable environment and will be able to adhere, spread, and function. In addition, ECM has been used to coat the elastomer scaffold, thus providing a biomimetic surface that will promote cell attachment and tissue regeneration (Hussain et al., 2013; Kim and Cho, 2016; Montero et al., 2020). These surface coatings go well with bioactive molecules like the growth factors, cytokines, or small-molecule drugs that can be incorporated onto or released in a controlled manner over the elastomer over time (Bhaskar et al., 2022; Ghosh et al., 2024b; Singh et al., 2022). These bioactive molecules can proliferate the cell, make it differentiate, and thus help the tissue hold the energy of regeneration. Cardiac-cell formation can be introduced to the processes that will guide the stem cells toward a cardiac lineage thus the tissue will gain contractile properties.

9.3.5 Electrical Stimulation

The heart's ability to keep a steady rhythm and contract in sync depends on a tuned network of CMs. These cells communicate through tiny connections known as gap junctions and specialized ion channels that manage the flow of ions in and out of the cells (Stoppel et al., 2016). When the electrical communication between cells breaks down, it can lead to irregular heartbeats or arrhythmias, which can be life-threatening if not treated. For regenerative medicine, when creating heart tissue replacements, it's essential to ensure that the new tissue can sync up electrically with the patient's own heart to avoid complications (Tandon et al., 2009). In adult heart tissue, electrical signals are carried by ion channels, which allow the movement of sodium and potassium ions, and this process is supported by gap junctions. Human cardiomyocytes derived from stem cells that don't express these ion channels fail to mature properly (Ruan et al., 2016; Stoppel et al., 2016; Xia et al., 2022; Zhao et al., 2021). In regenerative medicine, electrical stimulation has the potential to improve the integration of engineered cardiac tissues with the host's native tissue by enhancing the electrical and mechanical properties of the graft, reducing the risk of arrhythmias or asynchrony between the graft and the host tissue (Hernández et al., 2016; Liang et al., 2021a). These findings highlight the importance of ion channels in heart health and underscore the need to consider electrical signaling when designing heart tissue models for potential treatments.

9.4 ELASTOMERIC MATERIALS: PROPERTIES AND RELEVANCE IN CARDIAC APPLICATIONS

Elastomers are classified as a novel category of polymers known for their amazing elasticity hence they can undergo extensive deformation under stress and return to their original pattern if that stress is lifted (Ferrantini et al., 2019; Hiob et al., 2016; Webb et al., 2004). It is an ability that makes elastomers the best fit in a wide range of biomedical applications, especially in the CTE application. The heart is constantly active, with its cycles of excitation and relaxation during every heartbeat being the processes required in heart maintenance. Hence, the materials must possess the ability to absorb the mechanical stress without degrading (Chen et al., 2013). The properties of elastomers have the flexibility, durability, and mechanical resilience required to meet those challenges, making them ideal elastomers for CTE (Chen et al., 2013; Jawad et al., 2010; Ponniah et al., 2016).

The selection of the material is critical for fabricating elastomer actuators. The heart has an extremely variable mechanical environment. There is a need for the material to imitate the biomechanical properties of cardiac tissue so that it can support the proper function and integration of cardiac tissue (Payne et al., 2017; Zhou et al., 2016). Among the elastomers studied for CTE, the three that show the most promise are silicones, polyurethanes, and TPEs. Each of these materials provides specific properties that can be tweaked to suit the particular requirements of CTE.

9.4.1 Silicone Elastomers

Silicone elastomers have been a standard in medical applications for a long time due to their remarkable biocompatibility, chemical inertness, and versatility. In the tissue engineering of the heart, the role of these elastomers is quite crucial since the range of mechanical properties they exhibit can be thoroughly boosted (Kofod and Sommer-Larsen, 2005; Michel et al., 2010). This flexibility of design is critical in the creation of materials that reproduce the mechanical behavior of damaged tissue in the heart. This property of the material is important to help the healing of delivery cardiac constructs. Silicone elastomers are generally made up of silicon, oxygen, carbon, and hydrogen and provide a strong skeleton that remains stable in high temperatures and oxidative conditions (Kofod and Sommer-Larsen, 2005; Wu et al., 2021). They are also resistant to hydrolysis and have a low surface tension, making them safe to use in the body for prolonged periods where long-term stability and biocompatibility are the priority. They can produce silicone elastomer-based scaffolds with similar mechanical properties to those of the spontaneously contracting heart plush, which are suitable for this line of work (Carpi et al., 2009, 2010). An additional positive aspect of silicone elastomers in heart-related assignments is that they have good potential for being made into sophisticated shapes and structures (Hu et al., 2022). Different fabrication techniques such as molding, casting, or 3D printing can be used for elastomer actuators (Li et al., 2022). This property increases its ease of cultivation. The aforementioned properties such as flexibility and high surface area make silicones desirable in the process of cell attachment, proliferation, and differentiation (Hu et al., 2022; Michel et al., 2010).

9.4.2 Polyurethane Elastomers

Among the most materials explored in the realm of tissue engineering for heart repair are polyurethanes which are elastomers (Jo et al., 2010). These advanced materials demonstrate the delicate balance of several properties such as flexibility, toughness, and biocompatibility. These properties are important to copy the detectable mechanical properties of the heart (Hu et al., 2019; Ponniah et al., 2016). The polymeric structures are known to be highly elastic and strong, which are the main reasons for their success in mimicking the properties of the cardiac tissue. One of the important features of polyurethane foam can be produced from a copolymer type of synthetic polymer which contains both rubbery and hard segments (Okuzaki et al., 2014; Romasanta et al., 2015; Zhang et al., 2021a). Consequently, the soft/hard segment ratio can be varied for tuning the biocompatibility of the material. The materials can be customized in a way that they have the desired properties of stiffness, elasticity, and fatigue resistance that the heart requires for long-term use (Liang et al., 2021b; Renard et al., 2017). Polyurethane elastomers possess the most important preference, which is their long life under cyclic loading. This is equivalent to a number of millions of cycles over the lifetime of a patient. Thus, materials applied in the CTE have to bear this repetitive mechanical load without suffering any damage or deterioration of properties. Polyurethane elastomers are capable of keeping their mechanical properties constant for long periods (Bruschi et al., 2021; Hu et al., 2019; Renard et al., 2017). This makes them suitable materials for heart patches, valves, and other cardiac constructs used in medicine. Additionally, polyurethanes may be altered to increase their biological efficacy. The balance between mechanical strength and biological responsiveness to using polyurethane elastomers in tissue engineering to build a structure that resembles native tissue is a desirable approach (Bothe and Pretsch, 2013; Bruschi et al., 2021; Okuzaki et al., 2014).

9.4.3 Thermoplastic Elastomers

TPEs provide advanced possibilities in the fabrication of cardiac applications, especially in the aspect of flexibility fabrication (Spontak and Patel, 2000). Traditional elastomers necessitate crosslinking or vulcanization so as to achieve their ultimate characteristics; TPEs, in contrast, are able to be processed at low-temperature settings with no chemical crosslinking (Bothe and Pretsch, 2013; Spontak and Patel, 2000). The fast and scalable manufacturing routes, applicable to various adoption methods like extrusion, injection molding, and 3-D printing, are significantly influenced by this capability. Their detailed design and capability force reproducibility of the anisotropic nature of the cardiac tissue. Made up of both thermoplastic and elastomeric components, TPEs are endowed with a very special flexibility level and molding capacity (Armstrong and Spontak, 2018). In CTE, through manipulating TPEs scientists can achieve mechanical features similar to those found in native heart tissue, including stiffness, elasticity, and fatigue resistance. Furthermore, with easy handling, these materials are also suitable for the production of patient-specific implants or scaffolds, which is a very important consideration in personalized medicine (Busek et al., 2021; Weymann et al., 2023). Additionally, the capacity to modify TPEs via additives or copolymers is a key aspect of their versatility in improving biological functioning. For example, bioactive molecules like the growth factor or peptide could be embedded in the material to release them to engage cells followed by the cells undergoing cell division and tissue regeneration processes.

9.5 CHALLENGES AND OPPORTUNITIES IN CTE

Every kind of elastomer actuator has its specific merits but over and above that, they all experience the same problems of the transition from basic research to practical CTE. One of the widespread issues is the issue of biocompatibility and the minimization of immune response when the actuators are in vivo. The choice of materials must be carefully made in these actuators as otherwise, there may be some adverse immune reaction that can lead to either inflammation or device rejection. In this respect, surface alterations, such as the coating of the actuators with biocompatible materials or the use of bioinert scaffolds in conjunction with the actuators, are under examination to improve tissue compatibility. The scaling up of actuators to the size necessary for human hearts remains a challenge. While many elastomer types have been applied to small animals with great success, an essential aspect of the research work applied is the recreation of those results obtained in such a case for the human heart size without having an impact on its mechanical quality or the functioning of the actuators at the same time.

To ensure a long-lasting service both material fatigue, electrode detachment as well as electrical failures would be the potential shortcomings that must be mitigated. Elastomer actuators would also have a good chance to enter CTE. The integration of sensors with actuators could let them monitor the process in real time and influence the actions of the heart accordingly. It would allow more accurate synchronization of the actuator with the native heart tissue, leading potentially to the improvement of the patient's outcomes. Moreover, the progress in the technologies of 3D printing can provide new ways of custom-designed elastomer actuators that can meet individual patients' specific anatomical and functional needs.

Future directions in the development of elastomer actuators, among these pathways is the creation of self-healing elastomers, which have the characteristics of being able to heal themselves after being mechanically damaged or worn out over time. Through self-healing materials, actuators' lifespan in dynamic circumstances could be dramatically lengthened, and the risk of device malfunction could also be lessened by frequent replacements. Another promising area of research is the biohybrid actuators' use, which involves a combination of elastomeric materials with cells. These biohybrid systems are so ingeniously reliant on muscle cells, or cardiomyocytes, that they are cultured and implanted into the elastomeric scaffold.

Developments in nanotechnology will undoubtedly also usher in the future of elastomer actuators. The practice of connecting nanomaterials, carbon nanotubes, or graphene with elastomeric material to enhance the former's electrical conductivity, tensile strength, and stimulus-reactiveness will be well accepted too. The future development of such technologies will very likely lead to the utilization of elastomer actuators in advanced heart treatments that will be the next generation, restoring the heart's function and enhancing the quality of the patients.

REFERENCES

Allison, S., Ahumada, M., Andronic, C., McNeill, B., Variola, F., Griffith, M., Ruel, M., Hamel, V., Liang, W., Suuronen, E.J., Alarcon, E.I., 2017. Electroconductive nanoengineered biomimetic hybrid fibers for cardiac tissue engineering. J. Mater. Chem. B 5, 2402–2406. https://doi.org/10.1039/C7TB00405B

Almanza, M., Clavica, F., Chavanne, J., Moser, D., Obrist, D., Carrel, T., Civet, Y., Perriard, Y., 2021. Feasibility of a dielectric elastomer augmented aorta. Adv. Sci. 8, 1–13. https://doi.org/10.1002/advs.202001974

Armstrong, D.P., Spontak, R.J., 2018. Crystallization-directed anisotropic electroactuation in selectively solvated olefinic thermoplastic elastomers: A thermal and (electro)mechanical property study. Adv. Funct. Mater. 28, 1–12. https://doi.org/10.1002/adfm.201803467

Arumugam, R., Chinnadurai, R.K., Subramaniam, B.N., Devaraj, B., Subramanium, V., Sekhar, S.E., Nallani, S., 2018. Scalable novel PVDF based nanocomposite foam for direct blood contact and cardiac patch applications. J. Mech. Behav. Biomed. Mater. 88, 270–280. https://doi.org/10.1016/j.jmbbm.2018.08.020

Bar-Cohen, Y., Anderson, I.A., 2019. Electroactive polymer (EAP) actuators—Background review. Mech. Soft Mater. 1, 5. https://doi.org/10.1007/s42558-019-0005-1

Bar-Cohen, Y., Cardoso, V.F., Ribeiro, C., Lanceros-Méndez, S., 2017. Electroactive polymers as actuators. Advanced Piezoelectric Materials (2nd ed.). Woodhead Publishing, 319–352. https://doi.org/10.1016/b978-0-08-102135-4.00008-4

Barreto, S., Hamel, L., Schiatti, T., Yang, Y., George, V., 2019. Cardiac progenitor cells from stem cells: Learning from genetics and biomaterials. Cells 8, 1–55. https://doi.org/10.3390/cells8121536

Bhaskar, R., Kumar Gupta, M., Soon Han, S., 2022. Tissue engineering approaches for the in vitro production of spermatids to treat male infertility: A review. Eur. Polym. J. 174, 111318. https://doi.org/10.1016/j.eurpolymj.2022.111318

Bothe, M., Pretsch, T., 2013. Bidirectional actuation of a thermoplastic polyurethane elastomer. J. Mater. Chem. A 1, 14491–14497. https://doi.org/10.1039/c3ta13414h

Bruschi, A., Donati, D.M., Choong, P., Lucarelli, E., Wallace, G., 2021. Dielectric elastomer actuators, neuromuscular interfaces, and foreign body response in artificial neuromuscular prostheses: A review of the literature for an in vivo application. Adv. Healthc. Mater. 10, 1–15. https://doi.org/10.1002/adhm.202100041

Bu, K., Gong, X., Yu, C., Xie, F., 2022. Biomimetic aquatic robots based on fluid-driven actuators: A review. J. Mar. Sci. Eng. 10. https://doi.org/10.3390/jmse10060735

Bursac, N., Loo, Y., Leong, K., Tung, L., 2007. Novel anisotropic engineered cardiac tissues: Studies of electrical propagation. Biochem. Biophys. Res. Commun. 361, 847–853. https://doi.org/10.1016/j.bbrc.2007.07.138

Busek, M., Nøvik, S., Aizenshtadt, A., Amirola-Martinez, M., Combriat, T., Grünzner, S., Krauss, S., 2021. Thermoplastic elastomer (TPE)–poly(methyl methacrylate) (PMMA) hybrid devices for active pumping PDMS-free organ-on-a-chip systems. Biosensors 11. https://doi.org/10.3390/bios11050162

Calo, S., Chandler, J.H., Campisano, F., Obstein, K.L., Valdastri, P., 2020. A compression valve for sanitary control of fluid-driven actuators. IEEE/ASME Trans. Mechatron. 25, 1005–1015. https://doi.org/10.1109/TMECH.2019.2960308

Capulli, A.K., MacQueen, L.A., Sheehy, S.P., Parker, K.K., 2016. Fibrous scaffolds for building hearts and heart parts. Adv. Drug Deliv. Rev. 96, 83–102. https://doi.org/10.1016/j.addr.2015.11.020

Carpi, F., Frediani, G., De Rossi, D., 2009. Electroactive elastomeric haptic displays of organ motility and tissue compliance for medical training and surgical force feedback. IEEE Trans. Biomed. Eng. 56, 2327–2330. https://doi.org/10.1109/TBME.2009.2024691

Carpi, F., Raspopovic, S., Frediani, G., De Rossi, D., 2010. Real-time control of dielectric elastomer actuators via bioelectric and biomechanical signals. Polym. Int. 59, 422–429. https://doi.org/10.1002/pi.2757

Chen, Q., Liang, S., Thouas, G.A., 2013. Elastomeric biomaterials for tissue engineering. Prog. Polym. Sci. 38, 584–671. https://doi.org/10.1016/j.progpolymsci.2012.05.003

Deng, W., Zhou, Y., Libanori, A., Chen, G., Yang, W., Chen, J., 2022. Piezoelectric nanogenerators for personalized healthcare. Chem. Soc. Rev. 51. https://doi.org/10.1039/d1cs00858g

Eschenhagen, T., Didié, M., Heubach, J., Ravens, U., Zimmermann, W.H., 2002. Cardiac tissue engineering. Transpl. Immunol. 9, 315–321. https://doi.org/10.1016/S0966-3274(02)00011-4

Eschenhagen, T., Eder, A., Vollert, I., Hansen, A., 2012. Physiological aspects of cardiac tissue engineering. Am. J. Physiol. - Hear. Circ. Physiol. 303. https://doi.org/10.1152/ajpheart.00007.2012

Ferrantini, C., Pioner, J.M., Martella, D., Coppini, R., Piroddi, N., Paoli, P., Calamai, M., Pavone, F.S., Wiersma, D.S., Tesi, C., Cerbai, E., Poggesi, C., Sacconi, L., Parmeggiani, C., 2019. Development of light-responsive liquid crystalline elastomers to assist cardiac contraction. Circ. Res. 124, e44–e54. https://doi.org/10.1161/CIRCRESAHA.118.313889

Filippi, M., Buchner, T., Yasa, O., Weirich, S., Katzschmann, R.K., 2022. Microfluidic tissue engineering and bio-actuation. Adv. Mater. 34. https://doi.org/10.1002/adma.202108427

Gao, T., Liao, Q., Si, W., Chu, Y., Dong, H., Li, Y., Liao, Y., Qin, L., 2024. From fundamentals to future challenges for flexible piezoelectric actuators. Cell Rep. Phys. Sci. 5, 101789. https://doi.org/10.1016/j.xcrp.2024.101789

Ghai, P., Mayerhofer, T., Jha, R.K., 2020. Exploring the effectiveness of incorporating carbon nanotubes into bioengineered scaffolds to improve cardiomyocyte function. Expert Rev. Clin. Pharmacol. 13, 1347–1366. https://doi.org/10.1080/17512433.2020.1841634

Ghazanfarian, J., Mohammadi, M.M., Uchino, K., 2021. Piezoelectric energy harvesting: A systematic review of reviews. Actuators 10, 1–40. https://doi.org/10.3390/ACT10120312

Ghosh, S., Bhaskar, R., Mishra, R., Arockia Babu, M., Mohammad Abomughaid, M., Kumar Jha, N., Kumar Sinha, J., 2024a. Neurological insights into brain-targeted cancer therapy and bioinspired microrobots. Drug Discov. Today 29, 104105. https://doi.org/10.1016/j.drudis.2024.104105

Ghosh, S., Ghosh, S., Sharma, H., Bhaskar, R., Han, S.S., Sinha, J.K., 2024b. Harnessing the power of biological macromolecules in hydrogels for controlled drug release in the central nervous system: A review. Int. J. Biol. Macromol. 254, 127708. https://doi.org/10.1016/j.ijbiomac.2023.127708

Ghosh, S., Sinha, J.K., Ghosh, S., Sharma, H., Bhaskar, R., Narayanan, K.B., 2023. A comprehensive review of emerging trends and innovative therapies in epilepsy management. Brain Sci. 13. https://doi.org/10.3390/brainsci13091305

Golob, M., Moss, R.L., Chesler, N.C., 2014. Cardiac tissue structure, properties, and performance: A materials science perspective. Ann. Biomed. Eng. 42, 2003–2013. https://doi.org/10.1007/s10439-014-1071-z

Gomes, M.R., Castelo Ferreira, F., Sanjuan-Alberte, P., 2022. Electrospun piezoelectric scaffolds for cardiac tissue engineering. Biomater. Adv. 137, 212808. https://doi.org/10.1016/j.bioadv.2022.212808

Gu, J., Zhou, Z., Xie, Y., Zhu, X., Huang, G., Zhang, Z., 2024. A microactuator array based on ionic electroactive artificial muscles for cell mechanical stimulation. Biomimetics 9. https://doi.org/10.3390/biomimetics9050281

Hammoud, A., Liu, N., Le Gorrec, Y., Civet, Y., Perriard, Y., 2024. Energy-based modeling and robust position control of a dielectric elastomer cardiac assist device. 8th IFAC work. Lagrangian Hamiltonian Methods Nonlinear Control.

Hashem, R., Stommel, M., Cheng, L.K., Xu, W., 2021. Design and characterization of a bellows-driven soft pneumatic actuator. IEEE/ASME Trans. Mechatron. 26, 2327–2338. https://doi.org/10.1109/TMECH.2020.3037643

Hernández, D., Millard, R., Sivakumaran, P., Wong, R.C.B., Crombie, D.E., Hewitt, A.W., Liang, H., Hung, S.S.C., Pébay, A., Shepherd, R.K., Dusting, G.J., Lim, S.Y., 2016. Electrical stimulation promotes cardiac differentiation of human induced pluripotent stem cells. Stem Cells Int. 2016. https://doi.org/10.1155/2016/1718041

Hiob, M.A., Crouch, G.W., Weiss, A.S., 2016. Elastomers in vascular tissue engineering. Curr. Opin. Biotechnol. 40, 149–154. https://doi.org/10.1016/j.copbio.2016.04.008

Hu, P., Albuquerque, F.B., Madsen, J., Skov, A.L., 2022. Highly stretchable silicone elastomer applied in soft actuators. Macromol. Rapid Commun. 43, 1–9. https://doi.org/10.1002/marc.202100732

Hu, T., Wu, Y., Zhao, X., Wang, L., Bi, L., Ma, P.X., Guo, B., 2019. Micropatterned, electroactive, and biodegradable poly(glycerol sebacate)-aniline trimer elastomer for cardiac tissue engineering. Chem. Eng. J. 366, 208–222. https://doi.org/10.1016/j.cej.2019.02.072

Hussain, A., Collins, G., Yip, D., Cho, C.H., 2013. Functional 3-D cardiac co-culture model using bioactive chitosan nanofiber scaffolds. Biotechnol. Bioeng. 110, 637–647. https://doi.org/10.1002/bit.24727

Jahren, S.E., Martinez, T., Walter, A., Clavica, F., Heinisch, P.P., Buffle, E., Luedi, M.M., Hörer, J., Obrist, D., Carrel, T., Civet, Y., Perriard, Y., 2024. Novel para-aortic cardiac assistance using a pre-stretched dielectric elastomer actuator. Interdiscip. Cardiovasc. Thorac. Surg. 38. https://doi.org/10.1093/icvts/ivae027

Jawad, H., El Fray, M., Boccaccini, A.R., Harding, S.E., Wright, J.S., Chen, Q., Piegat, A., Ali, N.N., 2010. Nanocomposite elastomeric biomaterials for myocardial tissue engineering using embryonic stem cell-derived cardiomyocytes. Adv. Eng. Mater. 12, 664–674. https://doi.org/10.1002/adem.201080078

Jo, N.J., Lim, D.H., Bark, G.M., Chun, H.H., Lee, I.W., Park, H., 2010. Polyurethane-based actuators with various polyols. J. Mater. Sci. Technol. 26, 763–768. https://doi.org/10.1016/S1005-0302(10)60121-1

Kapat, K., Shubhra, Q.T.H., Zhou, M., Leeuwenburgh, S., 2020. Piezoelectric nanobiomaterials for biomedicine and tissue regeneration. Adv. Funct. Mater. 30. https://doi.org/10.1002/adfm.201909045

Kerativitayanan, P., Tatullo, M., Khariton, M., Joshi, P., Perniconi, B., Gaharwar, A.K., 2017. Nanoengineered osteoinductive and elastomeric scaffolds for bone tissue engineering. ACS Biomater. Sci. Eng. 3, 590–600. https://doi.org/10.1021/acsbiomaterials.7b00029

Kieda, J., Shakeri, A., Landau, S., Wang, E.Y., Zhao, Y., Lai, B.F., Okhovatian, S., Wang, Y., Jiang, R., Radisic, M., 2024. Advances in cardiac tissue engineering and heart-on-a-chip. J. Biomed. Mater. Res. - Part A 112, 492–511. https://doi.org/10.1002/jbm.a.37633

Kim, P.H., Cho, J.Y., 2016. Myocardial tissue engineering using electrospun nanofiber composites. BMB Rep. 49, 26–36. https://doi.org/10.5483/BMBRep.2016.49.1.165

Kofod, G., Sommer-Larsen, P., 2005. Silicone dielectric elastomer actuators: Finite-elasticity model of actuation. Sensors Actuat. A Phys 122, 273–283. https://doi.org/10.1016/j.sna.2005.05.001

Kralj, V., Brkic Bilos, I., 2013. Morbidity and mortality from cardiovascular diseases. Cardiol. Croat. 8, 373–378. https://doi.org/10.15836/ccar.2013.373

Lasher, R.A., Pahnke, A.Q., Johnson, J.M., Sachse, F.B., Hitchcock, R.W., 2012. Electrical stimulation directs engineered cardiac tissue to an age-matched native phenotype. J. Tissue Eng. 3, 1–15. https://doi.org/10.1177/2041731412455354

Leite-Moreira, A.M., Almeida-Coelho, J., Neves, J.S., Pires, A.L., Ferreira-Martins, J., Castro-Ferreira, R., Ladeiras-Lopes, R., Conceição, G., Miranda-Silva, D., Rodrigues, P., Hamdani, N., Herwig, M., Falcão-Pires, I., Paulus, W.J., Linke, W.A., Lourenço, A.P., Leite-Moreira, A.F., 2018. Stretch-induced compliance: A novel adaptive biological mechanism following acute cardiac load. Cardiovasc. Res. 114, 656–667. https://doi.org/10.1093/cvr/cvy026

Li, J., Wu, S., Zhang, W., Ma, K., Jin, G., 2022. 3D printing of silicone elastomers for soft actuators. Actuators 11. https://doi.org/10.3390/act11070200

Li, S., Bai, H., Shepherd, R.F., Zhao, H., 2019a. Bio-inspired design and additive manufacturing of soft materials, machines, robots, and haptic interfaces. Angew. Chemie - Int. Ed. 58, 11182–11204. https://doi.org/10.1002/anie.201813402

Li, Z., Gao, C., Fan, S., Zou, J., Gu, G., Dong, M., Song, J., 2019b. Cell nanomechanics based on dielectric elastomer actuator device. Nano-Micro Lett. 11, 1–19. https://doi.org/10.1007/s40820-019-0331-8

Liang, Y., Mitriashkin, A., Lim, T.T., Goh, J.C.H., 2021a. Conductive polypyrrole-encapsulated silk fibroin fibers for cardiac tissue engineering. Biomaterials 276, 121008. https://doi.org/10.1016/j.biomaterials.2021.121008

Liang, Y., Cui, T., Liu, L., 2021b. Effect of multi-armed chain extender on microphase morphology, stress-strain behavior and electromechanical properties of polyurethane elastomers. Polymer (Guildf) 235, 124279. https://doi.org/10.1016/j.polymer.2021.124279

Liau, B., Zhang, D., Bursac, N., 2012. Functional cardiac tissue engineering. Regen. Med. 7, 187–206. https://doi.org/10.2217/rme.11.122

Liu, Y., Yue, S., Tian, Z., Zhu, Z., Li, Y., Chen, X., Wang, Z.L., Yu, Z.Z., Yang, D., 2024. Self-powered and self-healable extraocular-muscle-like actuator based on dielectric elastomer actuator and triboelectric nanogenerator. Adv. Mater. 36, 1–11. https://doi.org/10.1002/adma.202309893

Lorenzon, L., Lucantonio, A., Costi, L., Zrinscak, D., Arleo, L., Cianchetti, M., 2024. Harnessing mechanical instabilities in the development of an efficient soft pump for an artificial heart ventricle simulator. IEEE/ASME Trans. Mechatron. 29, 936–946. https://doi.org/10.1109/TMECH.2023.3345529

Malik, S., Wong, N.D., Franklin, S.S., Kamath, T.V., L'Italien, G.J., Pio, J.R., Williams, G.R., 2004. Impact of the metabolic syndrome on mortality from coronary heart disease, cardiovascular disease, and all causes in United States adults. Circulation 110, 1245–1250. https://doi.org/10.1161/01.CIR.0000140677.20606.0E

Mc Namara, K., Alzubaidi, H., Jackson, J.K., 2019. Cardiovascular disease as a leading cause of death: How are pharmacists getting involved? Integr. Pharm. Res. Pract. 8, 1–11. https://doi.org/10.2147/iprp.s133088

Michel, S., Zhang, X.Q., Wissler, M., Löwe, C., Kovacs, G., 2010. A comparison between silicone and acrylic elastomers as dielectric materials in electroactive polymer actuators. Polym. Int. 59, 391–399. https://doi.org/10.1002/pi.2751

Montero, P., Flandes-Iparraguirre, M., Musquiz, S., Pérez Araluce, M., Plano, D., Sanmartín, C., Orive, G., Gavira, J.J., Prosper, F., Mazo, M.M., 2020. Cells, materials, and fabrication processes for cardiac tissue engineering. Front. Bioeng. Biotechnol. 8. https://doi.org/10.3389/fbioe.2020.00955

Morita, T., Nie, M., Takeuchi, S., 2024. Human induced pluripotent stem cell-derived cardiac muscle rings for biohybrid self-beating actuator. Lab Chip 24, 3377–3387. https://doi.org/10.1039/d4lc00276h

Nagayach, A., Bhaskar, R., Ghosh, S., Kumar, K., Soo, S., Kumar, J., 2024. Advancing the understanding of diabetic encephalopathy through unravelling pathogenesis and exploring future treatment perspectives. Ageing Res. Rev. 100, 102450. https://doi.org/10.1016/j.arr.2024.102450

Najjari, A., Mehdinavaz Aghdam, R., Ebrahimi, S.A.S., Suresh, S.K., Krishnan, S., Shanthi, C., Ramalingam, M., 2022. Smart piezoelectric biomaterials for tissue engineering and regenerative medicine: A review. Biomed. Tech. 67, 71–88. https://doi.org/10.1515/bmt-2021-0265

Narayanan, K.B., Bhaskar, R., Han, S.S., 2022. Recent advances in the biomedical applications of functionalized nanogels. Pharmaceutics 14. https://doi.org/10.3390/pharmaceutics14122832

Narayanan, K.B., Bhaskar, R., Sudhakar, K., Nam, D.H., Han, S.S., 2023. Polydopamine-functionalized bacterial cellulose as hydrogel scaffolds for skin tissue engineering. Gels 9, 1–16. https://doi.org/10.3390/gels9080656

Nejati, A., Mohammadi, H., 2024. A numerical framework for modeling 3D electrostrictive dielectric elastomer actuators. Comput. Struct. 303, 107495. https://doi.org/10.1016/j.compstruc.2024.107495

Nguyen, A.H., Marsh, P., Schmiess-Heine, L., Burke, P.J., Lee, A., Lee, J., Cao, H., 2019. Cardiac tissue engineering: State-of-the-art methods and outlook. J. Biol. Eng. 13, 1–21. https://doi.org/10.1186/s13036-019-0185-0

Okuzaki, H., Takagi, S., Hishiki, F., Tanigawa, R., 2014. Ionic liquid/polyurethane/PEDOT:PSS composites for electro-active polymer actuators. Sens. Actuat. B Chem. 194, 59–63. https://doi.org/10.1016/j.snb.2013.12.059

Payne, C.J., Wamala, I., Abah, C., Thalhofer, T., Saeed, M., Bautista-Salinas, D., Horvath, M.A., Vasilyev, N.V., Roche, E.T., Pigula, F.A., Walsh, C.J., 2017. An implantable extracardiac soft robotic device for the failing heart: Mechanical coupling and synchronization. Soft Robot. 4, 241–250. https://doi.org/10.1089/soro.2016.0076

Phan, P.T., Davies, J., Hoang, T.T., Thai, M.T., Nguyen, C.C., Ji, A., Zhu, K., Sharma, B., Nicotra, E., Hayward, C., Phan, H.P., Lovell, N.H., Do, T.N., 2024. Robotic cardiac compression device using artificial muscle filaments for the treatment of heart failure. Adv. Intell. Syst. 6. https://doi.org/10.1002/aisy.202300464

Ponniah, J.K., Chen, H., Adetiba, O., Verduzco, R., Jacot, J.G., 2016. Mechanoactive materials in cardiac science. J. Mater. Chem. B 4, 7350–7362. https://doi.org/10.1039/c6tb00069j

Pons, J.L., Rocon, E., Forner-Cordero, A., Moreno, J., 2007. Biomedical instrumentation based on piezoelectric ceramics. J. Eur. Ceram. Soc. 27, 4191–4194. https://doi.org/10.1016/j.jeurceramsoc.2007.02.126

Pushp, P., Bhaskar, R., Kelkar, S., Sharma, N., Pathak, D., Gupta, M.K., 2021. Plasticized poly(vinylalcohol) and poly(vinylpyrrolidone) based patches with tunable mechanical properties for cardiac tissue engineering applications. Biotechnol. Bioeng. 118, 2312–2325. https://doi.org/10.1002/bit.27743

Raman, R., 2024. Biofabrication of living actuators. Annu. Rev. Biomed. Eng. 26, 223–245. https://doi.org/10.1146/annurev-bioeng-110122-013805

Ramasamy, M.S., Bhaskar, R., Han, S.S., 2022. Piezoelectric biosensors and nanomaterials-based therapeutics for coronavirus and other viruses: A mini-review. Curr. Top. Med. Chem. 23, 115–127. https://doi.org/10.2174/1568026623666221226091907

Renard, C., Wang, D., Yang, Y., Xiong, S., Shi, C.Y., Dang, Z.M., 2017. Plasticized thermoplastic polyurethanes for dielectric elastomers with improved electromechanical actuation. J. Appl. Polym. Sci. 134, 1–10. https://doi.org/10.1002/app.45123

Ribeiro, C., Sencadas, V., Correia, D.M., Lanceros-Méndez, S., 2015. Piezoelectric polymers as biomaterials for tissue engineering applications. Colloids Surf. B Biointerfaces 136, 46–55. https://doi.org/10.1016/j.colsurfb.2015.08.043

Romasanta, L.J., Lopez-Manchado, M.A., Verdejo, R., 2015. Increasing the performance of dielectric elastomer actuators: A review from the materials perspective. Prog. Polym. Sci. 51, 188–211. https://doi.org/10.1016/j.progpolymsci.2015.08.002

Roshan, U., Mudugamuwa, A., Cha, H., Hettiarachchi, S., Zhang, J., Nguyen, N.T., 2024. Actuation for flexible and stretchable microdevices. Lab Chip 24, 2146–2175. https://doi.org/10.1039/d3lc01086d

Ruan, J.L., Tulloch, N.L., Razumova, M.V., Saiget, M., Muskheli, V., Pabon, L., Reinecke, H., Regnier, M., Murry, C.E., 2016. Mechanical stress conditioning and electrical stimulation promote contractility and force maturation of induced pluripotent stem cell-derived human cardiac tissue. Circulation 134, 1557–1567. https://doi.org/10.1161/CIRCULATIONAHA.114.014998

Sachdeva, P., Ji, S., Ghosh, S., Ghosh, S., Raghunath, M., 2023. Plausible role of stem cell types for treating and understanding the pathophysiology of depression. Pharmaceutics 15, 814. https://doi.org/10.3390/pharmaceutics15030814

Sachdeva, P., Narayanan, K.B., Sinha, J.K., Gupta, S., Ghosh, S., Singh, K.K., Bhaskar, R., Almutary, A.G., Zothantluanga, J.H., Kotta, K.K., Nelson, V.K., Paiva-Santos, A.C., Abomughaid, M.M., Kamal, M., Iqbal, D., Alharbi, M.H., Almutairi, A.A., Dewanjee, S., Nuli, M.V., Vippamakula, S., Jha, S.K., Ojha, S., Jha, N.K., 2024. Recent advances in drug delivery systems targeting insulin signalling for the treatment of Alzheimer's disease. J. Alzheimer's Dis. 98, 1169–1179. https://doi.org/10.3233/JAD-231181

Selvaraj, M., Takahata, K., 2020. Electrothermally driven hydrogel-on-flex-circuit actuator for smart steerable catheters. Micromachines 11. https://doi.org/10.3390/mi11010068

Li, J., Long, Y., Yang, F. and Wang, X., Degradable piezoelectric biomaterials for wearable and implantable bioelectronics. Current Opinion in Solid State and Materials Science, 24(1), 2020. https://doi.org/10.1016/j.cossms.2020.100806.

Sideris, E.A., de Lange, H.C., 2020. Pumps operated by solid-state electromechanical smart material actuators - A review. Sens. Actuat. A Phys. 307. https://doi.org/10.1016/j.sna.2020.111915

Singh, H., Purohit, S.D., Bhaskar, R., Yadav, I., Bhushan, S., Gupta, M.K., Mishra, N.C., 2022. Curcumin in decellularized goat small intestine submucosa for wound healing and skin tissue engineering. J. Biomed. Mater. Res. - Part B Appl. Biomater. 110, 210–219. https://doi.org/10.1002/jbm.b.34903

Singh, Y.P., Mishra, B., Gupta, M.K., Bhaskar, R., Han, S.S., Mishra, N.C., Dasgupta, S., 2023. Gelatin/monetite electrospun scaffolds to regenerate bone tissue: Fabrication, characterization, and in-vitro evaluation. J. Mech. Behav. Biomed. Mater. 137, 105524. https://doi.org/10.1016/j.jmbbm.2022.105524

Spontak, R.J., Patel, N.P., 2000. Thermoplastic elastomers: Fundamentals and applications. Curr. Opin. Colloid Interface Sci. 5, 333–340. https://doi.org/10.1016/s1359-0294(00)00070-4

Stehle, R., Iorga, B., 2010. Kinetics of cardiac sarcomeric processes and rate-limiting steps in contraction and relaxation. J. Mol. Cell. Cardiol. 48, 843–850. https://doi.org/10.1016/j.yjmcc.2009.12.020

Stoppel, W.L., Kaplan, D.L., Black, L.D., 2016. Electrical and mechanical stimulation of cardiac cells and tissue constructs. Adv. Drug Deliv. Rev. 96, 135–155. https://doi.org/10.1016/j.addr.2015.07.009

Swain, S., Bhaskar, R., Gupta, M.K., Sharma, S., Dasgupta, S., Kumar, A., Kumar, P., 2021. Mechanical, electrical, and biological properties of mechanochemically processed hydroxyapatite ceramics. Nanomaterials 11. https://doi.org/10.3390/nano11092216

Swain, S., Bhaskar, R., Mishra, B., Gupta, M.K., Sonia, Dasgupta, S., Kumar, P., 2022a. Microstructural, dielectric, mechanical, and biological properties of hydroxyapatite (HAp)/BZT-BCT (0.5Ba(Zr0.2Ti0.8)O3-0.5(Ba0.7Ca0.3)TiO3) bio-composites with improved mechano-electrical properties for bone repair. Ceram. Int. 48, 24505–24516. https://doi.org/10.1016/j.ceramint.2022.05.084

Swain, S., Bhaskar, R., Mishra, B., Kumar, M., Dasgupta, S., Kumar, P., 2022b. Microstructural, dielectric, mechanical, and biological properties of bio-composites with improved mechano-electrical properties for bone repair. Ceram. Int. https://doi.org/10.1016/j.ceramint.2022.05.084

Tandon, N., Cannizzaro, C., Chao, P.H.G., Maidhof, R., Marsano, A., Au, H.T.H., Radisic, M., Vunjak-Novakovic, G., 2009. Electrical stimulation systems for cardiac tissue engineering. Nat. Protoc. 4, 155–173. https://doi.org/10.1038/nprot.2008.183

Upendra, B., Panigrahi, B., Singh, K., Sabareesh, G.R., 2023. Recent advancements in piezoelectric energy harvesting for implantable medical devices. J. Intell. Mater. Syst. Struct. 35, 129–155. https://doi.org/10.1177/1045389X231200144

Wala, J., Maji, D., Das, S., 2017. Influence of physico-mechanical properties of elastomeric material for different cell growth. Biomed. Mater. 12. https://doi.org/10.1088/1748-605X/aa7e81

Wang, B., Wang, G., To, F., Butler, J.R., Claude, A., McLaughlin, R.M., Williams, L.N., De Jongh Curry, A.L., Liao, J., 2013. Myocardial scaffold-based cardiac tissue engineering: Application of coordinated mechanical and electrical stimulations. Langmuir 29, 11109–11117. https://doi.org/10.1021/la401702w

Wang, Y., Liao, W., Sun, J., Nandi, R., Yang, Z., 2022. Bioinspired construction of artificial cardiac muscles based on liquid crystal elastomer fibers. Adv. Mater. Technol. 7, 1–7. https://doi.org/10.1002/admt.202100934

Wang, J., Sarkar, D., Mohan, A., Lee, M., Ma, Z., Chortos, A., 2024a. Deep learning for strain field customization in bioreactor with dielectric elastomer actuator array. Cyborg Bionic Syst., 1–9. https://doi.org/10.34133/cbsystems.0155

Wang, L., Zhuo, J., Peng, J., Dong, H., Jiang, S., Shi, Y., 2024b. A stretchable soft pump driven by a heterogeneous dielectric elastomer actuator. Adv. Funct. Mater. 2411160, 1–8. https://doi.org/10.1002/adfm.202411160

Webb, A.R., Yang, J., Ameer, G.A., 2004. Biodegradable polyester elastomers in tissue engineering. Expert Opin. Biol. Ther. 4, 801–812. https://doi.org/10.1517/14712598.4.6.801

Weymann, A., Foroughi, J., Vardanyan, R., Punjabi, P.P., Schmack, B., Aloko, S., Spinks, G.M., Wang, C.H., Arjomandi Rad, A., Ruhparwar, A., 2023. Artificial muscles and soft robotic devices for treatment of end-stage heart failure. Adv. Mater. 35. https://doi.org/10.1002/adma.202207390

Wu, W., Zhang, S., Wu, Z., Qin, S., Li, F., Song, T., Cao, X., Wang, Z.L., Zhang, L., 2021. On the understanding of dielectric elastomer and its application for all-soft artificial heart. Sci. Bull. 66, 981–990. https://doi.org/10.1016/j.scib.2020.12.033

Xavier, M.S., Tawk, C.D., Zolfagharian, A., Pinskier, J., Howard, D., Young, T., Lai, J., Harrison, S.M., Yong, Y.K., Bodaghi, M., Fleming, A.J., 2022. Soft pneumatic actuators: A review of design, fabrication, modeling, sensing, control and applications. IEEE Access 10, 59442–59485. https://doi.org/10.1109/ACCESS.2022.3179589

Xia, G., Song, B., Fang, J., 2022. Electrical stimulation enabled via electrospun piezoelectric polymeric nanofibers for tissue regeneration. Research 2022, 1–23. https://doi.org/10.34133/2022/9896274

Xu, S., 2022. Sensing, Actuation, and Control of Soft Fluid-driven Robots by Liquid-elastomer Composite Sensors and Dielectric Elastomer Actuators. Harvard University ProQuest Dissertations & Theses, 29170181.

Yun, Z., Mei, C., Xu, K., Tang, X., Feng, Y., 2022. Design and mechanical performance of a fiber-constrained annular flexible actuator for direct ventricular assist devices. Appl. Sci. 12. https://doi.org/10.3390/app12115405

Zeng, Y., Jiang, L., He, Q., Wodnicki, R., Yang, Y., Chen, Y., Zhou, Q., 2021. Recent progress in 3D printing piezoelectric materials for biomedical applications. J. Phys. D. Appl. Phys. 55. https://doi.org/10.1088/1361-6463/ac27d2

Zhang, C., Wei, W., Sun, H., Zhu, Q., 2021a. Study on the properties of different dielectric elastomers applying to actuators. Sens. Actuat. A Phys 329, 112806. https://doi.org/10.1016/j.sna.2021.112806

Zhang, X., Li, L., Ouyang, J., Zhang, L., Xue, J., Zhang, H., Tao, W., 2021b. Electroactive electrospun nanofibers for tissue engineering. Nano Today 39, 101196. https://doi.org/10.1016/j.nantod.2021.101196

Zhao, G., Zhang, X., Lu, T.J., Xu, F., 2015. Recent advances in electrospun nanofibrous scaffolds for cardiac tissue engineering. Adv. Funct. Mater. 25, 5726–5738. https://doi.org/10.1002/adfm.201502142

Zhao, Y., Wang, P., Chen, Z., Li, M., Zhang, D., Yang, L., Li, H., 2021. Research progress of electrical stimulation in ischemic heart disease. Front. Cardiovasc. Med. 8, 1–11. https://doi.org/10.3389/fcvm.2021.761877

Zhou, Q., Lau, S., Wu, D., Kirk Shung, K., 2011. Piezoelectric films for high frequency ultrasonic transducers in biomedical applications. Prog. Mater. Sci. 56, 139–174. https://doi.org/10.1016/j.pmatsci.2010.09.001

Zhou, Z., Li, Q., Chen, L., Liu, C., Fan, S., 2016. A large-deformation phase transition electrothermal actuator based on carbon nanotube-elastomer composites. J. Mater. Chem. B 4, 1228–1234. https://doi.org/10.1039/c5tb02715b

Zolfagharian, A., Kouzani, A.Z., Khoo, S.Y., Moghadam, A.A.A., Gibson, I., Kaynak, A., 2016. Evolution of 3D printed soft actuators. Sens. Actuat., A Phys. 250, 258–272. https://doi.org/10.1016/j.sna.2016.09.028

Index

Note: Locators in *italics* represent figures and **bold** indicate tables in the text.

N

O

P

Q

R